EYE AND VISION RESEARCH DEVELOPMENTS

MYOPIA

OPTICS, CLINICAL PRESENTATION AND MANAGEMENT

EYE AND VISION RESEARCH DEVELOPMENTS

Additional books in this series can be found on Nova's website under the Series tab.

Additional e-books in this series can be found on Nova's website under the e-book tab.

EYE AND VISION RESEARCH DEVELOPMENTS

MYOPIA

OPTICS, CLINICAL PRESENTATION AND MANAGEMENT

DIEUDONNE KAIMBO WA KAIMBO

NOVA BIOMEDICAL

New York

For permission to use material from this book please contact us:
Telephone 631-231-7269; Fax 631-231-8175
Web Site: http://www.novapublishers.com

Library of Congress Cataloging-in-Publication Data

ISBN: 978-1-63117-506-0

Library of Congress Control Number: 2014938427

Published by Nova Science Publishers, Inc. † New York

Contents

Preface		**vii**
Acknowledgments		**ix**
Abstract		**xi**
Chapter I	Definition, Natural History, Pathogenesis, Genetics	**1**
Chapter II	Epidemiology and Risk Factors	**17**
Chapter III	Anatomy of the Eye	**37**
Chapter IV	Geometrical Optics	**99**
Chapter V	Physical Optics	**125**
Chapter VI	Biology of the Eye	**151**
Chapter VII	The Optics of Myopia	**161**
Chapter VIII	Diagnosing Myopia	**171**
Chapter IX	Myopia and Associations	**201**
Chapter X	Pathologic Complications Associated with Increasing Myopia	**227**
Chapter XI	Myopia and Management	**261**
Chapter XII	Myopia and Progression	**279**
Glossary		**295**
Author's Contact Information		**307**
Index		**309**

Preface

Myopia is the most common eye disease and is one of the leading causes of vision impairment worldwide. The book is written for all ophthalmologists, optometrists, refractionists, medical technicians, residents, fellows who pratique and prescribe treatment for refractive errors, especially for myopia. The objective is to provide practionners with an up-to-date information on myopia. Chapter I gives differents definitions, natural history, pathogenesis and genetic factors of myopia. Chaper II provides epidemiology and risk factors for myopia. Chapter III presents the anatomy of the eye with recent findings on cornea and choroid. Chapter IV presents the theory of geometrical optics with the application of theory in clinical practice; basic definitions are provided. Chapter V presents physical optics which deals with the nature of light itself. Chapter VI describes the optics of myopia, the refraction power of the eye. Chapter VII presents the biology of the eye as an optical system, explaining the components of refraction. Chapter VIII provides how diagnosing myopia with different processes. Chapter IX reports some associations between myopia and some diseases such as myelinated retinal nerve fibers, tilted disc syndrome, age related cataract,and glaucoma. Chapter X highlights pathologic complications in the eye with increasing myopia. Chapter XI presents the management of myopia by eye glasses, contact lenses and refractive surgery. Chapter XI gives techniques used to attempt to slow myopia.

Acknowledgments

I am grateful to Prof Dr Werner Spileers, head of the Department of Ophthalmology, KULeuven for giving me real opportunities and facilities to adequately perform my research proposal during my stay in Leuven, Belgium. I am particularly indebted to Prof Dr Fons Verdonck, Alumni KULeuven for his enthusiasm, guidance, advice, friendship, invaluable ideas and moral support. His invaluable help contributed to my research career. I wish to thank Prof Dr Luc Missotten, former head of the Department of Ophthalmology/KULeuven and Prof Karel Maertens who fostered my interest in ophthalmology and trained me as a general ophthalmologist and as a scientific leader in my country. I would like to thank Prof Dr Frank Buntinx who introduced me to clinical epidemiology. Special thanks go to Henri Yav and his wife Dr Anne Mutosh for friendship and many encouragements. I also want to express my gratitude to the Alumni of the KULeuven for their support. I thank Mirijam van Lameren and her family for their friendship. The collaboration of Mumba, chief of the nurses at the Department of Ophthalmology, University of Kinshasa, has been a never failing stimulus. Finally, special thanks to my mother, Mputu Hélène, my wife and children, Jacqueline Bambu, Jacques Michel Kaimbo, Trinka Kaimbo, Ornella Kaimbo for all their encouragements, support and love. Finally, I am grateful to (my) readers, my patients.

Abstract

Myopia is a common ocular condition affecting approximately 1.6 billion people worldwide. An increasing trend of myopia has been observed throughout the world and the prevalence of myopia is expected to increase to 2.5 billion by the year 2020. This book focuses on definition, mechanisms, optics, refraction, clinical presentation, complications and management of myopia in regards of recent advances.

Myopia (nearsightedness) is a refractive error (ametropia) that occurs when parallel rays of light entering the non-accommodating eye are not focused on the retina. As a result, images of distant objects are focused in front of the retina and thus appear blurred. Myopia is the most common eyesight problem in the World and is often mild and there are no serious problems. However, it may sometimes lead to blindness. Myopia can be corrected with spherical lenses, contact lenses or with refractive surgery. The book gives an overview of myopia from definition, etiology to surgical treatment. Contents are based on recent findings published in the medical literature and reflect the most advanced achievements in current clinical and experimental research on myopia. This book presents relevant information that students, optometrists, orthoptists, ophthalmologists as well as scientists involved in clinical and basic research on myopia need to know about this important topic.

Chapter I

Definition, Natural History, Pathogenesis, Genetics

1. Definitions

In normal eye, light rays from a distant object are focused sharply on the retina by the relaxed lens without the need of any accommodation effort. This condition is called emmetropia. A refractive error (ametropia) is a disorder that occurs when parallel rays of light entering the non-accommodating eye are not focused on the retina. Myopia refers to defocus due to light coming to focus anterior to the retinal plane (Abrams, 1993).

Myopia (nearsightedness) is a refractive error, a condition in which the cornea and lens of the nonaccommoding eye have too much plus power for the length of eye. As a result, images of distant objects are focused in front of the retina and thus appear blurred.

Myopia has been recognized as a distinct visual disability for millennia. Myopia has been known for more than 2000 years and was first described by the ancient Greeks (Donders, 1866; Hirschberg, 1985). It was probably the ancient Greeks who coined the term, using the roots myein (to close) and ops (eye) to characterize those individuals who narrow their eyelids to improve distance visual acuity, the pinhole effect. The focus of distant parallel rays of light falls anterior to the retinal plane and produces a blurred image in myopia. This situation can arise because either the primary refractive components are too powerful or the globe is too long. Thus, myopia can be due to increased corneal or lenticular curvature, or an increase in the lens index of refraction, as occurs with the development of nuclear sclerosis. More commonly, myopia is the result of axial elongation of the posterior segment of the eye. Previously used definitions of myopia have depended upon arbitrary criteria, as there is no common international consensus about the accepted definitions for myopia (Park and Congdon, 2004).

Definition of Myopia

Myopia is defined as that optical condition of the nonaccommodating eye in which parallel rays of light entering the eye are brought to a focus anterior to the retina. It also can be described as the condition in which the far point of focus is located at some finite distance in front of the cornea. For practical purposes, this is a distance of less than 6 meters, the distance at which visual acuity is normally tested. Thus, the uncorrected, nonaccommodating myopic eye has some point at a finite distance beyond which objects are not seen clearly. At this far point, an object is in clear focus, but with increasing distances beyond it, the image becomes progressively more indistinct. This far point also is defined as the focal point of the eye. The degree of myopia in diopters is found by determining the reciprocal of the far point or focal point of the eye measured in meters (Whitman and Curtin, 2006).

Refractive and Axial Myopia

Myopia can be characterized as refractive or axial, although a continuum of the two types exists. In refractive myopia, the overall refractive power of the eye as determined by cornea and crystalline lens power, modified by anterior chamber depth, is excessive in relation to an eye of normal axial length (21.5 to 25.5 mm). The axial length is normal because it is the product of normal growth. Axial myopia is the result of an excessive elongation of the eye with respect to its refractive components. In these eyes, there is added expansion due to stretching of the scleral wall. These differences in refraction components can have clinical effects. It is of some clinical importance to appreciate that equal amounts of myopic progression are produced by smaller increases in axial length in refractive myopia compared with axial myopia. For example, in refractive myopia, 0.34 mm of axial length change equals approximately 1 D of refractive error change, whereas in axial myopia, 0.4 mm of axial length change equals approximately 1 D of refractive error change (Balazs, 1961). The differences between axial and refractive myopia also can affect retinal image size (Whitman and Curtin, 2006).

Physiological (Physiologic) Myopia vs. Pathological (Pathologic) Myopia

Definition of Physiological (Physiologic) Myopia

Physiologic myopia is generally defined as that state in which the eye is rendered myopic by a combination of its components of refraction. In this situation, the refractive power of the eye (corneal power plus lens power slightly modified by anterior chamber depth) and the axial length are such that its posterior focal plane lies anterior to the retina. Each component has a value within its normal curve of distribution. These eyes demonstrate normal anatomy and physiology. Whether the absence of correlation among the elements of refraction occurs by chance or is a hereditable trait is unknown at present. Physiological (physiologic) myopia is also considered as low to moderate refractive errors defined as myopia less than 6.0 diopters (D),

Definition of Pathological Myopia

By definition, pathological myopia is also known as high, degenerative or malignant myopia. It refers to a condition in which individuals have an axial length exceeding a certain threshold (typically ≥ 25.5 or 26.50 mm), a corresponding refractive error (of at least –5.0 dpt) and which is accompanied by characteristic pathological changes (Curtin and Karlin,

1971; Soubrane, 2008; Silva, 2012). Posterior pole abnormalities typical of pathological myopia include tessellated fundus, lacquer cracks, diffuse atrophy, patchy atrophy, choroidal neovascularization (CNV), macular atrophy, posterior staphyloma but also straightened and stretched vessels, temporal peripapillary atrophic crescent, hemorrhages and tilting of the optic disk (Grossniklaus and Green, 1992; Hayashi et al., 2010). Although there is no universally agreed definition, pathological or degenerative myopia has been defined in recent studies as a spherical equivalent refractive error of at least −6 dioptres (D) accompanied by characteristic degenerative changes, with complications of pathological myopia being much more common when the refractive error is −8 D or worse (Yamamoto et al., 2007; Tano, 2002; Yotshida et al.,2002). As elongation of the globe is a key feature of pathological myopia (PM), an axial length of ≥26.5 mm has been adopted as a biometric definition in clinical trials (Verteporfin in Photodynamic Therapy Study Group, 2001), with recent studies reporting a mean of 29 mm (range 26.8–31.5 mm) (Yoshida et al., 2002; Yoshida et al., 2003). The limit of 25.5 mm of anteroposterior diameter of the eye is arbitrary and has been previously set as 25, 25.5 or 26.5 mm (Metge, 1994). The superposition of the myopic and emmetropic populations occurs between 25 and 26.7 mm (Pruett, 1994). From a refractive point of view, pathological myopia is defined by a refractive error with an inferior limit of -6 to -10 dpt. In the clinical practice we may consider pathological myopia as a refractive error greater than -6 dpt, provided that the average refractive power of the cornea is +43.5 dpt, in the absence of spherophakia or nuclear cataract. The definition of pathological myopia as a refractive error of -6 dpt is clinically useful, though it may exclude a number of eyes. Of greater interest is the determination of the best cut-off for high myopia. Criteria for high myopia that have been used in previous studies include -5.0D, -6.0D, -10.0D, and -12.0D and there is no universal definition for high myopia (Percival, 1987; Younan et al., 2002). It is thought that at this level, the risks of secondary complications, such as retinal detachment and glaucoma may increase (Younan et al., 2002; Tong et al., 2004; Saw et al., 2006). There may also be further deteriorations in visual field, central visual acuity (VA), increased risks of irregular astigmatism, keratoconus, and peripheral visual field defects.

Some authors have considered pathological myopia as refractive errors greater than –4 dpt in children less than 5 years of age (Tokoro, 1988). Pathological myopia usually starts in childhood between 5 and 10 years of age and progresses until the third decade or even later. Tokoro (Ruben and Rajpurohit, 1976) reported a prevalence of 0.1% in preschool children, 0.5% in high school students and 1.5% in university students.

School myopia vs. adult onset myopia

Myopia may be classified as "school myopia" or "adult onset myopia. School myopia develops during the school age and stabilizes around (Goldschmidt, 1990; Goss, 1982; Tokoro and Kabe, 1965) years of age, while adult onset myopia develops in young adults.

Functional Myopia vs Organic Myopia

Functional Myopia

Ciliary muscle spasm is a common effect of protracted near work in the adolescent and young adult. The resultant shifts in refraction towards myopia can be considerable in individual cases, but this phenomenon exists to a limited degree in many eyes that locate about the center of the distribution curve of refraction. This is dramatically demonstrated by the change in these curves when the same population is examined with and without cycloplegia. Two effects are seen to occur with cycloplegia; there is a shift towards hyperopia and a reduction in the excess at emmetropia. From this, ciliary muscle tone can be appreciated not only as a powerful emmetropizing force but also as a major cause of low myopia. Myopic persons outgrow their need for cycloplegic refraction considerably later than others. Other causes of ciliary spasm include medications that can be local, such as the cholinesterase inhibiting miotics, or systemic, like hydralazine and hydroxymethonium. Ocular trauma is also capable of producing ciliary spasm.

Organic Myopia

A large number of organic changes can produce myopia of either a transient or permanent nature. These are outlined as follows: an increased corneal power: decreased radius of curvature (e.g; keratoconus); an. increased lens power (decreased radii of curvature: lens hydration such as in diabetes, typhoid fever and with other dysenteries, drug effects. Ciliary edema: trauma, drug effects. Lens subluxation: developmental defect, trauma, secondary to systemic disease (syphilis, homocystinuria, Marfan syndrome). Increased index of refraction (nuclear cataract, diabetes).

Transient Drug-Induced Myopia

The effect of certain systemic drugs in producing a transient myopia is thought to be an idiosyncratic reaction and has been attributed to either lens hydration or, more likely, ciliary edema. Drugs known to produce this effect include sulfa drugs, acetazolamide (Diamox), ethoxzolamide (Cardrase), hydrochlorothiazide (Hydrodiuril), chlorthalidone (Hygroton), promethazine hydrochloride (Phenergan), prochlorperazine (Compazine), and oxytetracycline (Terramycin). Several treatment regimens used in toxoplasmic retinochoroiditis contain agents from the sulfonamide family which may cause transient myopia (Panday and Rhee, 2007). Ultra Biomicroscopy (UBM) explains this mechanism by demonstrating supraciliary choroidal effusion causing forward displacement of the ciliary body-lens-iris block and relaxation of zonular fibers leading to myopia, anterior chamber shallowing and angle closure glaucoma (Postel et al., 1996). The same mechanism can also occur when acetazolamide is used to treat inflammatory cystoid macular edema (CME), since this agent also belongs to the sulfonamide family (Fan et al., 1993; Krieg and Schipper, 1996). Several reports of a similar condition have been published following the use of topiramate, a sulfonamide derivative used for treatment of migraine headaches, seizures, alcohol abuse and other drug dependencies (Bhattachrayya and Busa, 2005; Rodriguez et al., 2012 ; Latini and Romano, 2012; Caglar et al., 2012; Muniesa etb al, 2012; Dorronzoro et al., 2011; van Issum et al., 2011 ; Kumar et al., 2012; Vilar Ventura et al., 2009; Gawley, 2009; Cruciani et al., 2009; Kerimoglu et al., 2009; Brandao et al., 2009; Boonyleephan et al., 2008; Mandal et al., 2008; Panday and Rhee, 2007; Guier, 2007). Transient myopia can also be caused by other drugs such as insulin (Penha et al., 2012; Lin et al., 2009; Feldkaemper et al., 2009; Zhu et al., 2007), methazolamide (Kwon et al., 2012), IGF1 and FGF2 (Ritchey et al., 2012), antithrombotic (Marcus et al., 2012), co-trimoxazole (Kamath et al., 2012), opiate (Paur et al., 2012), aripiprazole (Nair et al., 2012), amisulpride (Stratos et al., 2011), hydrochlorithiazide (Roh et al.,2011), psychotropic agents (Richa and Yazbek, 2010), acetazolamide (Szawar and Thompson, 2009), mefenamic acid

(Vishwakarma et al., 2009). Discontinuation of these medications leads to complete resolution of this anatomic shift.

Night Myopia

Other environmental effects upon the refraction include the "night myopia" associated with the shift from photoptic to scotoptic vision, and vision in the absence of normal visual stimuli, the "empty-field" myopia. Light rays at the edge of the human lens are refracted more than those at the center of the lens. Because our pupils are larger at night, more spherical aberration is present under lower light conditions. A refractive shift towards more myopia is needed to compensate for this increase in spherical aberration. Additionally, accommodation does not go to a neutral state under low light conditions. The visual system actually accommodates approximately 0.75D under low light conditions. These changes result in a need for more minus or less plus correction for those individuals, such as over the road truck drivers, who need to function with their highest visual clarity at night.

Other Myopia

Myopia secondary to restricted visual space, the counterpart of the laboratory studies cited previously, has been reported among both submarine and minutemen missile crews.

Malnutrition can produce a myopic error of some 1.25 D in children. This is thought to be a lens effect and is reversible. Special note should also be taken of the unusual course of refraction development in children with unilateral amblyopia. Under the effects of normal ocular use, the fixating eye has been found to undergo a steady drift towards myopia, whereas the refraction of the amblyopic fellow eye remains stable.

2. Natural History

The Distribution of Refractive Errors Changes with Age

Newborns average 3.0 D of hyperopia (Saunders, 1995). This may increase slightly in the first few months, but then it declines towards an average of 1.0 D of hyperopia by 1 year of age (Saunders, 1995). Fewer than 5% of infants have more than 3.0 D of hyperopia at age 1 (Saunders, 1995; Holmstrom and Larsson, 2005). This shift towards emmetropia is a complex process that involves changes in the power of the refractive components of the eye, including thinning of the crystalline lens (Zadnik et al., 1993). Visual stimulation appears to play a role in this process (Robb, 1977; Rabin et al., 1981).

Myopia typically appears between 6 and 12 years of age, but the onset age of myopia that is frequently mentioned is between 5 and 15 years, and a number of studies have been conducted to depict the prevalence rate of myopia worldwide and the mean rate of progression is approximately 0.5 D per year, based on studies of mostly Caucasian children (Grosvenor et al., 1987; Jensen, 1992; Parssinen et al., 1989). A recent study reported that progression of myopia varied by ethnicity and by age of the child (Hyman et al., 2005). In ethnic Chinese children, the rate of progression is higher (Fan et al., 2004; Fan et al., 2004; Saw et al., 2005; Shih et al., 1999; Shih et al., 2001; Zhao et al., 2002).

Individuals with high refractive errors are more likely to develop pathologic ocular changes over time. Highly myopic patients have an increased incidence of retinal thinning, peripheral retinal degeneration, retinal detachment (The Eye Disease Case-Control Study Group, 1993), cataract (Lim et al., 1999), and glaucoma (Grødum et al., 2001; Wong et al., 2003).

Normally, the axial length of the human eye increases from 17 mm at birth to 24 mm at 14 years of age. From an initial hypermetropia the refraction gradually changes toward emmetropia. It has been hypothesized that a growth-control mechanism exists, which can either accelerate or slow down axial growth in response to defocusing of the retinal image during the period of normal eye growth. Results from experimental myopia in mammals suggest that this mechanism works by regulating the scleral extensibility through complex changes in the synthesis and degradation of extracellular matrix components (McBrien and Gentle, 2003; Guggenheim and McBrien, 1996; Jobling et al., 2004; Trier et al., 2008).

In myopic children an excessive eye elongation is typically seen from age 6 years until 20 years. The axial length will then be in the range of 24–28 mm. Until the age of 14 years, the increase in myopia is approximately linear (Jones et al., 2005), after which a slow deceleration is seen (Thorn et al., 2005). With maturity, an increase in collagen cross-linking occurs (Baily et al., 1998), which probably explains the gradual stabilization of myopia. The myopic eye differs in shape from normal eyes, because the increase in length (0.35 mm per diopter) is greater than the increase in height (0.19 mm per diopter) and width (0.1 mm per diopter), resulting in the characteristic "egg-shape" of highly myopic eyes (Atchison et al., 2004). With increasing axial length there is an increased risk of potentially blinding complications later in life, such as retinal detachment, macular degeneration, or glaucoma. About 23% of all cases of retinal detachment occur in eyes with myopia of more than -6 dioptres (Polkinghome and Craig, 2004). This underlines the importance of finding an efficient and safe way to prevent excessive axial elongation (Trier et al., 2008).

3. Pathogenesis

The aetiology, pathogenesis, and treatment of myopia have been hotly debated in the ophthalmic community for decades (Mutti and Bullimore, 1999). There are several theories on the mechanism of development of myopia arising from disruption of the emmetropisation process. Emmetropisation is achieved when the optical power of the eye matches the axial length, resulting in a focused image of a distant object on the retina without accommodative effort (Troilo and Wallman, 1991). It has been proposed that overacting intraocular muscles may result in excessive accommodation and influence emmetropisation (Mutti et al., 1996). The two basic mechanisms by which animal myopia may be induced are form deprivation and optical defocus. Form deprivation myopia can be induced by the application of translucent occluders over the animal's eyes. Local retinal effects may occur and the resultant scleral growth modulated by chemicals such as dopamine, growth factors, and muscarinic antagonists (Laties and Stone, 1991; Stone et al., 1989; Troilo et al., 2000). Negative spectacle lenses in chicks induce compensatory axial elongation and myopia (Hung et al., 1995). Suitable therapeutic modalities such as pharmacological interventions and optical corrective devices that may retard the progression of myopia in myopic individuals have been reported. The overwhelming majority of these reports have been cited in optometry and not ophthalmology journals. The optical correction of myopia and optimal strategies to prevent the progression of myopia have been developed and prescribed largely by optometrists. On the other hand, issues regarding the causes and prevention of myopia have only gained interest among ophthalmologists in the recent decade.

The choroid is an integral structure in the eye that accounts for most of the ocular blood flow. Thus, the choroid is of paramount importance to retinal and visual function because it supplies nutrients to retinal pigment epithelial cells and the outer retina. In addition, the choroid also contributes to the blood supply of the prelaminar portion of the optic nerve. Compromised choroidal circulation may account for the retinal dysfunction and vision loss that is observed in highly myopic patients (Ho et al., 2013)

4. Genetics

Genetic Factors of Pathological Myopia (Silva, 2012)

It is well known that there is a higher prevalence of high myopia in Asian populations and a lower prevalence in African and Pacific island groups (Green et al., 1986; Munier et al., 1998; Krumpaszky et al., 1999; Buch et al., 2001; Cotter et al., 2006; Iwase et al., 2006; Xu et al., 2006). Myopia is a complex disease affected by both environmental and genetic factors (Jacobsen et al., 2008; Lyhne et al., 2008).

Determination of the genetic factors that predispose a person to myopia is challenging because myopia is a multigenetic condition involving several overlapping signaling pathways, each of which is associated with a group of distinct genetic profiles (Lin et al., 2010).

High myopia most commonly appears as a complex disease caused by a combination of genetic and environmental factors working together. However, it sometimes presents as one of the features in a wide variety of genetic disorders. Genes responsible for these syndromic genetic disorders with myopia as a consistent clinical finding have been identified: collagen 2A1 and 11A1 for Stickler syndromes type 1 and 2, respectively (Knowlton, 1989; Richards et al., 1996), lysyl-protocollagen hydroxylase for type 4 Ehler-Danlos syndrome, (Pousi et al., 1994), collagen 18A1 for Knobloch syndrome (Sertie et al., 2000), and fibrillin for Marfan syndrome (Dietz et al., 1991; Nijbroek et al., 1995).

Each of these genes is expressed in the sclera, demonstrating how knowledge of gene expression in the scleral wall is critical to our understanding of eye expansion and myopia (Young, 2004). Family studies in both Asian (Ashton, 1985; Yap et al., 1993; Edwards, 1998; Liang et al., 2004;) and Caucasian populations (Ashton, 1985, 53–57 Wold, 1949; Keller, 1973; Gwiazda et al., 1993; Goss and Jackson, 1996; Mutti et al., 2002) have demonstrated that the parental refractive status plays an important role in the refractive status of their offspring.

Large twin studies support the evidence that genetic factors play a critical role in the development of myopia, especially high myopia. High heritabilities of 84–86% (Hammond et al., 2000), 89–94% (Lyhne et al., 2001) and 75–88% (Dirani et al., 2006) were found. Myopia can be inherited as a complex trait or in a monogenic form. For the complex form, myopia appears to be the result of an interaction of multiple genes and environmental factors. Several loci have been identified by genome-wide association study as being responsible for complex myopia (Young et al., 1998; Andrew et al., 2008; Nakanishi et al., 2009; Li et al., 2010).

There is substantive evidence that genetic factors play a significant role in the development of nonsyndromic high myopia. It may be inherited in a monogenic form, in an autosomal dominant, autosomal recessive and Xlinked recessive manner (Martin and Martin, 1975). One of the first myopia loci to be mapped was on chromosome Xq28 (named MYP1) from a family with the X linked recessive form of myopia. The syndrome was later renamed as the Bornholm eye disease, and includes myopia, lazy eyes and red-green color blindness in its diagnosis (Schwartz et al., 1990).

Three autosomal dominant loci by linkage analysis were mapped in multiple independent families with nonsyndromic dominant high myopia (over –6 dpt): myopia-2 locus (MYP2) localized to chromosome 18p11.31, myopia-3 locus (MYP3) localized to chromosome 12q23.1–q24, myopia locus to chromosome 17q21–q22 (Young, 2004).

Several other genetic loci (MYP1–12) have been linked with myopia. These include the loci at 2q37.1 (MYP12)(66 Paluru et al., 2005), 4q22–27 (MYP11) (Zhang et al., 2005) and 7q36 (MYP4) (Young et al., 1998;), which are linked to high myopia (SphE –6.00 dpt). Zhu et al. (Zhu et al., 2008) have shown that axial length, a major endophenotype for refractive error, is highly heritable and is likely to be influenced by one or more genes on the long arm of chromosome 5. In addition, low/moderate (common) myopia (SphE –0.50 to –5.99 dpt) has been linked to 22q12 (MYP6) (Stambolian et al., 2004), 11p13 (MYP7), 3q36 (MYP8), 4q12 (MYP9) and 8q23 (MYP10) (Hammondd et al., 2004). There is now evidence to show that the high-myopia loci are heterogeneous (Paluru et al., 2005; Paluru et al., 2003; Young et al., 1998), and it has been speculated that some high-myopia loci may contribute to all degrees of myopia (Ibay et al., 2004; Mutti et al., 2002). However, studies that have attempted to achieve this have so far failed to replicate highmyopia loci (MYP2 and MYP3) when using the phenotype of common myopia (–1.00 or –0.75 dpt in each meridian) (Ibay et al., 2004; Mutti et al., 2002).

Several positional candidate genes were screened and found to be located at specific loci; these genes included *TGIF, EMLIN-2, MLCB* and *CLUL1*, and they map within the high-grade myopia-2 locus *(MYP2)* candidate interval (Young, 2004) and on the dermatan sulfate proteoglycan 3, decorin and *LUM* genes located on *MYP3* (Young et al., 1998). However, there is disagreement about the role of some of these candidate genes (Lin et al., 2010). For example, *TGIF* was proposed as a possible gene for *MYP2* -associated high myopia because of its location and possible involvement in scleral growth (Lam et al., 2003), but this finding was questioned by Scavello et al. (Scavello et al., 2004). Polymorphism in the *LUM* gene was also found to be associated with high myopia (Wang et al., 2006).

Results of case-control studies indicated that the single-nucleotide polymorphism of the *LUM* gene may be a risk factor for the pathogenesis of high myopia in Han Chinese, English and Finnish populations (Majava et al., 2007) and also in the Taiwanese population (Lin et al., 2010).

Until now, genetic linkage studies have mapped two dozen loci, while association studies have implicated more than 25 different genes in refractive variation. According to Wojciechowski (Wojciechowski, 2011), many of these genes are involved in common biological pathways known to mediate extracellular matrix composition and regulate connective tissue remodeling. Other associated genomic regions suggest novel mechanisms in the etiology of human myopia, such as mitochondrial-mediated cell death or photoreceptor-mediated visual signal transmission. Taken together, observational and experimental studies have revealed the complex nature of human refractive variation, which likely involves variants in several genes and functional pathways. Multiway interactions between genes and/or environmental factors may also be important in determining individual risks of myopia, and may help explain the complex pattern of refractive error in human populations (Jacobi and Pusch, 2010).

Instead of a simple 1-gene locus controlling the onset of myopia, a complex interaction of many mutated proteins acting in concert may be the cause. Instead of myopia being caused by a defect in a structural protein, defects in the control of these structural proteins might be the actual cause of myopia (Jacobi and Pusch, 2010).

References

Andrew T, Maniatis N, Carbonaro F, Liew SH, Lau W, Spector TD, et al. Identification and replication of three novel myopia common susceptibility gene loci on chromosome 3q26 using linkage and linkage disequilibrium mapping. *PLoS Genet* 2008; 4:e1000220.

Ashton GC. Segregation analysis of ocular refraction and myopia. *Hum Hered* 1985; 35: 232–239.

Atchison DA, Jones CE, Schmid KL, et al. Eye shape in emmetropia and myopia. *Invest Ophthalmol Vis Sci.* 2004; 45:3380–3386.

Baily AJ, Paul RG, Knott L. Mechanisms of maturation and ageing of collagen. Mech Age Dev. 1998;106:1–56.

Bhattachrayya KB, Basu S. Acute myopia induced by topiramate: report of a case and review of the literature. *Neurol India*2005; 53:108–109.

Boonyaleephan S. Bilateral *J Med Assoc Thai.* 2008 Dec;91(12):1904-1907.

Brandão MN, Fernandes IC, Barradas FF, Machado JF, Oliveira MT. [Acute myopia *Arq Bras Oftalmol.* 2009 Jan-Feb;72(1):103-105. Portuguese.

Buch H, Vinding T, Nielsen NV. Prevalence and causes of visual impairment according to World Health Organization and United States criteria in an aged, urban Scandinavian population: the Copenhagen City Eye Study. *Ophthalmology* 2001; 108: 2347-2357.

Caglar C, Yasar T, Ceyhan D. Topiramate induced bilateral angle-closure. *J Ocul Pharmacol Ther.* 2012 Apr;28(2):205 207. doi: 10.1089/jop.2011.0161. Epub 2011 Dec 8.

Cotter SA, Varma R, Ying-Lai M, Azen SP, Klein R, Los Angeles Latino Eye Study Group. Causes of low vision and blindness in adult Latinos: the Los Angeles Latino Eye Study. *Ophthalmology* 2006; 113: 1574-1582.

Cruciani F, Lorenzatti M, Nazzarro V, Abdolrahimzadeh S. Bilateral acute angle closure glaucoma and myopia induced topiramate. *Clin Ter.* 2009;160(3):215 216.

Curtin B, Karlin D. Axial length measurements and fundus changes of the myopic eye. *Am J Ophthalmol* 1971; 71: 42-53.

Dietz HC, Cutting GR, Pyeritz RE, Maslen CL, Sakai LY, Corson GM, et al. Marfan syndrome caused by a recurrent de novo missense mutation in the fibrillin gene. *Nature* 1991; 352: 337-339.

Dirani M, Chamberlain M, Shekar SN, Islam AF, Garoufalis P, Chen CY, et al. Heritability of refractive error and ocular biometrics: the Genes in Myopia (GEM) twin study. *Invest Ophthalmol Vis Sci* 2006; 47: 4756–4761.

Donders FC. Die Anomalien der Refraction und Accommodation des Auges. 1866:279–379.

Dorronzoro E, Santos-Bueso E, Vico-Ruiz E, Sáenz-Frances F, Argaya J, Gegúndez-Fernández JA. [Myopia and retinal striae *Arch Soc Esp Oftalmol.* 2011 Jan;86(1):24-26. doi: 10.1016/j.oftal.2010.10.009. Epub 2011 Feb 19. Spanish.

Edwards MH. Effect of parental myopia on the development of myopia in Hong Kong Chinese. *Ophthalmic Physiol Optics J Br Coll Ophthalmic Opticians* 1998; 18: 477–483.

Fan DS, Lam DS, Lam RF, et al. Prevalence, incidence, and progression of myopia of school children in Hong Kong. Invest Ophthalmol Vis Sci 2004;45:1071-1075.

Fan DS, Rao SK, Cheung EY, et al. Astigmatism in Chinese preschool children: prevalence, change, and effect on refractive development. *Br J Ophthalmol* 2004;88:938-941.

Fan JT, Johnson DH, Burk RR. Transient myopia, angle-closure glaucoma, and choroidal detachment after oral acetazolamide. *Am J Ophthalmol.* 1993;115:813–814.

Feldkaemper MP, Neacsu I, Schaeffel F. Insulin acts as a powerful stimulator of axial myopia *Invest Ophthalmol Vis Sci.* 2009 Jan;50(1):13-23. doi: 10.1167/iovs.08-1702. Epub 2008 Jul 3.

Gawley SD. Topiramate induced acute transient myopia *Cases J.* 2009 Jul 3;2:7430. doi: 10.4076/1757-1626-2-7430.

Goldschmidt E. Myopia in humans: can progression be arrested? *Ciba Found Symp* 1990;155:222-229.

Goss DA, Jackson TW. Clinical findings before the onset of myopia in youth. 4. Parental history of myopia. *Optometry Vision Sci* 1996; 73: 279-282.

Goss DA. Attempts to reduce the rate of increase of myopia in young people—a critical literature review. *Am J Optom Physiol Optics* 1982;59:828–841.

Green JS, Bear JC, Johnson GJ. The burden of genetically determined eye disease. *Br J Ophthalmol* 1986; 70: 696–699.

Grødum K, Heijl A, Bengtsson B. Refractive error and glaucoma. *Acta Ophthalmol Scand* 2001;79:560-566.

Grossniklaus H, Green W. Pathologic findings in pathologic myopia. *Retina* 1992; 12: 127–133.

Grosvenor T, Perrigin DM, Perrigin J, Maslovitz B. Houston Myopia Control Study: a randomized clinical trial. Part II. Final report by the patient care team. *Am J Optom Physiol Opt* 1987;64:482-498.

Guggenheim JA, McBrien NA. Form-deprivation myopia induces activation of scleral matrix metalloproteinase-2 in tree shrew. *Invest Ophthalmol Vis Sci.* 1996;37:1380–1395.

Guier CP. Elevated intraocular *Optom Vis Sci.* 2007 Dec;84(12):1070-1073.

Gwiazda J, Thorn F, Bauer J, Held R. Emmetropization and the progression of manifest refraction in children followed from infancy to puberty. *Clin Vis Sci* 1993; 8: 337–344.

Hammond CJ, Andrew T, Mak YT, Spector TD. A susceptibility locus for myopia in the normal population is linked to the PAX6 gene region on chromosome 11: a genome wide scan of dizygotic twins. *Am J Hum Genet* 2004; 75: 294–304.

Hammond CJ, Snieder H, Spector TD, Gilbert CE. Factors affecting pupil size after dilatation: the Twin Eye Study. *Br J Ophthalmol* 2000; 84: 1173-1176.

Hayashi K, Ohno-Matsui K, Shimada N, Moriyama M, Kojima A, Hayashi W, et al. Long-term pattern of progression of myopic maculopathy: a natural history study. *Ophthalmology* 2010; 117: 1595-1611.

Hirschberg J. The history of ophthalmology. The middle ages; the sixteenth and seventeenth centuries. West Germany, 1985;2:263–279.

Ho M, Liu DTL, Chan VCK, Lam DSC. Choroidal thickness measurement in myopic eyes by enhanced depth optical coherence tomography. *Ophthalmology* 2013;120:1909-1914.

Holmstrom GE, Larsson EK. Development of spherical equivalent refraction in prematurely born children during the first 10 years of life: a population-based study. *Arch Ophthalmol* 2005;123:1404-1411.

Hung LF, Crawford ML, Smith EL. Spectacle lenses alter eye growth and the refractive status of young monkeys. *Nat Med* 1995;1:761–765.

Hyman L, Gwiazda J, Hussein M, et al. Relationship of age, sex, and ethnicity with myopia progression and axial elongation in the correction of myopia evaluation trial. Arch Ophthalmol 2005;123:977-987.

Ibay G, Doan B, Reider L, Dana D, Schlifka M, Hu H, et al: Candidate high myopia loci on chromosomes 18p and 12q do not play a major role in susceptibility to common myopia. *BMC Med Genet* 2004; 5: 20.

Iuvone PM, Tigges M, Stone RA, et al. Effects of apomorphine, a dopamine receptor agonist, on ocular refraction and axial elongation in a primate model of myopia. *Invest Ophthalmol Vis Sci.* 1991;32:1674–1677.

Iwase A, Araie M, Tomidokoro A, Yamamoto T, Shimizu H, Kitazawa Y, et al. Prevalence and causes of low vision and blindness in a Japanese adult population: the Tajimi Study. *Ophthalmology* 2006; 113: 1354–1362.

Jacobi FK, Pusch CM. A decade in search of myopia genes. *Front Biosci* 2010; 15: 359–372.

Jacobsen N, Jensen H, Goldschmidt E: Does the level of physical activity in university students influence development and progression of myopia? A 2-year prospective cohort study. *Investigative Ophthalmol Vis Sci* 2008; 49: 1322–1327.

Jensen H. Myopia progression in young school children and intraocular pressure. *Doc Ophthalmol* 1992;82:249-255.

Jobling A, Nguyen M, Gentle A, et al. Isoform-specific changes in scleral TGF-β expression and the regulation of collagen synthesis during myopia progression. *J Biol Chem.* 2004;279:18121–18126.

Jones LA, Mitchell GL, Mutti DO, et al. Comparison of ocular component growth curves among refractive error groups in children. *Invest Ophthalmol Vis Sci.* 2005;46:2317–2327.

Kamath S, Acharya N, Nithyanandam S. Co-trimoxazole-induced myopia. *Int J STD AIDS.* 2012 Jan;23(1):71-2. doi: 10.1258/ijsa.2011.010476.

Keller JT: A comparison of the refractive status of myopic children and their parents. *Am J Optometry Arch Am Acad Optometry* 1973; 50: 206–211.

Kerimoglu H, Tokgoz M, Ozturk B, Gonul S, Pekel H. Topiramate-induced acute-onset myopia. *Can J Ophthalmol.* 2009 Apr;44(2):222-3. doi: 10.3129/i09-017.

Knowlton RG, Weaver EJ, Struyk AF, Knobloch WH, King RA, Norris K, et al. Genetic linkage analysis of hereditary arthro-ophthalmopathy (Stickler syndrome) and the type II procollagen gene. *Am J Hum Genet* 1989; 45: 681–688.

Krieg PH, Schipper I. Drug-induced ciliary body oedema: a new theory. *Eye* (Lond) 1996;10:121–126.

Krumpaszky HG, Ludtke R, Mickler A, Klauss V, Selbmann HK. Blindness incidence in Germany. A population-based study from Wurttemberg-Hohenzollern. *Ophthalmologica* 1999; 213: 176–182.

Kumar M, Kesarwani S, Rao A, Garnaik A. Macular folds: an unusual association in topiramate toxicity *Clin Exp Optom.* 2012 Jul;95(4):449-452. doi: 10.1111/j.1444-0938.2012.00722.x. Epub 2012 May 9.

Kwon SJ, Park DH, Shin JP. Bilateral transient myopia, angle-closure glaucoma, and choroidal detachment induced by methazolamide. *Jpn J Ophthalmol.* 2012 Sep;56(5):515-517. doi: 10.1007/s10384-012-0159-y. Epub 2012 Jul 12.

Lam DS, Lee WS, Leung YF, Tam PO, Fan DS, Fan BJ, et al. TGF beta-induced factor: a candidate gene for high myopia. *Invest Ophthalmol Vis Sci* 2003; 44: 1012–1015.

Laties AM, Stone RA. Some visual and neurochemical correlates of refractive development. *Vis Neurosci* 1991;7:125–128.

Latini MF, Romano LM. Topiramate-induced acute myopia. *Acta Neurol Belg* 2012 Mar;112(1):81-84. doi: 10.1007/s13760-012-0022-4. Epub 2012 Feb 3.

Li Y, Vinckenbosch N, Tian G, Huerta-Sanchez E, Jiang T, Jiang H, et al. Resequencing of 200 human exomes identifies an excess of low-frequency non-synonymous coding variants. *Nat Genet* 2010; 42: 969–972.

Liang CL, Yen E, Su JY, Liu C, Chang TY, Park N, et al: Impact of family history of high myopia on level and onset of myopia. *Invest Ophthalmol Vis Sci* 2004; 45: 3446–3452.

Lim R, Mitchell P, Cumming RG. Refractive associations with cataract: the Blue Mountains Eye Study. *Invest Ophthalmol Vis Sci* 1999;40:3021-3026.

Lin HJ, Kung YJ, Lin YJ, Sheu JJ, Chen BH, Lan YC, et al: Association of the lumican gene functional 3 _ -UTR polymorphism with high myopia. *Invest Ophthalmol Vis Sci* 2010; 51: 96–102.

Lin SF, Lin PK, Chang FL, Tsai RK. Transient hyperopia *Ophthalmologica* 2009;223(1):68-71. doi: 10.1159/000173714. Epub 2008 Nov 20.

Lyhne N, Sjolie AK, Kyvik KO, Green A: The importance of genes and environment for ocular refraction and its determiners: a population based study among 20–45 year old twins. *Br J Ophthalmol* 2001; 85: 1470–1476.

Majava M, Bishop PN, Hagg P, Scott PG, Rice A, Inglehearn C, et al. Novel mutations in the small leucine-rich repeat protein/proteoglycan (SLRP) genes in high myopia. *Hum Mutat* 2007; 28: 336–344.

Mandal A, Chatterjee S, Bose S, Ganguly G. Ocular adverse effects *Indian J Pharmacol.* 2008 Nov;40(6):278-280. doi: 10.4103/0253-7613.45156.

Marcus MW, Müskens RP, Ramdas WD, Wolfs RC, de Jong PT, Vingerling JR, Hofman A, Stricker BH, Jansonius NM. Antithrombotic medication *Invest Ophthalmol Vis Sci* 2012 Jun 20;53(7):3801-3805. doi: 10.1167/iovs.12-9604.

Martin NG, Martin PG. The inheritance of scholastic abilities in a sample of twins. I. Ascertainments of the sample and diagnosis of zygosity. *Ann Hum Genet* 1975; 39: 213–218.

McBrien NA, Gentle A. Role of sclera in the development and pathological complications of myopia. *Prog Ret Eye Res* 2003;22:307–38.

Metge, P: Definitions. Vol. La myopie forte. 1994, pp 14–17.

Munier A, Gunning T, Kenny D, O'Keefe M. Causes of blindness in the adult population of the Republic of Ireland. *Br J Ophthalmol* 1998; 82: 630–633.

Muniesa Royo MJ, Traveset Maeso A, Jurjo Campo C. [Topiramate-induced bilateral acute angle closure glaucoma. Med Clin (Barc). 2012 Apr 7;138(8):368-9. doi: 10.1016/j.medcli.2011.06.003. Epub 2011 Sep 21. Spanish.

Mutti DO, Bullimore MA. Myopia: an epidemic of possibilities? Optom Vis Sci 1999;76:257–258.

Mutti DO, Mitchell GL, Moeschberger ML,Jones LA, Zadnik K. Parental myopia, near work, school achievement, and children's refractive error. *Invest Ophthalmol Vis Sci* 2002; 43: 3633–3640.

Mutti DO, Semina E, Marazita M, Cooper M, Murray JC, Zadnik K. Genetic loci for pathological myopia are not associated with juvenile myopia. *Am J Med Genet* 2002; 112: 355–360.

Mutti DO, Zadnik K, Adams AJ. Myopia. The nature versus nurture debate goes on. *Invest Ophthalmol Vis Sci* 1996;37:952–957.

Nair AG, Nair AG, George RJ, Biswas J, Gandhi RA. Aripiprazole induced transient myopia *Cutan Ocul Toxicol* 2012 Mar;31(1):74-76. doi: 10.3109/15569527.2011.603106. Epub 2011 Aug 10.

Nakanishi H, Yamada R, Gotoh N, Hayashi H, Yamashiro K, Shimada N, et al: A genome-wide association analysis identified a novel susceptible locus for pathological myopia at 11q24.1. *PLoS Genet* 2009; 5:e1000660.

Nijbroek G, Sood S, McIntosh I, Francomano CA, Bull E, Pereira L, et al. Fifteen novel FBN1 mutations causing Marfan syndrome detected by heteroduplex analysis of genomic amplicons. *Am J Hum Genet* 1995; 57: 8–21.

Paluru P, Ronan SM, Heon E, Devoto M, Wildenberg SC, Scavello G, et al. New locus for autosomal dominant high myopia maps to the long arm of chromosome 17. *Invest Ophthalmol Vis Sci* 2003; 44: 1830–1836.

Paluru PC, Nallasamy S, Devoto M, Rappaport EF, Young TL: Identification of a novel locus on 2q for autosomal dominant highgrade myopia. *Invest Ophthalmol Vis Sci* 2005; 46: 2300–2307.

Panday VA, Rhee DJ. Review of sulfonamide-induced acute myopia and acute bilateral angle-closure glaucoma. *Compr Ophthalmol Update* 2007;8:271–276.

Parssinen O, Hemminki E, Klemetti A. Effect of spectacle use and accommodation on myopic progression: final results of a three-year randomised clinical trial among schoolchildren. *Br J Ophthalmol* 1989;73:547-551.

Paur R, Wallner C, Hermann P, Stöllberger C, Finsterer J. Neurological abnormalities in opiate addicts with and without substitution. *Am J Drug Alcohol Abuse* 2012 May;38(3):239-245. doi: 10.3109/00952990.2011.644001.

Penha AM, Burkhardt E, Schaeffel F, Feldkaemper MP. Effects of intravitreal insulin *Mol Vis* 2012;18:2608-2622. Epub 2012 Oct 20.

Polkinghorne PJ, Craig JP. North New Zealand rhegmatogenous retinal detachment study: epidemiology and risk factors. *Clin Exp Ophthalmol* 2004;32:159–163.

Postel EA, Assalian A, Epstein DL. Drug-induced transient myopia and angle-closure glaucoma associated with supraciliary choroidal effusion. *Am J Ophthalmol* 1996;122:110–112.

Pousi B, Hautala T, Heikkinen J, Pajunen L, Kivirikko KI, Myllyla R. Alu-Alu recombination results in a duplication of seven exons in the lysyl hydroxylase gene in a patient with the type VI variant of Ehlers-Danlos syndrome. *Am J Hum Genet* 1994; 55: 899–906.

Pruett R. Pathologic myopia; in Albert DM, Jakobiec JF (eds): Principles and Practice of Ophthalmology. Philadelphia, *Saunders Co*, 1994, pp 878–889.

Rabin J, Van Sluyters RC, Malach R. Emmetropization: a vision-dependent phenomenon. *Invest Ophthalmol Vis Sci* 1981;20:561-564.

Richa S, Yazbek JC. Ocular adverse effects. *CNS Drugs* 2010 Jun;24(6):501-26. doi: 10.2165/11533180-000000000-00000. Review.

Richards AJ, Yates JR, Williams R, Payne SJ, Pope FM, Scott JD, et al. A family with Stickler syndrome type 2 has a mutation in the COL11A1 gene resulting in the substitution of glycine 97 by valine in alpha 1 (XI) collagen. *Hum Mol Genet* 1996; 5: 1339–1343.

Risk factors for idiopathic rhegmatogenous retinal detachment. The Eye Disease Case-Control Study Group. *Am J Epidemiol* 1993;137:749-757.

Ritchey ER, Zelinka CP, Tang J, Liu J, Fischer AJ. The combination of IGF1 and FGF2 and the induction. *Exp Eye Res* 2012 Jun;99:1-16. doi: 10.1016/j.exer.2012.03.019.

Robb RM. Refractive errors associated with hemangiomas of the eyelids and orbit in infancy. *Am J Ophthalmol* 1977;83:52-58.

Rodríguez-Blanco M, Piñeiro A, Bande M, López-Valladares MJ. [Angle-closure. *Arch Soc Esp Oftalmol.* 2012 Apr;87(4):122-124. doi: 10.1016/j.oftal.2011.07.015. Epub 2012 Jan 13. Spanish.

Roh YR, Woo SJ, Park KH. Acute-onset bilateral myopia. *Korean J Ophthalmol.* 2011 Jun;25(3):214-217. doi: 10.3341/kjo.2011.25.3.214. Epub 2011 May 24.

Ruben M, Rajpurohit P. Distribution of myopia in aphakic retinal detachments. *Br J Ophthalmol* 1976; 60: 517–521.

Saunders KJ. Early refractive development in humans. *Surv Ophthalmol* 1995;40:207-16.

Saw SM, Tong L, Chua WH, et al. Incidence and progression of myopia in Singaporean school children. *Invest Ophthalmol Vis Sci* 2005;46:51-57.

Saw SM. How blinding is pathological myopia? *Br J Ophthalmol* 2006;90:525–526

Scavello GS, Paluru PC, Ganter WR, Young TL. Sequence variants in the transforming growth beta-induced factor (TGIF) gene are not associated with high myopia. *Invest Ophthalmol Vis Sci* 2004; 45: 2091–2097.

Schwartz M, Haim M, Skarsholm D: Xlinked myopia: Bornholm eye disease. Linkage to DNA markers on the distal part of Xq. *Clin Genet* 1990; 38: 281–286.

Sertie AL, Sossi V, Camargo AA, Zatz M, Brahe C, Passos-Bueno MR: Collagen XVIII, containing an endogenous inhibitor of angiogenesis and tumor growth, plays a critical role in the maintenance of retinal structure and in neural tube closure (Knobloch syndrome). *Hum Mol Genet* 2000; 9: 2051–2058.

Shih YF, Chen CH, Chou AC, et al. Effects of different concentrations of atropine on controlling myopia in myopic children. *J Ocul Pharmacol Ther* 1999;15:85-90.

Shih YF, Hsiao CK, Chen CJ, et al. An intervention trial on efficacy of atropine and multi-focal glasses in controlling myopic progression. *Acta Ophthalmol Scand* 2001;79:233-6.

Soubrane G. Choroidal neovascularization in pathologic myopia: recent developments in diagnosis and treatment. *Surv Ophthalmol* 2008; 53: 121–138.

Stambolian D, Ibay G, Reider L, Dana D, Moy C, Schlifka M, et al. Genomewide linkage scan for myopia susceptibility loci among Ashkenazi Jewish families shows evidence of linkage on chromosome 22q12. *Am J Hum Genet* 2004; 75: 448–459.

Stone RA, Lin T, Laties AM, et al. Retinal dopamine and form-deprivation myopia. *Proc Natl Acad Sci 1989;86:704–706.*

Stratos AA, Peponis VG, Portaliou DM, Stroubini TE, Skouriotis S, Kymionis GD. Secondary pseudomyopia induced by amisulpride. *Optom Vis Sci.* 2011 Nov;88(11):1380-2. doi: 10.1097/OPX.0b013e3182297d44.

Szawarski P, Hall-Thompson B. Acetazolamide-induced myopia. *Wilderness Environ Med. 2009* Fall;20(3):300-1. doi: 10.1580/08-WEME-LE-259R1.1

Tano Y. Pathologic myopia: where are we now? *Am. J Ophthalmol* 2002;134:645–660

Thorn F, Gwiazda J, Held R. Myopia progression is specified by a double exponential growth function. *Opt Vis Sci.* 2005;82:E286.

Tokoro T, Kabe S. Treatment of the myopia and the changes in optical components. Report II. Full or under correction of myopia by glasses. *Acta Soc Ophthalmol Jpn* 1965;69:140–144.

Tokoro T. On the definition of pathologic myopia in group studies. *Acta Ophthalmol Suppl* 1988; 185: 107–108.

Trier K, Olsen EB, Kobayashi T, et al. Biochemical and ultrastructural changes in rabbit sclera after treatment with 7- methylxanthine, theobromine, acetazolamide or L-ornithine. *Br J Ophthalmol.* 1999;83:1370–1375.

Trier K, Munk Ribel-Madsen S, Cui D, Brøgger Christensen S. Systemic 7-methylxanthine in retarding axial eye growth and myopia progression: a 36-month pilot study. *J Ocul Biol Dis Infor* 2008, 1(2-4):85-93.

Troilo D, Nickla DL, Wildsoet CF. Form deprivation myopia in mature common marmosets (Callithrix jacchus). *Invest Ophthalmol Vis Sci* 2000;41:2043–2049.

Troilo D, Wallman J. The regulation of eye growth and refractive state: an experimental study of emmetropization. *Vis Res* 1991;31:1237–1250.

van Issum C, Mavrakanas N, Schutz JS, Shaarawy T. Topiramate-induced acute bilateral angle closure *Eur J Ophthalmol.* 2011 Jul-Aug;21(4):404-409. doi: 10.5301 /EJO.2010.5979.

Verteporfin in Photodynamic Therapy Study Group. Photodynamic therapy of subfoveal choroidal neovascularization in pathologic myopia with verteporfin. 1-year results of a randomized clinical trial–VIP report no. 1. *Ophthalmology* 2001; 108:841–852

Vilar Ventura RM, Vilar Fabra C, Ramos Martí F. [Acute myopia] *Neurologia.* 2009 Jun;24(5):350. Spanish. No abstract available.

Vishwakarma P, Raman GV, Sathyan P. Mefenamic acid. *Indian J Ophthalmol.* 2009 Sep-Oct;57(5):398-400. doi: 10.4103/0301-4738.55066.

Wang IJ, Chiang TH, Shih YF, Hsiao CK, Lu SC, Hou YC, et al. The association of single nucleotide polymorphisms in the 5'-regulatory region of the lumican gene with susceptibility to high myopia in Taiwan. *Mol Vision* 2006, 12: 852–857.

Wojciechowski R: Nature and nurture: the complex genetics of myopia and refractive error. *Clin Genet* 2011; 79: 301–320.

Wold K. Hereditary myopia. *Arch Ophthalmol* 1949; 42: 225–237.

Wong TY, Klein BE, Klein R, et al. Refractive errors, intraocular pressure, and glaucoma in a white population. *Ophthalmology* 2003;110:211-217.

Xu L, Wang Y, Li Y, Wang Y, Cui T, Li J, et al. Causes of blindness and visual impairment in urban and rural areas in Beijing: the Beijing Eye Study. *Ophthalmology* 2006; 113 (7): 1134 e1–e11.

Yamamoto I, Rogers AH, Reichel E, Yates PA, Duker JS. Intravitreal bevacizumab (Avastin) as treatment for subfoveal choroidal neovascularisation secondary to pathological myopia. *Br J Ophthalmol* 2007;91:157–160

Yap M, Wu M, Liu ZM, Lee FL, Wang SH. Role of heredity in the genesis of myopia. *Ophthalmic Physiol Optics J Br Coll Ophthalmic Opticians* 1993; 13: 316–319.

Yoshida T, Ohno-Matsui K, Ohtake Y, Takashima T, Futagami S, Baba T, Yasuzumi K, Tokoro T, Mochizuki M. Long-term visual prognosis of choroidal neovascularization in high myopia: a comparison between age groups. *Ophthalmology* 2002; 109:712–719

Whitman WG, Curtin BJ. The optics of myopia. Chapter 42. In Duane's ophthalmology on CD-Rom, Tasman W and Jaeger EA, editors. Philadelphia: *Lippincott Williams & Wilkins,* 2006 edition

Yoshida T, Ohno-Matsui K, Yasuzumi K, Kojima A, Shimada N, Futagami S, Tokoro T, Mochizuki M. Myopic choroidal neovascularization: a 10-year follow-up. *Ophthalmology* 2003; 110:1297–1305

Young TL, Ronan SM, Alvear AB, Wildenberg SC, Oetting WS, Atwood LD, et al. A second locus for familial high myopia maps to chromosome 12q. *Am J Hum Genet* 1998; 63: 1419–1424.

Young TL, Ronan SM, Drahozal LA, Wildenberg SC, Alvear AB, Oetting WS, et al. Evidence that a locus for familial high myopia maps to chromosome 18p. *Am J Hum Gen* 1998; 63: 109–119.

Young TL. Dissecting the genetics of human high myopia: a molecular biologic approach. *Trans Am Ophthalmol Soc* 2004; 102: 423–445.

Zadnik K, Mutti DO, Friedman NE, Adams AJ. Initial cross-sectional results from the Orinda Longitudinal Study of Myopia. *Optom Vis Sci* 1993;70:750-758.

Zhang Q, Guo X, Xiao X, Jia X, Li S, Hejtmancik JF. A new locus for autosomal dominant high myopia maps to 4q22–q27 between D4S1578 and D4S1612. *Mol Vision* 2005; 11: 554–560.

Zhao J, Mao J, Luo R, et al. The progression of refractive error in school-age children: Shunyi district, China. *Am J Ophthalmol* 2002;134:735-743.

Zhu G, Hewitt AW, Ruddle JB, Kearns LS, Brown SA, Mackinnon JR, et al. Genetic dissection of myopia: evidence for linkage of ocular axial length to chromosome 5q. *Ophthalmology* 2008; 115: 1053–1057.

Zhu ZC, Zhang JS, Ji XY, Wang YF, Chen Y, Li XJ. [Insulin-like growth] *Zhonghua Yan Ke Za Zhi.* 2007 Dec;43(12):1125-1129. Chinese.

Chapter II

Epidemiology and Risk Factors

1. Epidemiology

Myopia is the most common eye disease and is one of the leading causes of vision impairment worldwide (Lin et al., 2004; Wang et al., 1988; Vitale et al., 2009; Bar Bayan et al., 2005; Klaver et al., 1998; Liu et al., 2001; Krumpaszky et al., 1999; Evans et al., 2004; Xu et al., 2006; Avisar et al., 2006; Yamada et al., 2010; You et al., 2011). The number of people with myopia is increasing (Wang et al., 1988; Vitale et al., 2009), particularly in developing countries (Lin et al., 2004; Bar Bayan et al., 2005; Klaver et al., 1998), and is reaching very high proportions.

Cross-sectional studies report wide variations in the prevalence of myopia among different populations (He et al., 2007;He et al., 2004; Maul et al., 2000; Murthy et al., 2002; Naidoo et al., 2003; Zhao et al., 2000; Saw et al., 2006).

The prevalence of refractive errors varies among the populations. The prevalence of myopia (spherical equivalent (SE), <-1.0 or -0.5 diopters (D)) ranged from 15% to 28% among white populations in Europe (Hofman et al., 1991; Kempen, 2004), the United States (Sperduto et al., 1983; Katz et al., 1997; Wang et al., 1994), and Australia (Wensor et al., 1999; Attebo et al., 1999; Hyams et al., 1977) and 17% in a Hispanic population (Tarczy-Hornoch et al., 2006). Myopia is reportedly less common among black populations (Katz et al., 1997; Kaimbo and Kaimbo and Missotten,1996). In East Asian countries, several recent population-based studies on refractive error have been carried out in developing and developed Asian countries and the prevalence of myopia often has been presumed to be much higher (Saw et al., 1996; Saw et al., 2002; Dandona et al., 2002; Dandona et al., 2002; Murthy et al., 2002; Wickremasinghe et al., 2004; Bourne et al., 2004; Tong et al., 2004; Lin et al., 2001; Wong et al., 2000; Cheng et al., 2003; Xu et al., 2005). The prevalence of myopia in elderly individuals exceeded 30% in Indonesia (Saw et al., 2002) and Singapore (Wong et al., 2000), whereas it was lower (17%–27%) in India (Dandona et al., 2002), Mongolia (Wickremasinghe et al., 2004), Bangladesh (Bourne et al., 2004), and China (Xu et al., 2005). In Japan, a developed country of East Asia the prevalence of myopia was 41.8%. (Sawada et al., 2008). In Korea, the prevalence of myopia was 96.54% (Jung et al., 2012) which is one of the highest prevalences of myopia in published reports to date.

Prevalence of myopia is significantly different among racial groups, although its worldwide prevalence is approximately 30% (3%–84%) (Edwards and Lam, 2004). The highest prevalence is found in East Asia, such as mainland China (78.4% in people aged 5–15 years) (He et al., 2004); Hong Kong (70% in people aged 17 years) (Edwards and Lam, 2004); Taiwan (84.0% in peopled aged 16–18 years) (Lin et al., 2004); Japan (65.6% in people aged 17 years) (Matsumura and Hirai, 1999) and in Korea (96.54%, in 19-year-old male conscripts). Mongolia has a markedly lower prevalence of myopia (17.2%), although this data was harvested from a group aged over 40 years (Wickremasinghe et al., 2004).

The prevalence of myopia in the US population was estimated in the early 1970s to be 25% in persons aged 12 to 54 years (Sperduto et al., 1983). A recent meta-analysis of population-based studies found a prevalence of 25% in persons over age 40 (Kempen et al.,2004).

Approximately three quarters of Americans over the age of 40 have ametropia of sufficient magnitude to require refractive correction (Kempen et al., 2004). It has been estimated that 93 million Americans aged 12 years and older use some form of eyewear to correct refractive errors in distance (Vitale et al., 2006). About 36 million people in the United States (US) used contact lenses in 2005 (Barr, 2006). It is estimated that over 8 million patients in the US have undergone refractive surgery since 1995 (Global refractive marlet report, 2006).

Two population-based studies in the US have reported that the prevalence of myopia in Latino persons aged 40 and older was 17% to 18% (Kempen et al., 2004; Tarczy-Hornoch et al., 2006). A similar pattern was reported in Australia (Attebo et al., 1999; Wensor and McCarty, 1999) and in populations of African descent in Baltimore and Barbados (Katz et al., 1997; Wu et al.,1999).

A number of population-based studies in different Asian countries indicate that the prevalence of myopia varies considerably: in elderly Taiwanese persons, the prevalence was 19% (≥65 years); in India, the prevalence was 37% (≥40 years) (Dandona et al., 2002); in Indonesia, the prevalence was 26% (Saw et al.,2002); and in Beijing, the prevalence was 23% (≥40 years) (Xu et al.,2005). Other studies of young adult Asian populations indicate that the prevalence of myopia is much higher than in their US counterparts, ranging from 56% in 15- to 19-year old Singaporean students (Quek et al., 2004) to 85% in 19- to 23-year old medical students in Singapore (Woo et al.,2004). In Lao People's, a landlocked country in South Asia, a low prevalence of myopia was found (Casson et al., 2012); there was an estimated 16% overall prevalence of refractive error (myopia and hyperopia combined), but the overall prevalence of refractive error was only 3.6% (95% CI, 2.6-4.7; 112 subjects). Correspondingly, few subjects were visually impaired, and only 5 subjects had moderate visual impairment.

The prevalence of myopia is considerably lower in western Asian regions (Dandona et al., 2002; Pokharel et al., 2000, Yekta et al., 2010) and white Australian children (Robael et al., 2006), and at its lowest in healthy indigenous Australian children (Taylor et al., 2010; Landers et al., 2010; Stocks et al., 1997). A nationwide study found that the prevalence of "low vision" (VA<20/40 but ≤20/200) in Australian aboriginal children aged 5 to 15 years was 1.5% (95% CI, 0.9-2.1), and only 15 of the 1694 children in the sample had low vision due to refractive error (Taylor et al., 2010). In schoolchildren (age range, 6 to 11 years) from Lao People (Casson et al., 2012), the prevalence of low vision was slightly lower than that in indigenous Australian children (1.2% (95% CI, 0.4-2.0)) and was also explained by the extremely low prevalence of myopia.

The prevalence of myopia in American children aged 12 to 17 was estimated at around 25% in the early 1970s (Sperduto et al., 1983). In a recent study, myopia (–0.75 D or more) was found in 9% of children aged 5 to 17 years (Kleinstein et al., 2003). Data from the Orinda, California, Longitudinal Study found that the prevalence of myopia of 0.5 D or more was about 3% among 5- to 7-year-olds, 8% among 8- to 10-year-olds, and 14% among 11- to 12-year-olds (Zadnik et al., 1993). Recent data suggest that ethnic Chinese children have much higher rates of myopia at all ages. A national survey in Taiwan found the prevalence was 12% among 6-year-old children and 84% among those 16 to 18 years old (Lin et bal, 1999). In a series of studies using similar methodology and definitions for myopia (–0.5 D or more) in children aged 7 to 15 years, prevalences of myopia varied widely by country and ethnicity: 4% in India (Dandona et al.,2002); 10% to 34% in Malaysia (Goh et al.,2005); 5% to 17% in southern China (He et al., 2004); 7% in New Delhi (Murthy et al., 2002); and 9% to 40% in Malaysia and Singapore (Saw et al., 2006). Similar rates have been found in Singapore (12% among 6- to 7-year-olds to 79% among 18-year-old males), and in Japan (44% among 12-year-olds to 66% among 17-year-olds) (Wu et al., 2001; Lin et al.,, 1988; Zhan et al., 2000; Matsumura and Hirai, 1999).

Pathologic Myopia - Myopic Retinopathy

Pathologic myopia is among the major causes of visual impairment and blindness worldwide, especially in East Asia. It is well known that prevalence of high myopia is higher in Asian populations than other racial populations (Sawada et al., 2008). According to the Tajimi Study, myopic macular degeneration is the third leading cause of low vision, and the leading cause of blindness in Japan (Iwase et al., 2006). In the Shihpai Eye Study, it was the second most frequent cause of visual impairment and blindness in Taiwan (Hsu et al., 2004). In the Beijing Eye Study, myopic macular degeneration was the second most common cause of low/blindness in China (Xu et al., 2006). Although myopia was found to be less prevalent in Western countries, myopic macular degeneration has also been reported to be second to fourth most frequent cause of blindness in Caucasians (Buch et al., 2004; Cedrone et al., 2003; Klaver et al., 1998, Krumpaszky et al., 1999; Cotter et al., 2006). Myopic retinopathy often has bilateral impacts, and patients are frequently middle-aged and working people (Hayashi et al., 2010, Vongphanit et al., 2002).

Previously, 2 population-based studies estimated the prevalence of myopic retinopathy. In the Blue Mountains Eye Study in Australia, which focused on a white population, the prevalence of myopic retinopathy was 1.2% (Vongphanit et al., 2012). In The Beijing Eye Study performed in a Chinese population the prevalence was 3.1% (Liu et al., 2010). It has been reported that high myopia is more common among Asian populations, especially in East Asian countries, than among white, black, or Hispanic people (Sawada et al., 2008). The prevalence of myopia (SE<0.5 diopters) in the Hisayama Study (Asakuma et al., 2012) performed in a general Japanese population was 37.7%., which is higher than that in the Beijing Eye Study (21.8%) and that in the Blue Mountains Eye Study (14.4%). In the Hisayama Study (Asakuma et al., 2012), the prevalence of high myopia (SE<-5.0 diopters) was 5.7%, which is still higher than that in the Beijing Eye Study (3.3%) and much higher than that in the Blue Mountains Eye Study (2.2%) (Vongphanit et al., 2012; Xu et al., 2005; Attebo et al., 1999).. The precise reason for racial differences in the prevalence of myopic retinopathy is unknown, but it could be related to differences in the characteristics of study participants (e.g., the age and proportion of either gender), differences in the methodology or study design (e.g., the definition of myopic retinopathy), or perhaps to genetic factors. Further investigations of other populations worldwide are expected.

2. Risk Factors

Research has been focused on factors associated with the development of myopia (Xu et al., 2007; Liu et al., 2010; Vongphanit et al., 2002). Both hereditary and environmental factors appear to play a role in the development of myopia. Studies suggest a higher concordance of myopia between monozygotic than dizygotic twins and between children and parents (Saw et al., 2001; Zadnik et al., 1994; Dirani et al., 2006). More recent studies have identified links between several gene regions, particularly chromosome 18p, and myopia (Farbrother et al., 2004; Hammond et al., 2004; Lam et al., 2003; Stambolian et al., 2004; Wojciechowski et al., 2005; Zhang et al., 2006), although other studies have either found no association (Ibay et al., 2004) or more complex relationships (Klein et al., 2005; Mak et al., 2006). More years of formal education have been strongly associated with a higher prevalence of myopia (Wu et al., 2001; Tan et al., 2000; Tan et al., 2000; Kinge et al., 2000). Some studies have reported that near work is associated with a higher prevalence and progression of myopia (Mutti et al., 2002; Saw et al., 2002; Saw et al., 2002), but subsequent studies have not, especially with respect to middle distance activities such as those that involve video display terminals (Kinge et al., 2000; Rechichi and Scullica, 1996; Saw et al., 2000). The use of night lights in children under age 2 years has been reported as a strong risk factor for myopia (Quinn et al., 1999); however, other studies that were able to adjust for parental refractive status did not find such an association (Saw et al., 2002; Zadnik et al., 2000). Studies of ethnic Chinese in Taiwan document an increase in the prevalence and severity of myopia over two generations (Lin et al., 1999; Lin et al., 1988; Wu et al., 1999; Lin et al., 2004). Genetics alone are unlikely to account for such a rapid change, although one study has speculated that genetic factors do not preclude such a change (Rose et al., 2002). A study of successive cohorts of enlistees in the Israeli army showed a marked increase in prevalence of myopia over a 13-year period (Dayan et al., 2005).

There had been epidemiological evidence that children who spend more time outside are protected from the development of myopia than those who spend more time doing near work (Saw et al., 2001).

Various hypotheses currently compete to explain the wide variation in school-age myopia prevalence, including near work during childhood (Ip et al., 2008; Saw et al., 2001; Saw et al., 2002), outdoor activity (Dirani et al., 2009; Low et al., 2010; Rose et al., 2008), urban versus rural living (Dandona et al., 2002; He et al., 2007; He et al., 2004; Murthy et al., 2002; Ip et al., 2008) and population density (Zhang et al., 2010). A predisposition to myopia seems to be particularly strong in those of Han Chinese descent, but to date, there is no convergence of evidence toward a unifying explanation, and the gene/environment interactions that underpin the development of school-age myopia remain poorly understood (Jacobi and Pusch,

2010; Wojciechowski, 2011). Myopia has been reported to affect approximately 37% of 13-year-old children living in rural southern China (He et al., 2004). Whether the trend to increasing rates of myopia is occurring in other less-developed parts of neighboring East Asia remains largely unknown (Casson et al., 2012).

Uncorrected refractive error (URE) is a leading cause of blindness worldwide as well as the primary cause of visual impairment in the United States (Resnikoff et al., 2008; Vitale et al., 2006). Studies have reported that among Unites States Latino populations, URE is associated with older age and socioeconomic factors such as lower levels of income and education (Schneider et al., 2010; Uribe et al., 2011; Muñoz et al., 2002).

Epidemiological studies found that the prevalence of myopic retinopathy significantly increased with advancing age. (Vongphanit et al., 2012; Liu et al., 2010; Lai et al., 2008; Asakuma et al., 2012). Histological studies have shown a decreased density of photo receptors, ganglion cells, retinal pigment epithelium and optic nerve fibers with age (Panda-Jonas et al., 1995; Gao and Hollyfield, 1992). In addition, several studies using OCT have shown a negative relationship between retinal thickness and age (Eriksson and Alm, 2009; Alamouti and Funk, 2003). Therefore, along with the axial elongation of the eyeball in highly myopic eyes, increasing age may contribute to the pathogenesis of myopic retinopathy by causing retinal thinning.

A number of population-based studies have shown that the prevalence of myopia decreases with age from about 40% among persons in their 40s to about 15% among persons in their 70s and 80s (Wang et al., 1994; Katz et al., 1997; The Framingham Offspring Eye Study Group, 1996). Individuals who develop nuclear sclerosis, tend to undergo a myopic shift over time (Lee et al., 1999; Mutti and Zadnik, 2000; Shufelt et al., 2005;).

In the Hisayama study, men had longer axial lengths than women ($P<0.001$ for both eyes), a higher prevalence of myopic retinopathy was found in women (2.2%) than in men (1.2%). After adjustment for age, gender, and axial length, a 3-fold increased risk of myopic retinopathy was shown in women. Similar findings were observed in a number of hospital-based studies (Shih et al.,2006; Ito-Ohara et al.,1998; Moriyama et al., 2011). For example, Hayashi et al. (Hayashi et al., 2010) showed that, of 429 consecutive patients with pathologic myopia, 147 were men and 282 were women, making the incidence in women approximately double than in men. Comparable findings were also observed in the Blue Mountains Eye Study and in the Beijing Eye Study. This suggests that not only greater axial length, but also other risk factors, such as genetic factors and lifestyle risk factors, may contribute to the pathogenesis of myopic retinopathy (Asakuma et al., 2012).

Recent investigations have revealed that the prevalence of myopia in children was associated with older age, female sex, urban region of habitation, and type of school attended, such as comprehensive public school, selective public schools, or private schools (Parssinen and Lyyar, 1992; Wong et al., 2000; Saw et al., 2002; Mutti et al., 2002; Jones et al., 2007; Ip et al., 2007; Rose et al., 2008; Ip et al., 2008; Low et al., 2010; Sharma et al., 2010). Some of these parameters, such as sex and age, cannot be altered to reduce the risk of the development of myopia. Research has, therefore, been concentrated to detect myopia-related environmental or behavioral factors that could be influenced to reduce the risk of the development of myopia (Saw et al., 2001; Saw et al., 2002; Loman et al., 2002; Saw et al., 2002; Saw et al., 2006; Ip et al., 2008; Lu et al., 2009; Rose et al., 2008b; Dirani et al., 2009; Williams et al., 2008; Lim et al., 2010; Guggenheim et al., 2012). In a recent study by Rose et al. (Rose et al., 2008b), a lower prevalence of myopia in Chinese children raised in Sydney compared with Chinese children living in Singapore was associated with increased hours of outdoor activities. Rose et al. (Rose et al., 2008) also hypothesized that another factor contributing to the differences in the prevalence of myopia between Chinese children from Sydney versus Singapore was the early educational pressures found in Singapore but not in Sydney.

The study by Rose et al. (Rose et al., 2008) was supported by an investigation of Guggenheim et al. (30 Guggenheim et al., 2012), who found that both less time spent outdoors and less physical activity were associated with incident myopia, with time outdoors having the larger effect. Guggenheim et al. concluded that time spent outdoors was predictive of incident myopia independent of the physical activity level. In the study by Guo et al.,(Guo et al., 2013), that question was readdressed including school children from Greater Beijing.

Recent studies of the myopic shift in the young generation of urban East Asian and Southeast Asian populations have focused on factors that potentially influenced the development of myopia in children. These studies revealed that myopia was associated with parental myopia (Saw et al., 2002; Mutti et al., 2002; Jones et al., 2007; Ip et al., 2007), near work (Mutti et al., 2002;), school achievements and other school-associated factors (Mutti et al., 2002; Rose et al., 2008; Saw et al., 2001) and other school-associated factors (Mutti et al.,2002; Rose et al., 2008; Saw et al., 2001) and less outdoor activity and time spent outdoors (Jones et al.,2007; Low et al.,2010; Rose et al., 2008b, Dirani et al., 2009; Guggenheim et al., 2012). The results of the study by Guo et al. (Guo et al., 2023) confirm these findings. The ocular axial length and ratio of AL/CC as surrogates for myopia were higher in children whose mother was myopic and who were taller, lived in the urban region of Beijing, or spent less time outdoors and more time indoors studying. Correspondingly, the children were more likely to be myopic if their mothers were myopic, they lived in the urban region of Beijing, and they spent less time outdoors and more time indoors studying. The statistical analysis showed that after inclusion of the area of habitation, risk factors such as the measures of outdoor activities were no longer significantly associated with the axial length and prevalence of myopia. This was most likely due to the 2 parameters being collinear to each other, that is, urban areas were characterized by lower levels of time outdoors and higher levels of indoors activities. This leads to the conclusion that less outdoor activity and more indoor studying, in addition to older age and maternal myopia, were associated with longer ocular axial length and myopia in grade 1 and grade 4 primary school children in Greater Beijing (Guo et al., 2013).

In the study by Guo et al. (Guo et al., 2013), the total time spent outdoors including the time spent outdoors with sports was associated with a longer ocular axial length and a lower prevalence of myopia. This is in agreement with the studies by Rose et al. (Rose et al.,2008) in which Chinese children raised in Sydney showed a markedly lower prevalence of myopia and spent a considerably longer time outdoors than Chinese children living in Singapore. In these studies, Rose et al. also hypothesized that another factor contributing to the differences in the prevalence of myopia between Chinese children from Sydney versus Singapore was the early educational pressures found in Singapore was the early educational pressures found in Singapore but not in Sydney. The studies by Rose et al. were supported by an investigation by Guggenheim et al. (Guggenheim et al., 2012), who found that both less time spent outdoors and less physical activity were associated with incident myopia, with time outdoors having the larger effect. They concluded that time spent outdoors was predictive of incident myopia independent of the physical activity level. Mutti et al. (Mutti et al., 2002) reported a protective effect of outdoor activities against myopia in a cross-sectional study, as did Jones et al. (Jones et al., 2007) in a longitudinal study. The finding of an association between outdoor activity and myopia also was reported for other ethnic groups, such as from Jordan (Khader et al., 2007) and Turkey (Onal et al., 2007). One may infer that in addition to differences in cultural parameters, the association between little time spent outdoors and development of myopia in children is independent of ethnicity. Because the amount of outdoor activity can be influenced, myopic parents may ask their children to spend more time outdoors to decrease the probability of the child developing myopia. An association between little time spent outdoors and myopia development is contradictory to a report on Chinese children in the Xichang Pediatric Refractive Error Study by Lu et al. (Lu et al., 2009), who did not find such an association. The current study, therefore, suggests that a correlation between myopia development and intensive indoor study and little time spent outdoors as reported for Chinese children from Singapore also may be valid for Chinese children from mainland China (Guo et al., 2013).

The total time spent outdoors was higher in the Beijing study population (Guo et al., 2013) (11.3 hours/week) than in the Singaporean study population (3.1 hours/week) in the investigation by Rose et al. (Rose et al.,2008) and shorter than in the study population from Sydney (13.75 hours/week) in the study by Sharma et al. (Sharma et al.,2010). These differences correlate with differences in the prevalence of myopia, with the lowest value in the Singaporean study population group (29.1%) for 6 and 7 year old children (Rose et al., 2008).

Rose et al. (Rose et al., 2008) suggested that bright light outdoors might prevent myopia by increasing the release of dopamine from the retina; dopamine has been known to be an inhibitor of axial elongation (Iuvone et al., 1991; Dong et al., 2011). It was shown that bright light prevented the development of myopia in animal models and that this prevention was dopamine-dependent (Ashby et al., 2009). The results of these experimental studies support the findings obtained in studies by Rose et al. (Rose et al., 2008), Guggenheim et al. (Guggenheim et al., 2012), and others (Jones et al., 2007; Low et al., 2010; Dirani et al., 2009), because outdoor activity is associated with the exposure to bright light. This hypothesis may be strengthened by a recent study by French et al. (French et al., 2012), who found that European Caucasian children in Northern Ireland (with less sunlight) had a greater prevalence of myopia (and hyperopia and astigmatism) when compared with children living in Sydney (with more intense sunlight) (Guo et al., 2013).

The self-reported time spent with playing electronic gadgets was not related to the presence of myopia or to axial length; however, because the self-reported time spent with electronic gadgets was relatively short (0.1±0.3 hours) and much shorter than the time spent studying (5.3±0.9 hours), the data may not allow statements on whether playing with electronic gadgets influences the development of myopia in children (Guo et al., 2013).

The time reportedly spent watching television was negatively associated with the presence of myopia and axial length. After adjustment for age and maternal myopia, axial length was longer and prevalence of myopia was lower in children who spent more time watching television. The reason for this finding may be the correlation between more time spent watching television and less time spent studying. It also has remained unclear why the effect of maternal myopia seemed to be dominant over that of parental myopia in the association with the children's myopia. None of the previous studies found such an effect. Perhaps there is a statistical artifact in the sense that 2 parameters correlated with each other, of which one dropped out in the multivariate regression, when both may be important, that is, genetic factors or educational parameters, because mothers usually were more involved than fathers in the education of the children (Guo et al., 2013).

The study by Guo et al. (Guo et al., 2013) found that less outdoor activity, more indoor studying, older age, maternal myopia, and urban region of habitation were associated with longer ocular axial length and myopia. More outdoor activity (e.g., in the schools) may be helpful to reduce the high prevalence of myopia in Beijing (Guo et al., 2013).

Cross-sectional studies of school-aged children have shown that there is a higher prevalence of myopia and correspondingly less prevalent hyperopia in older children compared with younger children (Dandona et al., 2002; Maul et al., 2000; Murthy et al., 2002; Naidoo et al., 2003; Pokharez et al., 2000; Goh et al., 2005; Hasheni et al., 2004; Rezvan et al., 2012; Grönlund et al., 2006; Zadnik et al., 2003; O'Donoghue et al., 2010; Czepita et al., 2008; Kleinstein et al., 2003; Mutti et al., 2002; Logan et al., 2011; Villarreal et al., 2000; Ip et al., 2008; Ojaimi et al., 2005; Czepita et al., 2007; Zhao et al., 2000; He et al., 2004; Quek et al., 2004; Saw et al., 2006). These studies have also highlighted large differences in the prevalence of refractive errors between locations. The prevalence of myopia is generally highest in populations of East Asian ethnicity from East and Southeast Asia (Zhao et al., 2000; He et al., 2004; Quek et al., 2004; Saw et al., 2006; Lin et al., 2004; Zhan et al., 2000; Fan et al., 2004; Pi et al., 2010; He et al., 2007; Jung et al., 2012), particularly in urban locations such as Guangzhou (He et al., 2004), Hong Kong (Fan et al., 2004), Taiwan (Lin et al., 2004), and Korea (Jung et al., 2012).

Uncorrected refractive error is the leading cause of visual impairment worldwide (Dandona and Dandona, 2002) and in school-aged children in both industrialized and developing regions (Dandona et al., 2002; Goh et al., 2005; He et al., 2007;He et al., 2004; Maul et al., 2000; Murthy et al., 2002;Naidoo et al., 2003; Pokharel et al., 2000; Robael et al., 2006; Taylor et al., 2010; Zhao et al., 2000; Saw et al., 2006; Wong et al., 2006).

The prevalence of myopia in certain regions, particularly urban East Asian regions, is high (Wong et al., 2006). Existing evidence, albeit limited, indicates that the prevalence of myopia has dramatically increased in certain urbanized Asian regions, particularly Singapore (Wong et al., 2006) and Taiwan (Seet et al., 2001; Shih et al., 2010), but not in Australia (Junghans and Crewther, 2005), and only weakly in the United States (Lee et al., 2002).

The prevalence of myopia is considerably lower in western Asian regions (Dandona et al., 2002; Pokharel et al., 2000, Yekta et al., 2010) and white Australian children (Robael et al., 2006), and at its lowest in healthy indigenous Australian children (Taylor et al., 2010; Landers et al., 2010; Stocks et al., 1997). A recent nationwide study found that the prevalence of "low vision" (VA<20/40 but ≤20/200) in Australian aboriginal children aged 5 to 15 years was 1.5% (95% CI, 0.9-2.1), and only 15 of the 1694 children in the sample had low vision due to refractive error (Taylor et al., 2010). In the study of schoolchildren from Lao People's Democratic Republic (Casson et al., 2012), the prevalence of low vision was slightly lower than that in indigenous Australian children (1.2% (95% CI, 0.4-2.0)) and was also explained by the extremely low prevalence of myopia. The age range of the children from Lao People's was 6 to 11 years. The upper age limit was younger than the typical 5- to 15-year age range reported in other studies; thus, it would expect the overall prevalence of myopia and visual impairment to be lower in the Lao People's children (Casson et al., 2012).

It is well known that age has been highly correlated with the prevalence of refractive errors. For myopia, both population and nonpopulation-based studies have reported that the prevalence generally follows a bimodal pattern in adults, initially declining with age and then increasing in the higher age groups (Katz et al., 1997; Wang et al., 1994; Wensor et al., 1999; Wong et al., 2000), which also is seen in the current results.

Although the exact rationale for a bimodal aging pattern in the prevalence of myopia is still controversial, two theories have been forwarded: a true decrease in the prevalence of myopia in older people compared with younger persons (Wong et al., 2000; Mutti et al., 1996) and changes in the refractive index gradient of the lens with age (Wong et al., 2000; Cheng et al., 2003; Hemenger et al., 1995; Slataper, 1950). The former should be the result of both cohort and aging effects. The latter is supported by the current finding that the prevalence of myopia increased with age in eyes with cataract graded as moderate or severe but decreased in eyes without it.

Education level has been known to be associated with the prevalence of myopia (Sperduto et al., 1983; Wensor et al., 1999; Wong et al., 2000). The possible mechanism is that people with higher education spend more time doing nearwork activities, which is a known risk factor for the development of myopia (Rosner and Belkin, 1987; Saw et al., 2001; Jung et al., 2012).

Myopia was not associated with height ($P = 0.159$); weight ($P = 0.571$); or BMI ($P= 0.323$).

Multivariate linear regression models revealed that the refractive error was associated with education level (regression coefficient -0.246, P value < 0.001) and was not associated with height, weight, or BMI.

The prevalence of myopia is increasing at an ''epidemic'' rate, particularly in East Asia. This may be related to changing environmental factors, in particular the demands of near work (Saw et al., 2002). Many 19-year-old males in Seoul spend large amounts of time studying for university entrance examinations. Higher educational attainment and excessive near-focus work are wellknown risk factors for myopia development (Rosner and Belkin, 1987; Saw et al., 2001; Saw et al., 2002). The prevalence of myopia is also known to be higher in urban populations than in rural population (He et al., 2009) and our study population resided in a metropolitan area. One particular concern is that over 20% of our population had a high prevalence of myopia (worse than -6.0 D). This figure is higher than that in reports from any other population worldwide. The prevalence of high myopes in the Baltimore Eye Study was approximately 1.4%, and 8.2% in the Tajimi study in Japan (Sawada et al., 2008).

As mentioned above, educational status has been among the most frequently noted socioeconomic associations of myopia (Sperduto et al., 1983; Wensor et al., 1999, Wong et al., 2000). High educational levels were associated with myopia (Jung et al., 2012). These associations may be an indicator of near work and support the use-abuse theory for myopia. In the National Health and Nutrition Examination Survey, the prevalence of myopia increased with educational level (Sperduto et al., 1983). Both the Baltimore and Beaver Dam studies showed a monotonic relationship between education and myopia (Wang et al., 1994; Katz et al., 1997).

There have been several studies on the balance between genes and environment as the etiology of myopia. A recent study has shown that ocular refraction is a complex phenotype that is influenced by both environmental factors and genetic predisposition, although environmental exposures play crucial roles in ocular growth and refractive development (Wojciechowski, 2001). Another study suggested that environmental change appears to be a major factor in increasing the prevalence of myopia around the world, while there may be a small genetic contribution to school myopia (Morgan and Rose, 2005). This hypothesis was supported by a study showing an association between myopia and academic achievements (Jung et al., 2012). No relationship between measurements of body stature (height, weight, and BMI) and myopia was demonstrated in one study (Jung et al., 2012) which showed similar results as in the previous study that myopia was not associated with height or weight in 106,926 Israeli military recruits (Rosner et al., 1995). Some studies have found a correlation between myopic prevalence and height (Saw et al., 2002; Wong et al., 2001). A recent study including the twin eyes of Chinese children showed a significant association between height and axial length (Zhang et al., 2011). Another study reported that height was inversely associated with refractive error among Chinese boys, although no such association was observed among girls (Sharma et al., 2010). A population-based Finnish study found that myopic males were 1.9 cm taller on average than nonmyopic males (Teikari, 1987). Among Danish recruits, myopes were 0.8 cm taller on average than emmetropes, and hypermetropes were 0.2 cm shorter than emmetropes (Teasdale and Goldschmidt, 1988). The discrepancies in the results of the major studies examining the association between height and myopia suggested that axial length is significantly correlated with height, whereas refractive error may not be. One possible reason is that emmetropization can adjust axial length by flat cornea to produce emmetropic refraction. The results of measuring refractive error might be affected by emmetropization (Jung et al., 2012).

Several studies have reported a higher prevalence of myopia in females compared with males (Vitale et al., 2008; Kempen et al., 2004). This sex difference is often attributed to females having more nearwork and less outdoor activities during a young age. Thus, our data of Jund et al. (Jung et al., 2012) had the possibility of underestimation in the prevalence of myopia compared with the general population. Another limitation of that study (Jung et al., 2012) was a lack of evaluation of axial length, which is essential to evaluate the cause of the myopia. Prevalence of myopia without axial length measurement might be affected by the process of emmetropization that may reduce the impact of bigger eyes with the flatter corneas and longer axial length on refractive status by matching the axial length of the eye to the corneal power to produce an approximately emmetropic refraction. However, many studies have reported the prevalence of myopia without axial length measurement (Edwards and Lam, 2004; He et al., 2004; Lin et al., 2004; Wang et al., 1994; Vitale et al., 2008; Kempen et al., 2004). It might be due to the technical and economical difficulty of these studies with regard to ocular epidemiology. Recently, a new environmental factor having protective effects against the development of myopia has been discovered (Morgan et al., 2012; Pan et al., 2012). Increased amounts of time spent outdoors protects against the development of myopia, whereas near work or having myopic parents is less associated with the risk of developing myopia. Indoor sports and engagement in specific sports were found to have no association with the development of myopia (Rose et al., 2008). The postulated mechanism is that the increased light intensity outdoors may have protective effects owing to the increased release of dopamine, which is known to reduce eye growth (McCarthy et al., 2007).

Jacobsen and colleagues (Jacobsen et al., 2007) describe a well-designed retrospective study that describes the current prevalence of myopia among 4,681 Danish military recruits.

The authors quantify the prevalence of myopia as well as analyze associations with level of education, IQ scores, and a variety of physical attributes. In addition to the internal results of the study, the authors compared their results to studies completed 40 and 122 years previously. Among the conscripts studied, the prevalence of myopia was 12.8% less than -0.5 D, 7.7% less than -1.5 D, and 0.3% less than -6.5 D. There was a trend towards higher myopia in conscripts with more education, but this finding was not statistically significant. The authors describe an interesting positive correlation between IQ scores and degree of myopia, even when duration of ducation was considered. This is consistent with prior studies. No correlation was observed between physical characteristics (height, weight, BWI) and myopia. Compared to the study performed 40 years prior, the authors describe a decrease in the prevalence of low myopia (<-1.5 D). Potential explanations offered center around the impact of education on myopia, including commonality, age initiated, duration, and structure. Additionally, a significantly lower prevalence of high myopia (<-6.5 D) is reported, possibly secondary to differences in patient inclusion/exclusion criteria.

The findings of this study are interesting because they describe a relatively low prevalence of myopia among Danish conscripts, as well as an apparent decline in the prevalence of low and high myopia in this population, despite a marked increase in schooling over this time, and similar studies in other countries that have described an increasing prevalence of myopia over time. The specific reasons for these findings are not clear and warrant further investigation.

References

Abrams D. Duke-Elder's Practice of Refraction, 10th ed. London: Churchill Livingstone, 1993; Chap 6:65.

American Academy of Ophthalmology Basic and Clinical Science Course Subcommittee. Basic and Clinical Science Course. Section 3: Clinical Optics, 2007-2008. San Francisco, CA: American Academy of Ophthalmology; 2007:117-118.

American Academy of Ophthalmology Basic and Clinical Science Course Subcommittee. Basic and Clinical Science Course. Section 3: Clinical Optics, 2007-2008. San Francisco, CA: American Academy of Ophthalmology; 2007:118.

American Academy of Ophthalmology Cataract/Anterior Segment Panel. Preferred Practice Pattern® Guidelines. Cataract in the Adult Eye. San Francisco, CA: American Academy of Ophthalmology; 2006. Available at: http://www.aao.org/ppp.

American Academy of Ophthalmology Pediatric Ophthalmology/Strabismus Panel. Preferred Practice Pattern® Guidelines. Pediatric Eye Evaluations. San Francisco, CA: American Academy of Ophthalmology; 2007. Available at: http://www.aao.org/ppp.

American Academy of Ophthalmology Preferred Practice Patterns Committee. Preferred Practice Pattern® Guidelines. Comprehensive Adult Medical Eye Evaluation. San Francisco, CA: American Academy of Ophthalmology; 2005. Available at: http://www.aao.org/ppp.

Asakuma T, Yasuda M, Ninomiya T, Noda Y, Arakawa S, Hashimoto S, Ohno Matsui K, Kiyohara Y, Ishibashi T. d risk factors for myopic retinopathy in a Japanese population. The Hisayama Study. *Ophthalmology* 2012; 119:1760-1765.

Attebo K, Ivers RQ, Mitchell P. Refractive errors in an older population: the Blue Mountains Eye Study. *Ophthalmology* 1999;106:1066-1072.

Avisar R, Friling R, Snir M, et al. Estimation of prevalence and incidence rates and causes of blindness in Israel, 1998-2003. *Isr Med Assoc J* 2006;8:880–881.

Bar Dayan Y, Levin A, Morad Y, et al. The changing prevalence of myopia in young adults: a 13-year series of population-based prevalence surveys. *Invest Ophthalmol Vis Sci* 2005;46:2760–2765.

Barr JT. Annual report: Contact lenses 2005. Contact Lens Spectrum January 2006. Available at: http://www.clspectrum.com/article.aspx?article=12913. 2006 global refractive market report. Market Scope October 2006:10-11.

Bourne RR, Dineen BP, Ali SM, et al. Prevalence of refractive error in Bangladeshi adults. Results of the National Blindness and Low Vision Survey of Bangladesh. *Ophthalmology* 2004; 111:1150–1160.

Casson RJ, Kahawita S, Kong A, Muecke J, Sisaleumsak, Visonnavong V. Exceptionally low prevalence of refractive error and visual impairment in schoolchildren from Lao People's Democratic Republic. *Ophthalmology* 2012;119:2021-2027.

Cheng CY, Hsu WM, Liu JH, et al. Refractive errors in an elderly Chinese population in Taiwan: the Shihpai Eye Study. *Invest Ophthalmol Vis Sci* 2003;44:4630-4638.

Czepita D, Mojsa A, Ustianowska M, et al. Prevalence of refractive errors in schoolchildren ranging from 6 to 18 years of age. *Ann Acad Med Stetin* 2007;53:53– 56.

Czepita D, Mojsa A, Zejmo M. Prevalence of myopia and hyperopia among urban and rural schoolchildren in Poland. *Ann Acad Med Stetin* 2008;54:17–21.

Dandona R, Dandona L, Srinivas M, et al. Population-based assessment of refractive error in India: the Andhra Pradesh eye disease study. *Clin Experiment Ophthalmol* 2002;30:84-93.

Dandona R, Dandona L, Srinivas M, et al. Refractive error in children in a rural population in India. *Invest Ophthalmol Vis Sci* 2002;43:615-622.

Dayan YB, Levin A, Morad Y, et al. The changing prevalence of myopia in young adults: a 13-year series of population-based prevalence surveys. *Invest Ophthalmol Vis Sci* 2005;46:2760-2765.

Dirani M, Chamberlain M, Shekar SN, et al. Heritability of refractive error and ocular biometrics: the Genes in Myopia (GEM) twin study. *Invest Ophthalmol Vis Sci* 2006;47:4756-4761.

Edwards MH, Lam CS. The epidemiology of myopia in Hong Kong. *Ann Acad Med Singapore.* 2004;33:34–38.

Evans JR, Fletcher AE, Wormald RP. MRC Trial of Assessment and Management of Older People in the Community. Causes of visual impairment in people aged 75 years and older in Britain: an add-on study to the MRC Trial of Assessment and Management of Older People in the Community. *Br J Ophthalmol* 2004;88:365–370.

Eye Diseases Prevalence Research Group, Kempen JH, Mitchell P, et al. The prevalence of refractive errors among adults in the United States, Western Europe, and Australia. *Arch Ophthalmol* 2004;122:495–505.

Familial aggregation and prevalence of myopia in the Framingham Offspring Eye Study. The Framingham Offspring Eye Study Group. *Arch Ophthalmol* 1996;114:326-332.

Fan DS, Lam DS, Lam RF, et al. Prevalence, incidence, and progression of myopia of school children in Hong Kong. *Invest Ophthalmol Vis Sci* 2004;45:1071–1075.

Farbrother JE, Kirov G, Owen MJ, et al. Linkage analysis of the genetic loci for high myopia on 18p, 12q, and 17q in 51 U.K. families. *Invest Ophthalmol Vis Sci* 2004;45:2879-2885.

French AN, O'Donoghue L, Morgan IG, Saunders KJ, Mitchell P, Rose KA. Comparison of refraction and ocular biometry in European Caucasian children living in Northern Ireland

and Sidney, Autralia. *Invest Ophthalmol Vis Sci* 2012; 53(7):4021-4031. Doi: 10.1167/iovs.12-9556.

Goh PP, Abqariyah Y, Pokharel GP, Ellwein LB. Refractive error and visual impairment in school-age children in Gombak District, Malaysia. *Ophthalmology* 2005;112:678 – 685.

Grødum K, Heijl A, Bengtsson B. Refractive error and glaucoma. *Acta Ophthalmol Scand* 2001;79:560-566.

Grönlund MA, Andersson S, Aring E, et al. Ophthalmological findings in a sample of Swedish children aged 4 –15 years. *Acta Ophthalmol Scand* 2006;84:169 –176.

Grosvenor T, Perrigin DM, Perrigin J, Maslovitz B. Houston. Myopia Control Study: a randomized clinical trial. Part II. Final report by the patient care team. *Am J Optom Physiol Opt* 1987;64:482-498.

Hammond CJ, Andrew T, Mak YT, Spector TD. A susceptibility locus for myopia in the normal population is linked to the PAX6 gene region on chromosome 11: a genomewide scan of dizygotic twins. *Am J Hum Genet* 2004;75:294-304.

Hashemi H, Fotouhi A, Mohammad K. The age- and gender-specific prevalences of refractive errors in Tehran: the Tehran Eye Study. *Ophthalmic Epidemiol* 2004;11:213–225.

He M, Huang W, Li Y, Zheng Y, Yin Q, Foster PJ. Refractive error and biometry in older Chinese adults: the Liwan eye study. *Invest Ophthalmol Vis Sci* 2009;50(11):5130-5136. Doi. 10.1167/iovs.09-3455.

He M, Huang W, Zheng Y, et al. Refractive error and visual impairment in school children in rural southern China. *Ophthalmology* 2007;114:374 – 382.

He M, Zeng J, Liu Y, et al. Refractive error and visual impairment in urban children in southern China. *Invest Ophthalmol Vis Sci* 2004;45:793–799.

He M, Zeng J, Liu Y, Xu J, Pokharel GP, Ellwein LB. Refractive error and visual impairment in urban children in southern China. *Invest Ophthalmol Vis Sci.* 2004;45:793-799.

Hemenger RP, Garner LF, Ooi CS. Change with age of the refractive index gradient of the human ocular lens. *Invest Ophthalmol Vis Sci* 1995;36:703–707.

Hofman A, Grobbee DE, de Jong PT, van den Ouweland FA. Determinants of disease and disability in the elderly: the Rotterdam Elderly Study. *Eur J Epidemiol* 1991;7:403–422.

Holmstrom GE, Larsson EK. Development of spherical equivalent refraction in prematurely born children during the first 10 years of life: a population-based study. *Arch Ophthalmol* 2005;123:1404-1411.

Hyams SW, Pokotilo E, Shkurko G. Prevalence of refractive errors in adults over 40: a survey of 8102 eyes. *Br J Ophthalmol* 1977;61:428 –432.

Hyman L, Gwiazda J, Hussein M, et al. Relationship of age, sex, and ethnicity with myopia progression and axial elongation in the correction of myopia evaluation trial. *Arch Ophthalmol* 2005;123:977-987.

Ibay G, Doan B, Reider L, et al. Candidate high myopia loci on chromosomes 18p and 12q do not play a major role in susceptibility to common myopia. *BMC Med Genet* 2004;5:20.

Ip JM, Huynh SC, Robaei D, et al. Ethnic differences in refraction and ocular biometry in a population-based sample of 11-15-year-old Australian children. *Eye* (Lond) 2008;22: 649 –656.

Iwase A, Suzuki Y, Araie M, et al. The prevalence of primary open-angle glaucoma in Japanese. The Tajimi Study. *Ophthalmology* 2004;111:1641– 1648.

Jacobsen N, Hensen H, Goldschmidt E: Prevalence of myopia in Danish conscripts. *Acta Ophthalmol Scand* 2007; 85:165-170.

Jensen H. Myopia progression in young school children and intraocular pressure. *Doc Ophthalmol* 1992;82:249-255.

Jung S-K, Lee JH, Kakizaki H, Jeel D. Prevalence of myopia and its association with body stature and educational level in 19-year-old male conscripts in Seoul, South Korea. *Invest Ophthalmol Vis Sci* 2012;53:5579–5583.DOI:10.1167/iovs.12-10106.

Kaimbo Wa Kaimbo D, Missotten L. [Refractive errors in Zalre]. *Bull Soc Belge Ophtalmol* 1996;261:101-105.

Katz J, Tielsch JM, Sommer A. Prevalence and risk factors for refractive errors in an adult inner city population. *Invest Ophthalmol Vis Sci.* 1997;38:334–340.

Kempen JH, Mitchell P, Lee KE, et al. The prevalence of refractive errors among adults in the United States, Western Europe, and Australia. *Arch Ophthalmol* 2004;122:495-505.

Kinge B, Midelfart A, Jacobsen G, Rystad J. The influence of near-work on development of myopia among university students. A three-year longitudinal study among engineering students in Norway. *Acta Ophthalmol Scand* 2000;78:26-29.

Klaver CC, Wolfs RC, Vingerling JR, et al. Age-specific prevalence and causes of blindness and visual impairment in an older population: the Rotterdam Study. *Arch Ophthalmol* 1998;116:653–658.

Klein AP, Duggal P, Lee KE, et al. Support for polygenic influences on ocular refractive error. *Invest Ophthalmol Vis Sci* 2005;46:442-446.

Kleinstein RN, Jones LA, Hullett S, et al., Collaborative Longitudinal Evaluation of Ethnicity and Refractive Error Study Group. Refractive error and ethnicity in children. *Arch Ophthalmol* 2003;121:1141–1147.

Kleinstein RN, Jones LA, Hullett S, et al. Refractive error and ethnicity in children. *Arch Ophthalmol* 2003;121:1141-1147.

Krumpaszky HG, Lüdtke R, Mickler A, et al. Blindness incidence in Germany. A population-based study from Württemberg-Hohenzollern. *Ophthalmologica* 1999;213:176–182.

Lam DS, Tam PO, Fan DS, et al. Familial high myopia linkage to chromosome 18p. *Ophthalmologica* 2003;217:115-118.

Lee KE, Klein BE, Klein R. Changes in refractive error over a 5-year interval in the Beaver Dam Eye Study. *Invest Ophthalmol Vis Sci* 1999;40:1645-1649.

Lim R, Mitchell P, Cumming RG. Refractive associations with cataract: the Blue Mountains Eye Study. *Invest Ophthalmol Vis Sci* 1999;40:3021-3026.

Lin LL, Chen CJ, Hung PT, Ko LS. Nation-wide survey of myopia among schoolchildren in Taiwan, 1986. *Acta Ophthalmol Suppl* 1988;185:29-33.

Lin LL, Shih YF, Hsiao CK, Chen CJ. Prevalence of myopia in Taiwanese schoolchildren: 1983 to 2000. *Ann Acad Med Singapore* 2004;33:27–33.

Lin LL, Shih YF, Hsiao CK, et al. Epidemiologic study of the prevalence and severity of myopia among schoolchildren in Taiwan in 2000. *J Formos Med Assoc* 2001;100:684 – 691.

Lin LL, Shih YF, Tsai CB, et al. Epidemiologic study of ocular refraction among schoolchildren in Taiwan in 1995. *Optom Vis Sci* 1999;76:275-281.

Liu JH, Cheng CY, Chen SJ, Lee FL. Visual impairment in a Taiwanese population: prevalence, causes, and socioeconomic factors. *Ophthalmic Epidemiol* 2001;8:339–350.

Logan NS, Shah P, Rudnicka AR, et al. Childhood ethnic differences in ametropia and ocular biometry: the Aston Eye Study. *Ophthalmic Physiol Opt* 2011;31:550 – 558.

Mak W, Kwan MW, Cheng TS, et al. Myopia as a latent phenotype of a pleiotropic gene positively selected for facilitating neurocognitive development, and the effects of environmental factors in its expression. *Med Hypotheses* 2006;66:1209-1215.

Matsumura H, Hirai H. Prevalence of myopia and refractive changes in students from 3 to 17 years of age. *Surv Ophthalmol.* 1999;44(suppl 1):S109–S115.

Maul E, Barroso S, Munoz SR, et al. Refractive Error Study in Children: results from La Florida, Chile. *Am J Ophthalmol* 2000;129:445–454.

McCarthy CS, Megaw P, Devadas M, Morgan IG. Dopaminergic agents affect the ability of brief periods of normal vision to prevent form-deprivation myopia. *Exp Eye Res.* 2007;84:100–107.

Morgan I, Rose K. How genetic is school myopia? *Prog Retin Eye Res.* 2005;24:1–38.

Morgan IG, Ohno-Matsui K, Saw SM. Myopia. *Lancet.* 2012; 379:1739–1748.

Murthy GV, Gupta SK, Ellwein LB, et al. Refractive error in children in an urban population in New Delhi. *Invest Ophthalmol Vis Sci* 2002;43:623–631.

Murthy GV, Gupta SK, Ellwein LB, et al. Refractive error in children in an urban population in New Delhi. *Invest Ophthalmol Vis Sci* 2002;43:623–631.

Mutti DO, Mitchell GL, Moeschberger ML, et al. Parental myopia, near work, school achievement, and children's refractive error. *Invest Ophthalmol Vis Sci* 2002;43:3633-3640.

Mutti DO, Zadnik K, Adams AJ. Myopia: the nature versus nurture debate goes on. *Invest Ophthalmol Vis Sci* 1996;37: 952–957.

Mutti DO, Zadnik K. Age-related decreases in the prevalence of myopia: longitudinal change or cohort effect? *Invest Ophthalmol Vis Sci* 2000;41:2103-2107.

Naidoo KS, Raghunandan A, Mashige KP, et al. Refractive error and visual impairment in African children in South Africa. *Invest Ophthalmol Vis Sci* 2003;44:3764 –3770.

O'Donoghue L, McClelland JF, Logan NS, et al. Refractive error and visual impairment in school children in Northern Ireland. *Br J Ophthalmol* 2010;94:1155–1159.

Ojaimi E, Rose KA, Morgan IG, et al. Distribution of ocular biometric parameters and refraction in a population-based study of Australian children. *Invest Ophthalmol Vis Sci* 2005; 46:2748 –2754.

Pan CW, Ramamurthy D, Saw SM. Worldwide prevalence and risk factors for myopia. *Ophthalmic Physiol Opt.* 2012;32:3–16.

Park DJ, Congdon NG. Evidence for an ''epidemic'' of myopia. *Ann Acad Med Singapore.* 2004;33:21–26.

Parssinen O, Hemminki E, Klemetti A. Effect of spectacle use and accommodation on myopic progression: final results of a three-year randomised clinical trial among schoolchildren. *Br J Ophthalmol* 1989;73:547-551.

Pi LH, Chen L, Liu Q, et al. Refractive status and prevalence of refractive errors in suburban school-age children. *Int J Med Sci* 2010;7:342–353.

Pokharel GP, Negrel AD, Munoz SR, Ellwein LB. Refractive Error Study in Children: results from Mechi Zone, Nepal. *Am J Ophthalmol* 2000;129:436 – 444.

Quek TPL, Chua CG, Chong CS, et al. Prevalence of refractive errors in teenage high school students in Singapore. *Ophthalmic Physiol Opt* 2004;24:47–55.

Quinn GE, Shin CH, Maguire MG, Stone RA. Myopia and ambient lighting at night. *Nature* 1999;399:113-114.

Rabin J, Van Sluyters RC, Malach R. Emmetropization: a vision-dependent phenomenon. *Invest Ophthalmol Vis Sci* 1981;20:561-564.

Rechichi C, Scullica L. Trends regarding myopia in video terminal operators. *Acta Ophthalmol Scand* 1996;74:493-496.

Rezvan F, Khabazkhoob M, Fotouhi A, et al. Prevalence of refractive errors among school children in Northeastern Iran. *Ophthalmic Physiol Opt* 2012;32:25–30.

Risk factors for idiopathic rhegmatogenous retinal detachment. The Eye Disease Case-Control Study Group. *Am J Epidemiol* 1993;137:749-757.

Robb RM. Refractive errors associated with hemangiomas of the eyelids and orbit in infancy. *Am J Ophthalmol* 1977;83:52-58.

Rose KA, Morgan IG, Ip J, et al. Outdoor activity reduces the prevalence of myopia in children. *Ophthalmology.* 2008;115: 1279–1285.

Rose KA, Morgan IG, Smith W, Mitchell P. High heritability of myopia does not preclude rapid changes in prevalence. *Clin Experiment Ophthalmol* 2002;30:168-172.

Rosner M, Belkin M. Intelligence, education, and myopia in males. *Arch Ophthalmol.* 1987;105:1508–1511.

Rosner M, Laor A, Belkin M. Myopia and stature: findings in a population of 106,926 males. *Eur J Ophthalmol.* 1995;5:1–6.

Saunders KJ. Early refractive development in humans. *Surv Ophthalmol* 1995;40:207-16.

Saw SM, Chew SJ. Myopia in children born premature or with low birth weight. *Acta Ophthalmol Scand* 1997;75:548-550.

Saw SM, Chua WH, Hong CY, et al. Height and its relationship to refraction and biometry parameters in Singapore Chinese children. *Invest Ophthalmol Vis Sci.* 2002;43:1408–1413.

Saw SM, Chua WH, Hong CY, et al. Nearwork in early-onset myopia. *Invest Ophthalmol Vis Sci.* 2002;43:332–339.

Saw SM, Gazzard G, Koh D, et al. Prevalence rates of refractive errors in Sumatra, Indonesia. *Invest Ophthalmol Vis Sci* 2002;43:3174-3180.

Saw SM, Gazzard G, Shih-Yen EC, Chua WH. Myopia and associated pathological complications. *Ophthalmic Physiol Opt.* 2005;25:381–391.

Saw SM, Goh PP, Cheng A, et al. Ethnicity-specific prevalences of refractive errors vary in Asian children in neighbouring Malaysia and Singapore. *Br J Ophthalmol* 2006;90: 1230 –1235.

Saw SM, Hong CY, Chia KS, Stone RA, Tan D. Nearwork and myopia in young children. *Lancet.* 2001;357:390.

Saw SM, Katz J, Schein OD, Chew SJ, Chan TK. Epidemiology of myopia. *Epidemiol Rev.* 1996;18:175–187.

Saw SM, Nieto FJ, Katz J, et al. Factors related to the progression of myopia in Singaporean children. *Optom Vis Sci* 2000;77:549-554.

Saw SM, Nieto FJ, Katz J, et al. Familial clustering and myopia progression in Singapore school children. *Ophthalmic Epidemiol* 2001;8:227-236.

Saw SM, Shih Yen EC, Koh A, Tan D. Interventions to retard myopia progression in children: an evidence-based update. *Ophthalmology* 2002;109:415-421; *discussion* 422-424; quiz 425-426, 443.

Saw SM, Tong L, Chua WH, et al. Incidence and progression of myopia in Singaporean school children. *Invest Ophthalmol Vis Sci* 2005;46:51-57.

Saw SM, Zhang MZ, Hong RZ, et al. Near-work activity, night-lights, and myopia in the Singapore-China study. *Arch Ophthalmol* 2002;120:620-627.

Sawada A, Tomidokoro A, Araie M, Iwase A, Yamamoto T. Tajimi Study Group. Refractive errors in an elderly Japanese population. The Tajimi Study. *Ophthalmology* 2008;115:363-370.

Sharma A, Congdon N, Gao Y, et al. Height, stunting, and refractive error among rural Chinese schoolchildren: the See Well to Learn Well project. *Am J Ophthalmol.* 2010;149:347–353.e1.

Shih YF, Chen CH, Chou AC, et al. Effects of different concentrations of atropine on controlling myopia in myopic children. *J Ocul Pharmacol Ther* 1999;15:85-90.

Shih YF, Hsiao CK, Chen CJ, et al. An intervention trial on efficacy of atropine and multi-focal glasses in controlling myopic progression. *Acta Ophthalmol Scand* 2001;79:233-236.

Shufelt C, Fraser-Bell S, Ying-Lai M, et al. Refractive error, ocular biometry, and lens opalescence in an adult population: the Los Angeles Latino Eye Study. *Invest Ophthalmol Vis Sci* 2005;46:4450-4460.

Slataper FJ. Age norms of refraction and vision. *Arch Ophthalmol* 1950;43:466–481.

Sperduto RD, Seigel D, Roberts J, Rowland M. Prevalence of myopia in the United States. *Arch Ophthalmol.* 1983;101:405–407.

Stambolian D, Ibay G, Reider L, et al. Genomewide linkage scan for myopia susceptibility loci among Ashkenazi Jewish families shows evidence of linkage on chromosome 22q12. *Am J Hum Genet* 2004;75:448-459.

Tan GJ, Ng YP, Lim YC, et al. Cross-sectional study of near-work and myopia in kindergarten children in Singapore. *Ann Acad Med Singapore* 2000;29:740-744.

Tan NW, Saw SM, Lam DS, et al. Temporal variations in myopia progression in Singaporean children within an academic year. *Optom Vis Sci 2000*;77:465-472.

Tarczy-Hornoch K, Ying-Lai M, Varma R, Los Angeles Latino Eye Study Group. Myopic refractive error in adult Latinos: the Los Angeles Latino Eye Study. *Invest Ophthalmol Vis Sci* 2006;47:1845–1852.

Taylor HR, Xie J, Fox S, Dunn RA, Arnold AL, Keeffe JE. The prevalence and causes of vision loss in indigenous Australians: the National Indigenous Eye Health Survey. *Med J Austr* 2010;192(6):312-318.

Teasdale TW, Goldschmidt E. Myopia and its relationship to education, intelligence and height. Preliminary results from an on-going study of Danish draftees. *Acta Ophthalmol Suppl. 1988;185:41–43.*

Teikari JM. Myopia and stature. *Acta Ophthalmol* (Copenh). 1987;65:673–676.

Tong L, Saw SM, Chia KS, Tan D. Anisometropia in Singapore school children. *Am J Ophthalmol* 2004;137:474 –479.

Villarreal MG, Ohlsson J, Abrahamsson M, et al. Myopisation: the refractive tendency in teenagers. Prevalence of myopia among young teenagers in Sweden. *Acta Ophthalmol Scand* 2000;78:177– 181.

Vitale S, Cotch MF, Sperduto R, Ellwein L. Costs of refractive correction of distance vision impairment in the United States, 1999-2002. *Ophthalmology* 2006;113:2163-2170.

Vitale S, Ellwein L, Cotch MF, Ferris FL III, Sperduto R. Prevalence of refractive error in the United States, 1999-2004. *Arch Ophthalmol.* 2008;126:1111–1119.

Vitale S, Sperduto RD, Ferris FL, III. Increased prevalence of myopia in the United States between 1971–1972 and 1999–2004. *Arch Ophthalmol* 2009;127:1632–1639.

Wang Q, Klein BE, Klein R, Moss SE. Refractive status in the Beaver Dam Eye Study. *Invest Ophthalmol Vis Sci.* 1994;35: 4344–4347.

Wensor M, McCarty CA, Taylor HR. Prevalence and risk factors of myopia in Victoria, Australia. *Arch Ophthalmol.* 1999;117:658–663.

Wickremasinghe S, Foster PJ, Uranchimeg D, et al. Ocular biometry and refraction in Mongolian adults. *Invest Ophthalmol Vis Sci.* 2004;45:776–783.

Wickremasinghe S, Foster PJ, Uranchimeg D, et al. Ocular biometry and refraction in Mongolian adults. *Invest Ophthalmol Vis Sci* 2004;45:776–783.

Wojciechowski R, Congdon N, Bowie H, et al. Heritability of refractive error and familial aggregation of myopia in an elderly American population. *Invest Ophthalmol Vis Sci* 2005;46:1588-1592.

Wojciechowski R. Nature and nurture: the complex genetics of myopia and refractive error. *Clin Genet.* 2011;79:301–320.

Wong TY, Foster PJ, Hee J, et al. Prevalence and risk factors for refractive errors in adult Chinese in Singapore. *Invest Ophthalmol Vis Sci.* 2000;41:2486–2494.

Wong TY, Foster PJ, Johnson GJ, Klein BE, Seah SK. The relationship between ocular dimensions and refraction with adult stature: the Tanjong Pagar Survey. *Invest Ophthalmol Vis Sci.* 2001;42:1237–1242.

Wong TY, Klein BE, Klein R, et al. Refractive errors, intraocular pressure, and glaucoma in a white population. *Ophthalmology* 2003;110:211-217.

Woo WW, Lim KA, Yang H, et al. Refractive errors in medical students in Singapore. *Singapore Med J* 2004;45:470-474.

Wu HM, Seet B, Yap EP, et al. Does education explain ethnic differences in myopia prevalence? A population-based study of young adult males in Singapore. *Optom Vis Sci* 2001;78:234-239.

Wu MM, Edwards MH. The effect of having myopic parents: an analysis of myopia in three generations. *Optom Vis Sci* 1999;76:387-392.

Wu SY, Nemesure B, Leske MC. Refractive errors in a black adult population: the Barbados Eye Study. *Invest Ophthalmol Vis Sci* 1999;40:2179-2184.

Xu L, Li J, Cui T, et al. Refractive error in urban and rural adult Chinese in Beijing. *Ophthalmology* 2005;112:1676-1683.

Xu L, Wang Y, Li Y, et al. Causes of blindness and visual impairment in urban and rural areas in Beijing: the Beijing Eye Study. *Ophthalmology* 2006;113:1134. e1–e11.

Yamada M, Hiratsuka Y, Roberts CB, et al. Prevalence of visual impairment in the adult Japanese population by cause and severity and future projections. *Ophthalmic Epidemiol* 2010;17:50–57.

You QS, Xu L, Yang H, et al. Five-year incidence of visual impairment and blindness in adult. Chinese: the Beijing eye study. *Ophthalmology* 2011;118:1069–1075. Epub 2011.

Yuzawa M, Tamakoshi A, Kawamura T, et al. Report on the nationwide epidemiological survey of exudative age-related macular degeneration in Japan. *Int Ophthalmol* 1997;21:1–3.

Zadnik K, Jones LA, Irvin BC, et al. Myopia and ambient night-time lighting. CLEERE Study Group. Collaborative Longitudinal Evaluation of Ethnicity and Refractive Error. *Nature* 2000;404:143-144.

Zadnik K, Manny RE, Yu JA, et al., Collaborative Longitudinal Evaluation of Ethnicity and Refractive Error (CLEERE) Study Group. Ocular component data in schoolchildren as a function of age and gender. *Optom Vis Sci* 2003;80:226 –236.

Zadnik K, Mutti DO, Friedman NE, Adams AJ. Initial cross-sectional results from the Orinda Longitudinal Study of Myopia. *Optom Vis Sci* 1993;70:750-758.

Zadnik K, Satariano WA, Mutti DO, et al. The effect of parental history of myopia on children's eye size. *JAMA* 1994;271:1323-1327.

Zhan MZ, Saw SM, Hong RZ, et al. Refractive errors in Singapore and Xiamen, China–a comparative study in school children aged 6 to 7 years. *Optom Vis Sci* 2000;77:302– 308.

Zhang J, Hur YM, Huang W, Ding X, Feng K, He M. Shared genetic determinants of axial length and height in children: the Guangzhou twin eye study. *Arch Ophthalmol.* 2011;129: 63–68.

Zhang Q, Guo X, Xiao X, et al. Novel locus for X linked recessive high myopia maps to Xq23-q25 but outside MYP1. *J Med Genet* 2006;43:e20.

Zhao J, Pan X, Sui R, et al. Refractive Error Study in Children: results from Shunyi District, China. *Am J Ophthalmol* 2000; 129:427–435.

Chapter III

Anatomy of the Eye

The ability to see is produced by the actions of various parts of the eye, nerve cells, and the brain. Structures surrounding the eye, such as the lids and lashes, protect and assist this organ in its visual function. If any component of the visual system fails to operate properly, sight may be impaired. This chapter describes in detail the anatomy (structure) of the eye as the primary organ of vision and its surrounding structures

The eye is the organ of sight situated in the orbital cavity. It is almost spherical in shape and is about 2.5 cm in diameter. The volume of an eyeball is approximately 7 cc. The space between the eye and the orbital cavity is occupied by fatty tissue. The bony wall of the orbit and the fat help to protect the eye from injury. Struturally, the two eyes are separate but they function as a pair. It is possible to see with only one eye, but three-dimensional vision is impaired when only one eye is used specially in relation to the judgment of distance.

1. The Adnexa

The tissues and structures surrounding the eye are called the adnexa. They include the orbit, the extraocular muscles, the eyelids, and the tear-producing and tear-draining lacrimal apparatus. These structures serve to protect and support the globe.

Orbit

The orbit is defined as the bony cavity containing the globe, extraocular muscles, fat, nerves and blood vessels. Although the orbit is often described as pyramidal in shape, the space is actually pear-shaped, with its largest horizontal and vertical diameters lying 1 cm past the orbital rim and adjacent to the equator of the globe. Average orbital volume is approximately 25-30 cc, of which the globe occupies approximately 7 cc of space. The lateral walls are oriented about 90° to one another and run 40 to 45 mm in length to the apex. The medial walls of each orbit run parallel to each other and measure 45 to 50 mm in length. The optical axes themselves are also parallel to the course of the medial walls, rather than the diverging central axes of the orbits. Therefore, each globe is tonically held in adduction by the extraocular muscles to maintain ocular alignment (Mallajosyula, 2009).

Orbital Osteology

The orbital rim is roughly in the shape of a spiral, with its starting and end points at the anterior and posterior lacrimal crests (Whitnall, 1932). There are seven bones which make up the four orbital walls: the frontal, sphenoid (greater and lesser wings), ethmoid, lacrimal, maxillary, palatine, and zygomatic bones. The roof of the orbit is composed of the frontal bone anteriorly, and the lesser wing of the sphenoid bone posteriorly. The overall thgickness of the roof is significantly greater than that of either the medial wall or obital floor and therefore, relatively resistant to fracture. The medial wall includes the ethmoid, maxillary, and lacrimal bones, as well as the lesser wing of the sphenoid. The anterior ethmoidal foramen is typically located approximately 24 mm posterior to the orbital rim and the posterior ethmoidal foramen lies approximately 36 mm posterior to the rim. The optic foramen, in turn, is located approximately 6 mm posterior to the posterior ethmoidal foramen (Mallajosyula S., 2009).

The floor of the orbit consists of the maxillary, zygomatic and palatine bones. The maxillary bone forms the bulk of the floor while the zygomatic bone contributes anterolaterally and the palatine bone contributes to the posterior floor. The lateral wall contains the zygomatic bone and the greater wing of the sphenoid which separates the posterolateral orbit from the middle cranial fossa. The posterior borders of the lateral wall are defined by the superior and inferior otbital fissures. The boundary between the lateral wall and roof is formed by the frontosphenoid suture, which transmits the recurrent meningeal artery. The anterior part of the lateral wall is comprised of the zygoma.

The Orbital Apex

The orbital apex is the region in which many critical orbital structures converge and communicate with other important, periorbital spaces. Cranial nerves II through VI, major orbital vessels, and all of the extraocular muscles excluding the inferior oblique sit in tight proximity within the apex, and pathology in this region can produce profound deficits in vision and ocular motility (Yeh and Foroozan, 2004; Lenzi and Fieschi, 1977)

The apex is defined by only three walls; the floor is absent in the far posterior orbit (Whitnall SE. The anatomy of the human orbit and accessory organs of vision, 2nd ed. NewYork: Oxford University Press; 1932.)(Whitnall, 1932) The major bony landmarks include the superior orbital fissure, inferior orbital fissure, and the optic canal. The superior orbital fissure divides the sphenoid into the freater (lateral) and lesser (medial) wings and lies inferiorly and laterally to the optic foramen. This fissure measures approximately 20-22 mm in overall lenth and is eparated into superolateral and inferomedial sections by the tendon of the lateral rectus muscle.

The Extraocular Muscles

The extraocular (extrinsic) muscles of the eye are the four recti and the two oblique muscles. (The ciliary muscles and the sphincter pupillae and dilatator pupillae muscles are the intrinsic muscles). The recti muscles are (1) the medial rectus muscle, (2) the lateral rectus muscle, (3) the superior rectus muscle, and (4) the inferior rectus muscle. The four rectus muscles originate at the annulus of Zinn, within the orbital apex. Specifically, the superior and medial recti originate adjacent to the lesser wing of the sphenoid, next to the optic canal.

The inferior rectus originates from a portion of the annulus which extends from the body of the sphenoid bone to its great wing. The lateral rectus has a bifid origin from a tendinous segment of the annulus which extends across the superior orbital fissure from the greater to the lesser sphenoid wing and a more inferior portion which extends directly from the greater wing itself.

The superior oblique muscle also begins along the annulus of Zinn, superomedially and extends forward superiorly and along the junction between the orbital roof and the medial orbital wall. As it courses toward the anterior orbit, the muscle belly transitions to a tendinous segment as it reaches the trochlea, a pulley-like cartilaginous structure which lies approximately 6-10 mm posterior to the superomedial orbital rim(Helveston et al, 1982; Sacks, 1984)

The inferior oblique, unlike the other extraocular muscles, does not originate at the annulus, but from the periosteum of the znterior, inferomedial orbit on the maxillary bone.

The extraaocular muscles approximate a spiral in the distance between their individual insertions and the corneal limbus, the so-called spiral of Tillaux. Beginning with the medial, each successive muscle inserts farther from the limbus. Although there is individual variation, the average distances are: medial rectus, 5.5 mm; inferior rectus, 6.5 mm, lateral rectus, 6.9 mm, and superior rectus, 7.7 mm (Apt, 1988)

Innervation to the extraocular muscles is largely carried by the oculomotor nerve (third cranial nerve), which supplies the medial, inferior, and superior rectus muscles, the inferior oblique, as well as the levator palpebrae superioris. The superior oblique and lateral rectus receive innervation from the trochlear nerve (fourth cranial nerve) and the abducens nerve (sixth cranial nerve), respectively. The blood supply to the muscles is carried by muscular branches of the ophthalmic artery.

Eyelids

The eyelids are thin the curtains of skin, muscle, fibrous tissue, and mucous membrane that protect the eye from external irritation, interrupt and limit the amount of light entering the eye, and distribute tears over the surface of the globe. The upper eyelid is mimited above by the eyebrow; the lower eyelid merges with the cheek. Each eyelid is divided by a horizontal furrow (sulcus) into an orbital and a tarsal portion. The upper furrow is formed by skin insertions of the levator palpebrae superioris muscle. The lower furrow is poorly defined and is formed by a few cutaneous connections from the orbicularis

The normal interpalpebral fissure height is 10-12 mm and the average length is 28-30 mm. oculi muscles. The corneoscleral limbus is covered above and below by the eyelids.

When open, the eyelids form an elliptic opening, the palpebral fissure, which measures about 12 by 30 mm. Laterally the fissure forms a 60° angle; medially it is rounded. In blacks and whites the lateral margin (canthus) is about 2 mm higher than the medial; in orinetals it may be 5 mm higher. In blacks and whites the fissure is widest at the junction of the inner one third with the outer two thirds. In orientals the fissure is widest at the junction of the inner one half with the outer one half. In orientals the medial canthus is obscured by a characteristic vertical skin fold (epicanthus), which, when present in whites, may cause the eyes to appear to be turned in pseudostrabimus.

Each eyelid margin is 2 mm thick and 30 mm long.

The distance between the upper lid crease and lid margin measures approximately 8-11 mm at the pupillary axis. The highest point of the upper lid contour rests just nasal to the center of the pupil and the upper lid margin is typically located 1-2 mm below the superior limbus in adults. The lateral canthal angle sits approximately 2 mm higher than the medial canthus.

Both the upper and lower eyelids can be divided into the skin, orbicularis, orbital septum, orbital fat, lid retractors, tarsus, and conjunctiva.

The Conjunctiva

The conjunctiva is a thin, transparent mucous membrane that lines the inner surface of the eyelids and covers the anterior portion of the sclera. Its epithelium is continuous with that of the cornea and with the lacrimal drainage system through the puncta. The conjunctiva is divided into three areas: (1) the palpebral conjunctiva, (2) the conjunctiva of the superior and inferior fornices, and (3) the bulbar conjunctiva.

The palpebral conjunctiva is divided into marginal tarsal and orbital portions. The tarsal portion is closely adherent to the tarsal plate, from which it can be removed only with difficulty. The orbital portion is thrown into folds.

The conjunctiva of the superior and inferior fornices forms transitional areas between the palpebral and bulbar conjunctivae. It is but loosely attached to the underlying tissue and may become markedly swollen.

The bulbar conjunctiva is closely adherent to the sclera, which can be seen as the “white” of the eye through the transparent conjunctival tissue.

Lacrimal Apparatus

The lacrimal apparatus consists of a secretory and a collecting portion. The secretory portion is composed of the lacrimal gland and the accessory lacrimal glands of Krause and Wolfring. The collecting portion consists of the canaliculi with their orifices (the puncta), the lacrimal sac, and the lacrimal duct, which has its opening in the inferior nasal meatus.

2. The Eye, the Eyeball or the Globe

The eye rests in the front half of the cavity of the orbit upon a fascial hammock surrounded by ocular muscles, fat, and connective tissue. Only its anterior aspects is exposed, and it is protected by the bony orbital rim. As mentioned above, attached to the eye are four recti and two oblique muscles. These are innervated by oculomotor (N III), trochlear (N IV, superior oblique muscle), and abducent (N VI, lateral muscle) cranial nerves, which enter the orbit through the superior orbital fissure in the posterior orbit. The ophthalmic branch of the trigeminal nerve (N V) that transmits sensory fibers from the upper face and the eye also enters the cranial cavity through the superior orbital fissure. The optic nerve leaves the orbit through the optic foramen, which also transmits the ophthalmic artery and the sympathetic innervation of the eye. The exposed anterior one third of the eye consists of a central transparent portion, the cornea, and a surrounding white portion, the sclera. The sclera is covered with the bulbar conjunctiva, which is continuous with the palpebral conjunctiva lining the inner surface of the protective tissue curtains, the eyelids. The lacrimal gland is located in the upper outer portion of the bony orbit (Newell, 1986).

The anterior pole of the eye is the center of curvature of the cornea. The posterior pole marks the center of the posterior curvature of the globe, and it is located slightly temporal to the optic nerve. The geometric axis is a line connecting these two poles. The equator encircles the eye midway between the two poles.

The average size globe measures approximately 23.5 mm in the horizontal meridian and 23 mm vertically, with an antero-posterior dimension of about 24 mm. Its overall volume is about 7 cc. The anteroposterior diameter of the normal eye, measured by ultrasonic methods, is about 22 to 27 mm. The circumference is between 69 and 85 mm. In the average eye (24 mm in diameter), the equator is on the surface of sclera 16 mm posterior to the corneoscleral limbus. The posterior pole is 32 mm behind the corneoscleral limbus. Internally the anterior termination of the sensory retina (ora serrate) is approximately 5.75 to 6.5 mm posterior to the terminantion of the Descemet membrane of the cornea (Schwalbe line).

The prominence of the globes is dependent on orbital volume, globe size, orbital fat volume, and structure of the eyelids and conjunctiva, all of which vary between individuals and shows significant differences between ethnicities. Based on a study of 681 individuals with no history of orbital or endocrine disease, high myopia, or buphthalmos, Migliori and Gladstone found that white men had a mean protrusion value measured from the lateral orbital rim of 16.5 mm compared to 18.5 mm in black men, and 15.4 mm in white women compared to 17.8 mm in black women (Migliori and Gladstone, 1984).

Kaimbo wa Kaimbo (Kaimbo Wa Kaimbo and Kayembe, 1994), in a study of 95 black normal subjects aged from 15 to 18 years (mean age±SD, 17 years±3), found a mean±SD proptosis performed with the Hertel exophthalmoeter of 17.6 mm±2 for the ight eye and 17.2 mm±m2.1 for the left eye. No statistically significant difference was observed between boys and girls or between right and left eyes.

The globe has three main layers, each of which is further divided. The outer supporting coat consists of the transparent cornea, the opaque sclera, and their junction, the corneo-scleral limbus or sulcus. The middle layer, or the uvea, consists of the choroid, the ciliary body, and the iris, which contains a central opening, the pupil. The inner layer consists of the retina, which is composed of two parts, a sensory portion and the layer of retinal pigment epithelium.

The lens is a transparent structure located immediately behind the iris and supported in position by a series of fine fibers, the zonule. These are attached to the ciliary and the capsule of the lens.

The eye encloses three chambers: (1) the vitreous cavity, (2) the posterior chamber, and (3) the anterior chamber. The *vitreous cavity*, by far the largest, is olocated behind the lens and zonule and is adjacent to the sensory retina. The *posterior chamber* is minute in size and is bounded by the lens and zonule behind and the iris in front. The *anterior chamber* is located between the iris and the posterior surface of the cornea and communicates with the posterior chamber through the pupil. Aqueous humor is secreted by the ciliary processes into the posterior chamber and passes through the pupil into the anterior chamber. The aqueous humor leaves the anterior chamber through the trabecular meshwork that opens into the canal of schlemm, an endothelium-lined channel that encircles the anterior chamber.

Outer Coat

The outer coat of the eye consists of relatively tough fibrous tissues shaped as segments of two spheres: the sclera, with a radius of curvature of about 13 mm, and the cornea, with a radius of curvature of about 7.5 mm. The white, opaque sclera constitutes the posterior five sixths of the globe, and the transparent cornea provides the anterior onr sixth of the globe. The junction of the cornea and the sclera, the corneoscleral limbus, contains the trabecular meshwork and the aqueous humor drainange system, the canal od Schlemm, which is an important functional and anatomic area.

Anatomy of the Eyeball (McCaa, 1982)

The eye consists of a retinal-lined fibrovascular sphere which contains the aqueous humor, the lens and the vitreous body.. The retina is the essential component of the eye and serves the primary purpose of photoreception. All other structures of the eye are subsidiary and act to focus images on the retina, to regulate the amount of light entering the eye or to provide nutrition, protection or motion. The retina may be considered as an outlying island of the central nervous system, to which it is connected by a tract of nerve fibers, the optic nerve. As in the case of the brain and the spinal cord, the retina is within two coats of tissue which contribute protection and nourishment. On the outside of the sphere, corresponding to the dura mater, a layer composed of dense fibrous tissue serves as a protective envelope, the fibrous tunic. The posterior part of the fibrous tunic, the sclera, is white and opaque. Although it retains its protective function, the anterior portion, the cornea, is clear and transparent. Immediately internal to the sclera, and between it and the retina, lies the uvea, a vascular tunic analogous to the pia-arachnoid of the central nervous system. Primarily, the uvea provides nutrients to the eye. The posterior portion of the uvea is the choroid, a tissue composed almost entirely of blood vessels. A second portion of the uvea, the ciliary body, lies just anterior to the choroid and posterior to the corneoscleral margin and provides nutrients by forming intraocular fluid, the aqueous humor. In addition, the ciliary body contains muscles which provide a supporting and focusing mechanism for the lens. The most anterior portion of the uveal tract, the iris, is deflected into the interior of the eye. The iris acts as a diaphragm with a central rounded opening, the pupil, which dilates to allow more light to the retina in dim lighting and constricts in bright lighting. The iris also has some degree of nutritive function, since it acts to help regulate the fluid flow in the eye.

The lens, the focusing mechanism of the eye, is located immediately behind the iris and is supported from the ciliary body by a suspensory ligament, the zonule. The space between the iris and the lens is called the posterior chamber. The anterior chamber consists of the space between the iris and the cornea. Behind the lens is the vitreous, a gel-like, transparent body which occupies the space between the lens and the retina (McCaa, 1982).

The globe is surrounded by a loose fascial sheath, or Tendon's capsule, which is interconnected to the sclera by fine fibrous bands. The potential space between these layers is the episcleral space, and the areas of greatest adherence between them are approximately 1.5 mm from the limbus anteriorly, and posteriorly, at the optic nerve sheath. Tenon's capsule is suspended inside the orbit by interconnections with fine connective tissue septae within the surrounding orbital fat. This sheath must be traversed by the nerves and blood vessels which supply the globe. Likewise, the extraocular muscles must penetrate Tenon's layer to attach to the globe.

3. Cornea and Sclera

The Cornea

The cornea forms the anterior one-sixth of the eye. The cornea is a transparent avascular connective tissue that acts as the primary infectious and structural barrier of the eye. Together with the overlying tear film, it also provides a proper anterior refractive surface for the eye. It is the main refracting surface of the eye. The diopter power is +43 to +45 D. Its clarity is the result of many factors including the structural anatomy and physiology of its cellular components (Derek et al., 2011).

In the average adult, the horizontal diameter of the cornea is 11.5 to 12.0 mm (Rüfer et al, 2005) and about 1.0 mm larger than the vertical diameter. It is approximately 0.5 mm thick at the center and gradually increases in thickness toward the periphery. The shape of the cornea is prolated flatter in the periphery and steeper centrally which creates an aspheric optical system. Corneal shape and curvature are governed by the intrinsic biomechanical structure and extrinsic environment. Anterior corneal stromal rigidity appears to be particularly important in maintaining the corneal curvature (Müller et al, 2001). Organizational differences in the collagen bundles of the anterior stroma may contribute to a tighter cohesive strength in this area and may also explain why the anterior curvature resists change to stromal hydration much more than the posterior stroma, which tends to more easily develop folds. Stromal hydration also appears to affect the cornea's response to strain and shear forces (Simon and Ren, 1994). The cornea, the window of the eye, is unique because of its transparency. Corneal transparency is dependent on a special arrangement of cells and collagenous fibrils in an acid mucopolysaccharide environment, to an absence of blood vessels, and to deturgescence (the state of relative dehydration of corneal tissue) (Derek et al., 2011).

Structure of the Cornea

The cornea is composed of six distinct layers: (1) epithelium, (2) Bowman's membrane, (3) stroma, (4) Pre-Descemet's layer (Dua's layer) (5) Descemet's membrane and (6) endothelium. In addition, a tear film always covers the cornea of a healthy eye.

The Tear Film. The tear film is made up of three layers. The portion immediately next to the epithelium is rich in glycoprotein produced by the goblet cells of the conjunctival epithelium; a middle, watery layer is secreted by the lacrimal glands; an outside oily layer is produced by the meibomian glands and the glands of Moll and Zeis of the lid. The tear film is essential for the maintenance of the proper optical qualities of the cornea.

Corneal Epithelium

The epithelial surface of the cornea creates the first barrier to the outside environment and is an integral part of the tear film–cornea interface that is critical to the refractive power of the eye. It is a stratified, nonkeratinizing squamous layer characterized by extreme uniformity from limbus to limbus. Embryologically, the corneal epithelium is derived from surface ectoderm between 5 and 6 weeks of gestation. It is composed of nonkeratinized, stratified squamous epithelium that is 4 to 6 cell layers thick (40 mm to 50 mm) (Farjo et al, 2008). As mentioned above, the epithelium is covered with a tear film, which is optically important in smoothing out microirregularities of the anterior epithelial surface. The air–tear film interface, together with the underlying cornea, provides two thirds of the total refractive power of the eye. The corneal epithelium and overlying tear film have a symbiotic relationship both anatomically and physiologically. The mucinous layer of the tear film, which is in direct contact with the corneal epithelium, is produced by the conjunctival goblet cells and interacts closely with the corneal epithelial cell glycocalyx to allow hydrophilic spreading of the tear film with each eyelid blink. It has been suggested that the epithelium itself may contribute to this mucinous layer, but this is unproven (Gipson et al, 1992). Loss of the glycocalyx from injury or disease results in loss of tear-film stability and subsequent breakdown of the ocular optical system. The tear film is the primary protector of the corneal surface from microbial invasion, as well as from chemical, toxic, and foreign-body damage. The tear film also supplies immunological and growth factors that are critical for epithelial health, proliferation, and repair (Cameron, 2005). Corneal epithelial cells have an average lifespan of 7 to 10 days (Hanna et al, 1961) and routinely undergo orderly involution, apoptosis (programmed cell death), and desquamation. This process results in complete turnover of the corneal epithelial layer every week as deeper cells replace the desquamating superficial cells in an orderly, apically directed fashion. The most superficial corneal epithelial cells form a mean of 2 to 3 layers of flat polygonal cells. These cells have extensive apical microvilli and microplicae, which in turn are covered by a fine, closely apposed, charged glycocalyceal layer (Farjo et al, 2008). This layer's apical membrane projections increase the surface area of contact and adherence between the tear film's mucinous layer and the cell membrane. As discussed earlier, this is critical for a smooth and clear optical system. These surface cells maintain tight junctional complexes between their neighbors, which prohibit tears from entering the intercellular spaces. This can be demonstrated clinically by observing a healthy epithelial surface's ability to repel dyes such as fluorescein and rose bengal. This barrier also prevents toxins and microbes from entering deeper corneal layers. Beneath the superficial cell layer and just anterior to the deepest basal layer of the epithelium are the suprabasal or wing cells. This layer is 2 to 3 cells deep and consists of cells that are less flat than the overlying superficial cells but possess similar tight lateral intercellular junctions.

The deepest cellular layer of the corneal epithelium is the basal layer, which comprises a single cell layer of columnar epithelium approximately 20 mm tall. Besides the stem cells and transient amplifying cells, basal cells are the only corneal epithelial cells capable of mitosis (Wiley et al, 1991). They are the source of wing and superficial cells and possess lateral intercellular junctions characterized by gap junctions and zonulae adherens. The basal cells are attached to the underlying basement membrane by a hemidesmosomal system. This strong attachment is what prevents the epithelium from separating from the underlying corneal layers. Abnormalities in this bonding system may result clinically in recurrent corneal erosion syndromes or non healing epithelial defects. Epithelial stem cells, which serve as an important source of new corneal epithelium, have been localized to the limbal basal epithelium. As the cells migrate to the central cornea, they differentiate into transient amplifying cells (cells capable of multiple but limited cellular division) and basal cells (Li et al, 2007).

The epithelial basement membrane, approximately 0.05 mm thick, comprises type IV collagen and laminin secreted by the basal cells. If damaged, fibronectin levels increase and the process of healing can take up to 6 weeks. During this time, the epithelial bond to the underlying, newly laid basement membrane tends to be unstable and weak.

Bowman Layer (Bowman's Membrane)

Bowman layer (or Bowman membrane) lies just anterior to the stroma and is not a true membrane but rather the acellular condensate of the most anterior portion of the stroma. This smooth layer is approximately 15 mm thick and helps the cornea maintain its shape. When disrupted, it will not regenerate and can form a scar.

Corneal Stroma

The corneal stroma provides the bulk of the structural framework of the cornea and comprises roughly 80% to 90% of its thickness. Embryologically, it is the result of a second wave of neural crest migration that occurs in the seventh week of gestation, after establishment of the primitive endothelium. The stroma differs from other collagenous structures in its transparency, which is the result of precise organization of the stromal fibers and extracellular matrix (ECM) (Maurice, 1970; Boote et al, 2003). The collagen fibers are arranged in parallel bundles called fibrils, and these fibrils are packed in parallel arranged layers or lamellae. It consists of alternating lamellae of collagenous tissue parallel to the surface of the cornea. The stroma of the human eye contains 200 to 250 distinct lamella, each layer arranged at right angles relative to fibers in adjacent lamellae (Maurice, 1970). The peripheral stroma is thicker than the central stroma, and the collagen fibrils may change direction to run circumferentially as they approach the limbus (Meek and Boote, 2004). This highly organized network reduces forward light scatter and contributes to the transparency and mechanical strength of the cornea. An additional feature of the stroma is that the ultrastructure within the organization of the lamella appears to vary based on the depth within the stroma. Deeper layers are more strictly organized than superficial layers, and this difference accounts for the greater ease of surgical dissection in a particular plane as one approaches the posterior depths of the corneal stroma. This variation in stromal organization also accounts for the differences in response to corneal edema, as mentioned previously. Descemet folds are the result of asymmetric swelling of the posterior stroma imposed by the structurally more rigid anterior cornea and structural restriction imposed by the limbus (Gipson and Joyce, 2008). Stromal swelling is therefore directed posteriorly and results in relative flattening of the posterior surface, which can push Descemet membrane into multiple folds that become visible as striae. Stromal collagen fibrils are composed of type I collagen in a heterodimeric complex with type V collagen to obtain their unique and narrow diameter (Fini and Stramer, 2005). These complexes are surrounded by specialized proteoglycans, consisting of keratan sulfate or chondroitin sulfate/dermatan sulfate side chains, which help regulate hydration and structural properties. Keratocytes are the major cell type of the stroma and are involved in maintaining the ECM environment. They are able to synthesize collagen molecules and glycosaminoglycans while also creating matrix metalloproteases (MMPs) - all crucial in maintaining stromal homeostasis. Most of these keratocytes reside in the anterior stroma and contain corneal"crystallins," representing 25% to 30% of soluble protein in the cells. These crystallins appear to be responsible for reducing backscatter of light from the keratocytes and maintaining corneal transparency (Jester et al, 1999).

Dua's Layer

A novel pre-Descemet's layer (Dua's layer) exists, a well-defined, acellular, strong layer in the pre-Descemet's cornea.

Descemet's Membrane

Beginning in utero at the 8-week stage, endothelial cells continuously secrete Descemet membrane. The anterior 3 mm secreted prior to birth has a distinctive banded appearance when viewed by electron microscopy, but Descemet membrane produced after birth is unbanded and has an amorphous ultrastructural texture. Descemet can accumulate up to 10 mm in thickness with age.

Corneal Endothelium

The endothelial layer of the cornea maintains corneal clarity by ensuring it remains in a relatively deturgesced state. The intact human endothelium is a monolayer, which appears as a honeycomb-like mosaic when viewed from the posterior side. In early embryogenesis, the posterior cornea is lined with a neural crest-derived monolayer of orderly arranged cuboidal cells (Beebe and Coats, 2000). Over time, these cells flatten and become tightly adherent to one another. Immediately anterior to the flattened layer is a discontinuous homogeneous acellular layer, which in time becomes Descemet membrane (Watsky et al, 1989). At birth, the endothelial monolayer is approximately 10 mm thick and consists of a uniform thickness layer of cells that spans the entire posterior corneal surface and fuses with the cells of the trabecular meshwork (Watsky et al, 1989). Similarly, Descemet membrane becomes continuous and uniform, fusing peripherally with the trabecular beams (Watsky et al, 1989). The fusion site, known as Schwalbe line, is a gonioscopic landmark that defines the end of Descemet membrane and the start of the trabecular meshwork. The individual cells continue to flatten over time and stabilize at approximately 4 mm in thickness in adulthood. Adjacent cells share extensive lateral interdigitations and possess gap and tight junctions along their lateral borders. The lateral membranes contain a high density of NaC, KC-ATPase pump sites (Stiemke et al, 1991). The basal surface of the endothelium contains numerous hemidesmosomes that promote adhesion to Descemet membrane.

Endothelial cell density and topography continue to change throughout life. From the second to eighthdecades of life, the cell density declines from 3000 to 4000 cells/mm^2 to around 2600 cells/mm^2, and the percentage of hexagonal cells declines from approximately

75% to approximately 60% (Yee et al, 1985). The central endothelial cell density decreases at an average rate of 0.6% per year in normal corneas (Bourne et al, 1997). As mentioned, the stroma is maintained in a relatively deturgesced state (78% water content) by the activity of the endothelial cells (Geroski et al, 1985). This dehydration is mediated by a pump–leak process as fluid egresses from the corneal stroma down the osmotic gradient from a relatively hypo-osmotic stroma toward a relatively hypertonic aqueous humor. This passive bulk fluid movement requires no energy but is fueled by the energy-requiring processes of transporting ions to generate the osmotic gradient. The 2 most important ion transport systems are the membrane-bound NaC and KC-ATPase sites and the intracellular carbonic anhydrase pathway. Activity in both these pathways produces a net flux of ions from the stroma to the aqueous humor. The barrier portion of the endothelium is unique in that it is permeable to some degree, permitting the ion flux necessary to establish the osmotic gradient (Watsky et al, 1989).

Endothelial cells have no mitotic activity in vivo; however, humans are born with a significant reserve. Cell density is approximately 3500 cells/mm^2 at birth, but this number decreases gradually throughout life at approximately 0.6% per year. It has been observed that eyes with endothelial cell counts below 500 cells/mm^2 may be at risk for the development of corneal edema. Endothelial cell morphology (size and shape) also appears to correlate with pump function. An increase in cell size (polymegathism) and an increase in variation of cell shape (pleomorphism) correlate to reduced ability of the endothelial cells to deturgesce the cornea (Polse et al, 1990). The number of endothelial cells decreases with age, trauma, inflammation, and other disease processes (ie, Fuchs endothelial dystrophy), but the remaining cells have the capacity to "stretch" and take over the space of the degenerated endothelial cells. As this process occurs, the remaining cells grow in size (polymegathism) and lose their hexagonal shape (pleomorphism).

Blood Supply of the Cornea

Although the normal human cornea is avascular, it relies on components of the blood to remain healthy. These components are supplied by tiny vessels at the outermost edge of the cornea as well as components supplied by end branches of the facial and ophthalmic arteries via the aqueous humor and tear film.

Nerve Supply of the Cornea

The cornea is one of the most heavily innervated and most sensitive tissues in the body. Corneal nerves and sensation are derived from the nasociliary branch of the first (ophthalmic) division of the trigeminal nerve. In the superficial cornea, the nerves enter the stroma radially in thick trunks forming plexiform arrangements, which eventually perforate Bowman membrane to provide a rich plexus beneath the basal epithelial layer (Oliveira-Soto and Efron, 2001). The cornea also contains autonomic sympathetic nerve fibers.

Corneal Epithelium

The corneal epithelium consists of five or six layers of cells which rest on a basement membrane. It is replaced by growth from its basal cells with perhaps greater rapidity than any other stratified epithelium (1).

Bowman's Membrane

Bowman's membrane is not a true basement membrane but is a clear acellular layer which is a modified portion of the superficial stroma. It is a homogenous layer without cells and has no capacity to regenerate if injured.

Corneal Stroma

The stroma makes up approximately 90% of the thickness of the cornea. The corneal cells, or keratocytes, are relatively few and lie within the collagen lamellae (1). Descemet's Membrane. Descemet's membrane is a strong, homogeneous true basement membrane. It is produced by the endothelial cells and can be regenerated if injured. Descemet's membrane is elastic and is more resistant than the remainder of the cornea to trauma and disease.

Corneal Endothelium

The corneal endothelium consists of a single layer of flattened cuboidal cells. The endothelium does not regenerate and is essential for maintaining dehydration of corneal tissue. Therefore, chemical or physical damage to the endothelium of the cornea is far more serious than epithelial damage. Destruction of the endothelial cells may cause marked swelling of the cornea and result in loss of its transparency.

4. Aging

Numerous anatomic changes occur in the eye with age (Grossniklaus et al, 2013). These changes generally include loss and attenuation of cells, such as the corneal endothelium and RPE; degenerative processes, such as vitreous liquefaction; and accumulations of materials, such as drusen. As the eye ages, the cornea flattens (Spencer, 1996). The thickness of Bowman's layer, 8 to 10 μm, remains constant throughout life. There is a tendency for calcific deposition at the periphery of Bowman's layer with aging. Arcus senilis, a deposition of lipid near the limbus, also may occur with aging. The stromal keratocyte density appears higher in children than adults. Arcus senilis appears in the peripheral cornea with aging in some patients (Cogan and Kuwabara, 1959). The thickness of Descemet's membrane increases with aging (Johnson et al, 1982). There is a decrease in corneal endothelial cell density that occurs with aging (Edelhauser, 2006). The most precipitous decrease in cell density occurs in the first five years of life. In general, the corneal endothelial cell density decreases from approximately 5000 cells/mm^2 at birth to 3000 cells/mm^2 in older age. There is a direct correlation between histologic corneal endothelial cell number and specular microscopic endothelial cell density (Williams et al, 1992). The corneal endothelial cell density is not uniform, with an increased endothelial cell density in the paracentral and peripheral regions of the cornea, which declines with age at a rate of between 0.2% and 0.6% per year (Amann et al, 2003). There is some evidence that endothelial stem cells are present in a regenerative zone near Schwalbe's line which give rise to a paracentral storage zone of cells (Amann et al, 2003; Whikehart et al, 2005).

The Sclera

The sclera is hydrated and has large collagen fibrils arranged haphazardly; therefore, it is opaque and white rather than clear. The sclera has three layers: the episclera, the outer layer; the sclera; and the melanocytic layer, the inner lamina fusca. The episclera, a highly vascular connective tissue, attaches Tenon's capsule to the sclera. The sclera proper is relatively avascular and contains considerable elastic tissue. The sclera is approximately 1 mm thick posteriorly and gradually thins to about 0.3 mm just posterior to the insertions of the recti muscles. Therefore, these sites posterior to the insertion of the muscles are the areas of the eye which are most liable to rupture with trauma to the globe.

Scleral Anatomy (Mrejen and Spaide, 2013)

The sclera is thickest (1.0 mm) at the posterior pole around the optic nerve and thinnest (0.3 mm) beneath the insertions of the rectus muscles, measuring 0.5 mm at the equator. The sclera is organized in three layers: outer episclera, scleral stroma, and inner lamina fusca. The superficial episclera is a connective tissue that contains melanocytes, a few fibroblasts, lymphocytes, and relatively numerous blood vessels. The scleral stroma is the largest portion of the sclera and is composed of branching bundles of collagen fibers, together with numerous elastic fibers, extracellular matrix, and a few fibroblasts. The lamina fusca, the innermost layer, can be distinguished by its brownish color, due to the presence of numerous embedded melanocytes, and blends with the suprachoroidal and supraciliary lamellae of the uveal tract. Collagen in the lamina fusca is arranged in thin, small bundles. This layer also contains elastic fibers. The sclera, like the cornea, is essentially an avascular fibrous structure, except for the vessels of the superficial episcleral plexus (Portnoy et al, 2006) and the intrascleral vascular plexus located just posterior to the limbus. A number of channels, or emissaria, penetrate and break the continuity of the sclera for the perforating ciliary nerves, short and long posterior ciliary arteries, anterior ciliary arteries, and vortex veins. Interesting variations of the sclera are associated with myopia, particularly high myopia. Eyes with high myopia have thinning of the sclera, with a decrease in the amount of collagen in the sclera. The distribution of collagen fibrils is different from that of emmetropic subjects, with an increased proportion of smaller diameter collagen fibrils (Curtin et al, 1979; McBrien et al, 2001; Rada et al, 2006) and the sclera is more elastic (McBrien et al, 2009).

The sclera forms five-sixths of the outer tunic of the eye, consists of dense fibrous tissue, and contains openings and canals for the various vessels and nerves entering and exiting the globe. Its mechanical properties and limited distensibility help contain the intraocular pressure and prevent deformations of the globe during extraocular movement. It is relatively avascular and principally composed of collagen with scant fibrocytes and ground substance. Externally it is white, whereas internally it is slightly brown because of the presence of pigmented melanocytes. This most interior layer of the sclera, adjacent to the uvea, is called the lamina fusca, whereas the most exterior layer of the sclera, consisting of delicate fibrous and elastic tissue connecting the bulbar fascia and the sclera, is called the episcleral tissue. If the sclera is thin, as in childhood, or its hydration content decreases to less than 40% or increases to more than 80%, the sclera becomes more lucent, such that it appears blue or slate grey. As the sclera thins, the underlying uvea absorbs more light and the scattering of shorter wavelength light by the scleral collagen imparts a blue hue.

The scleral thickness varies considerably in the anteroposterior dimension. It is thickest near the optic nerve, measuring 1 to 1.35 mm, and gradually thins anteriorly, where it measures 0.4 to 0.6 mm in thickness at the equator. The sclera is thinnest beneath the tendonous insertions of the extraocular muscles, where it measures approximately 0.3 mm in thickness (Bron et al, 1997; Maurice, 1969). At the limbus (the transitional area between cornea and sclera), the sclera thickness is approximately 0.825 mm. In older individuals, it is unclear whether the apparently thinner sclera is caused by age-related atrophy (Vannas and Teir, 1960) or changes in scleral hydration (Weale, 1982).

The anterior scleral foramen is defined by a zone in which the scleral fibers merge with the collagen fibrils of the corneal stroma. Usually the sclera is beveled internally to overlap the cornea anteriorly in the sagittal meridian, making the cornea appear as an ellipse. For this reason, the external diameter of the cornea averages 10.6 mm vertically and 11.6 mm horizontally (Maurice, 1969). Internally, the anterior scleral foramen is more nearly circular, with a diameter of 11.6 mm. Both the external and internal margins of the sclera at the sclerocorneal junction extend slightly anteriorly, creating an external and internal annular groove, called the external and internal scleral sulcus, respectively. The external scleral sulcus is approximately 1 mm in depth. However, most of this is filled in by the attachments of the conjunctiva and Tenon's fascia as they blend into the limbus, and thus is less apparent. The external scleral sulcus is more prominent nasally than temporally. The internal scleral sulcus is circular with an internal groove formed by the slight anterior projection of the sclera near the limbus. It is bound anteriorly by Schwalbe's ring, posteriorly by the scleral spur, and contains Schlemm's canal, externally, and the corneoscleral meshwork, internally. Along its inner surface, inserts the anterior tendons of the longitudinal ciliary muscles (Tripathi and Tripathi, 1982). The posterior margin of internal scleral sulcus extends anteriorly as the scleral spur and is the attachment for the ciliary muscle. At the base of the sulcus is Schlemm's canal. A so-called pectinate ligament can occasionally be found to bridge the internal scleral sulcus.

The posterior scleral foramen allows the ganglion cell axons to exit the globe and enter the orbital segment of the optic nerve. It is a short canal located 3 mm nasal to the vertical meridian and 1 mm inferior to the horizontal meridian in the posterior hemisphere. It has an internal diameter of 1.5 to 2.0 mm and an external diameter of 3.0 to 3.5 mm. It is approximately 0.7 mm long and exits the globe in a nasal direction at an oblique angle. The network of collagenous and elastic scleral fibers that traverse the foramen in the innermost one-third of the foramen is referred to as the lamina cribosa. It provides mechanical strength and anchorage points for the neural and vascular elements as they traverse the canal. The inner surface of the lamina cribosa is concave (Hayreh and Vrabee, 1966) and is displaced posteriorly in the presence of sustained ocular hypertension. Fibroelastic fibers from the outer two-thirds of the sclera turn outward to merge with the dural sheath of the optic nerve.

Emissary channels allow the passage of nerves and vessels through the scleral tunic. These can be divided into anterior, middle, and posterior emissary channels.

The anterior emissary channels are located near the limbus, through which the anterior ciliary arteries and veins and the ciliary nerves traverse. The anterior ciliary arteries travel with the rectus muscles, two in each muscle with the exception of the lateral rectus, which has one artery. Each artery enters the sclera just anterior to the insertions and travels obliquely to supply the ciliary body and feed the major arterial circle of the iris. Smaller branches turn externally toward the limbus, where they anastamose with subconjunctival vessels to form the episceral plexus. These recurrent branches of the limbal vessels supply the perilimbal conjunctiva within 3 to 6 mm of the limbus. The anterior ciliary veins leave the ciliary body and travel in a channel that is frequently shared with a branch of the posterior ciliary nerve, which passes close to the surface before looping into the ciliary body. This neurovascular loop is called the nerve loop of Axenfeld and is present in approximately 12% of individuals (Stevenson, 1963). Clinically, it appears as 1- to 2-mm dome-shaped gray area, that is often pigmented.

The middle emissary channels are located several millimeters posterior to the geometric equator and transmit the vortex veins. Their position can be somewhat variable. Temporally, these veins are closer to the sagittal meridian, and nasally they are farther away from this meridian. Internally, their position relative to the sclera varies from the equator to 6.36 mm posterior to the equator, with the most common position being 3 mm posterior to the equator (Fuchs, 1894; Rutin, 1967). Externally, their exit position from the sclera varies from 13.75 to 25 mm posterior to the limbus. The superotemporal and superonasal veins exit more posteriorly (20.2 mm and 19.3 mm from the limbus, respectively) than the inferotemporal and inferonasal veins (17.4 mm and 18 mm from the limbus, respectively). The superotemporal vein exits the sclera approximately 8 mm, the superonasal vein 7 mm, the inferotemporal vein 5.5 mm, and the inferonasal vein 6 mm posterior to the equator. The distance each vein travels in the sclera is variable and ranges from 1.25 to 8.5 mm. When they exit the sclera, the vortex veins travel loosely between it and the bulbar fascia for 5 to 10 mm, with the superior temporal vein having the longest episcleral course.

The sclera becomes more rigid as a person ages. There may be relative dehydration, especially anterior to the insertion of recti muscles, resulting in calcium salt deposition. The midportion of the involved sclera in this area contains a calcified plaque.57 A similar age-related process may occur posteriorly, thus resulting in posterior scleral calcification (Grossniklaus et al, 2013).

5. The Lens

The lens is a biconvex, transparent, and avascular structure. It is suspended behind the iris by the zonule of Zinn, a suspensory ligament, which connects it with the ciliary body. The lens capsule is a semipermeable membrane which will admit water and electrolytes. A subcapsular epithelium is present anteriorly. Subepithelial lamellar fibers are continuously produced throughout life. The nucleus and cortex of the lens are made up of long concentric lamellae each of which contains a flattened nucleus in the peripheral portion of the lens near the equator.

Function of the Lens

The lens acts to focus light rays upon the retina. To focus light from a near object, the ciliary muscle contracts, pulling the choroid forward and releasing the tension on the zonules.

The elastic lens capsule then molds the pliable lens into a more spherical shape with greater refractive power. This process is known as accommodation. With age, the lens becomes harder and the ability to accommodate for near objects is decreased.

Composition of the Lens

The lens consists of about 65% water and about 35% protein (the highest protein content of any tissue of the body). Potassium is more concentrated in the lens than in most body tissues and ascorbic acid and glutathione are both present in the lens. It contains no nerve fibers or blood vessels; therefore, its nutrition is derived from the surrounding fluids. Mechanical injury to the lens or damage from altered nutrient concentration in the aqueous may result in cataract formation.

Lens and Zonule

The Crystalline Lens

The lens is a vital refractive element of the human eye. The adult human lens is an asymmetric oblate spheroid that does not possess nerves, blood vessels, or connective tissue (Kuszak and Brown, 1994) The crystalline lens is a grossly transparent, biconvex structure, located directly behind the iris and pupil in the anterior compartiment of the eye, and anterior to a shallow depression in the vitreous face, the lenticular fossa.It is responsible for 15-20 diopters of convergent refractive of the eye. It is held (it is suspended within the eye by a complex ring of zonular fibers originating in the ciliary body and inserting on the anterior and posterior lens capsule) in position by its suspensory ligament, the zonule. It is approximately 10 mm in diameter and 4 mm thick. The center of curvature of the anterior surface is the anterior pole, the posterior pole is the corresponding point on the posterior surface. The anterior surface has a radius of curvature of 10 mm. The posterior pole has a radius of curvature of 6.0 mm. The equator is separated from the free edge of the processes of the ciliary body by a distance of 0.5 mm. The zonular fibers insert into the anterior and posterior lens capsule near the equator and extend further over the anterior than the posterior surface.

The lens forms new fibers throughout life (The lens grows continuously throughout life). In humans old fibers are compressed centrally to form an increasingly larger inelastic lens nucleus. At birth, it measures 6.4 mm equatorially and 3.5 mm anteroposteriorly and weighs approximately 90 mg. The adult lens measures 9mm equatorially and 5 mm anteroposteriorly and weighs approximately 255 mg. The relative thickness of the cortex increases with age. At the same time, the lens adopts an increasingly curved shape, so that older lenses have more refractive power. However, the index of refraction decreases with age, probably as a result of the increasing presence of insoluble protein particles. Thus, the aging eye may become either hyperopic or myopic with age, depending upon the balance of these opposing changes.

As the lens ages, it increases in mass and thickness and decreases in accommodative power. As new layers of cortical fibers form concentrically, the lens nucleus undergoes compression and hardening (nuclear sclerosis). Chemical modification and proteolytic cleavage of crystallins (lens proteins) result in the formation of high-molecular-mass protein aggregates. These aggregates may become large enough to cause abrupt fluctuations in the local refractive index of the lens, thereby scattering light and reducing transparency. Chemical modification of lens nuclear proteins also increases pigmentation, such that the lens becomes increasingly yellow or brown with advancing age. Other age-related changes include decreased concentrations of glutathione and potassium and increased concentrations of sodium and calcium in the lens cell cytoplasm (American Academy of Ophthalmology (AAO), 2011).

A very common cause of visual impairment in older adults is age-related cataract, the pathogenesis of which is multifactorial and not completely understood. There are 3 main types of age-related cataracts: nuclear, cortical, and posterior subcapsular. In many patients, components of more than one type are present.

Although the lens appears brilliantly transparent when viewed grossly, biomicroscopy discloses minute opacities and concentric areas with different indices of refraction.

Histologically the lens consists of three major components the lens is composed of (1) a lens capsule that envelops the entire lens, (2) an anterior lens epithelium located immediately beneath the anterior lens capsule, and (3) a lens substance consisting of the cortex (newly formed soft lens fibers with nuclei) and the nucleus (a dense central area of fibers that have lost their nuclei).

Lens Capsule

The lens is ensheated by an elastic acellular envelope, which serves to contain the epithelial cells and fibers as a structural unit and allows the passage of small molecules both into and out the lens. The lens capsule is a smooth, homogenous, acellular structure (envelope). It is an elastic, transparent basement membrane composed of type IV collagen laid down by the epithelial cells.This capsule contains the lens substance and is capable of molding it during accommodative changes. The lens capsule is composed of a number of lamellae stacked on top of each other. The lamellae are narrowest near the outside of the capsule and widest near the cell mass (Sealand, 1992) Major structural proteins and a small amount of fibronectin are found within the lamellae (Phelps Brown and Bron, 1996). This structure is continuously synthesized and represents one of the thickest basement membrane in the body. The capsule is produced anteriorly byb the lens epithelium and posteriorly by the elongating fiber cells.The outer layer of the lens capsule, the zonular lamella, also serves as the point of attachment for the zonular fibers. . The lens capsule) is thickest on the anterior and posteror surfaces just central (pre-equatorial zones) to the insertion of the zonular fibers and is thinnest in the region of the central posterior pole, where it may be as thin as 2-4 μm. The anterior lens capsule is the basement membrane of the anterior lens epithelium and is the thickest basement membrane in the body. It is considerably thicker than the posterior capsule at birth and increases in thickness throughout life. The thickness of the capsule depends upon the region of the capsule being measured and, except for the posterior capsule, increases with the age of the individual (Saude, 1993; Snell and Lemp, 1989; Forrester et al, 1996)

The anterior surface is in contact with the aqueous on the corneal side; the posterior surface is in contact with the vitreous. The anterior pole of the lens and the front of the cornea are separated byapproximately 3.5 mm

The posterior capsule is the basement membrane of lens cells that have their nuclei in the nuclear bow.

Epithelial Cells (The Lens Epithelium)

The anterior lens epithelial cells consist of a single row of cuboidal cells of irregular shape with numerous interdigitations.

The lens substance consists of elongated lens cells (fibers). The less mature fibers have nuclei at the lens equator in the nuclear bow. Their posterior processes extend to their basement membrane, the posterior capsule. Mature lens fibers have lost their nuclei and are no longer in contact with the posterior capsule. These form most of the lens substance of the lens. They are packed into an increasingly dense, central nucleus. The nuclei of young cells migrate inward from the lens equator towardthe center of the lens to form a nuclea bow zone. In fetal life, the apices of lens processes join at the anterior central area and maintain junctions with cells extending from corresponding cells of the opposite side to form the upright, anterior Y-suture of the lens. When cells lose their nuclei, the posterior fibers are detached from the posterior capsule and are pushed deeper into the central zone to form the inverted Y-shaped posterior suture. After the fetal nucleus forms, the developing lens fibres form more complicated junctions than the Y-sutures. Lens fibers are curved, narrow, membranous cylindeers that have numerous ridges and socket invaginations to receive knobs., especially in their lateral edges. Their apical ends are flat with lobulated edges.

The Zonule. Zonular Fibers.

The lens zonule (zonule of Zinn, or suspensory ligaments of the lens) are a series of fibrillin rich fibers that converge in a circular zone on the lens. The lens zonule supports the lens in position and connects the lens to the ciliary muscle. Experimental evidence suggests that the zonular fibers are secreted by the ciliary epithelium, although how these fibers insert into the lens capsule is not known. The zonular fibers begin to develop at the end of the third month of gestation. It is composed of a series of fine fibrils modified of collagenous tissue on the outer surface of the lens capsule. The zonules attach to the lamellar portion of the lens capsule on either side of the equator and to the basement membrane of the ciliary epithelium in the valleys between the ciliary processes. The ciliary attachment is long, and fibers may extend to the pars plana of the ciliary body. Other fibers attach to the anterior vitreous face. The lens insertion extends about 2 mm in front and 1 mm behind the lens equator.

Lens and Aging

The shape of the crystalline lens in histologic sections changes with age. In infants, the lens assumes a reniform configuration, whereas in adults, it is more oval (Folberg, 1996; Eagle and Spencer, 1996). The lens increases in weight from approximately 90 mg at birth to 150 mg at age 20 years, 190 mg at age 40 years, and 240 mg at age 80 years (Van Heynigen, 1976). Cataracts are associated with aging and are manifest with color changes in the lens due to oxidation of lens proteins. The most common age-related histologic cataractous changes are equatorial and posterior cortical degeneration (Eagle and Spencer, 1996). These changes result in inward turning of equatorial cortical fibers, and a difference in staining with hematoxylin and eosin between the lens nucleus and cortex. This may be accompanied by posterior migration of the lens epithelium (Eagle and Spencer, 1996). These cells may lie along the inner surface of the posterior capsule, and become balloon-like and swollen (Wedl cells) (Eagle and Spencer, 1996). A proliferation of these cells along the posterior capsule results in posterior subcapsular cataract (Streeten and Eshaghian, 1978). Eosinophilic fluid may appear between lens cortical cells with age, and when the cells eventually break down with aging, the released protein from the cells results in Morgagnian globules and eventual liquefaction of the cortex, with the lens nucleus floating in a sea of liquefied cortex (Morgagnian cataract) (Eagle and Spencer, 1996).

The Iris and Pupil

The iris is a diaphragm that lies in front of the lens and ciliary body and separates the anterior chamber from the posterior chamber. It rests upon the lens, and without this support the iris is tremulous (iridodonesis). The iris inserts into the scleral spur through the anterior chamber face of the ciliary body. Located slightly to its nasal side is a circular aperture, the pupil, which controls the amount of light entering the eye.

The anterior iris surface is divided into a central pupillary zone, from which the anterior border layer is absent, and a peripheral ciliary zone. These are divided by a curcular ridge, the collarette that marks the site of the minor vascular circle of the iris from which the pupillary membrane originated in embryonic life. Atrophy of the pupillary membrane begins inn the seventh gestational month and is usually completed by 8 ½ months, sometimes leaving behind a ferw delicate strands that extend from the collarette to the anterior lens capsule.

The pupillary zone of the iris is relatively flat with its width varying with the amount of atrophy of the anterior border layer and the degree of pupillary dilation. The ciliary zone is marked by more radial interlacing ridges, giving a gossamerlike appearance. In blue irises concentric contraction furrows may be seen. The color of the iris depends on the amount of melanin in the anterior border layer. If slight, reflection from the pigment of the pigmented epithelium causes scattering and thus a blue color. If there is a moderate amount of melanin, the iris is hazel; if there is a large amount, the iris is brown.

Structure

The iris consists of two layers: (1) stroma, located anteriorly and originating from mesoderm and (2) pigmented epithelium, located posteriorly and originating from neural ectoderm. The stroma may be divided into an anterior border layer and a deeper stroma proper. The anterior border layer of the iris is a loose collagen tissue in which pigmented or nonpigmented cells are densely packed. The layer develops maximally about the seventh month of fetal life. Thereafter generalized atrophy occurs in the pupillary zone. Irregular atrophy in the ciliary zones forms iris crypts. In brown irises the surface is smooth and heavily pigmented and in blue or hazel irises it is irregular with crypts. The anterior border layer ends abruptly at the iris root, but spokelike processes may continue as iris processes to the line of Schwalbe.

The stroma proper has a similar appearance irrespective of the color of the iris. It is visible in the pupillary zone and in the depth of iris crypts. It consists of bundles of collagen fibrils arranged in columns around blood vessels and nerves, pigment and nonpigmented cells, all enmeshed in a hyaluronidase-sensitive glycosaminoglycans. The stroma proper contains more elastic tissue and fewer pigment cells than the anterior border layer. Its capillaries are nonfenestrated with a structure similar to that of other nonfenestrated capillaries.

The iris pigmented epithelium consists of two layers of cells that constitute a fusion of the two layers of the primitive optic vesicle. They are densely packed with melanin. The anterior layer opf pigment cells intermingles with the dilatator pupillae muscle and is absent in the region of the sphincter pupillae muscle. The posterior layer of epithelium is covered on its lenticular surface wqith a basement membrane continuous with that of the retina and the ciliary body. Often the pupillary margin has a pigment frill continuous with the ectodermal pigmeneted epithelium that constitutes the anterior extremity of the optic cup.

The sphincter pupillae muscle is located in the pupillary zone of the posterior stroma. It is a smooth muscle about 1 mm wide that forms a sphincter surrounding the pupillary margin. The dilatator pupillae muscle is a thin sheet of smooth muscle (myoepithelium) located between the stroma and the posterior layer of the pigmented epithelium. It extends from the iris root at the ciliary body as far as the sphincter pupillae muscle. Both muscles are derived from neural ectoderm from the outer layer of the optic cup.

Blood supply. The blood supply of the iris is provided by radial vessels in the stromal layer that extend from the major arterial circle of the iris (circulus arteriosus iridis major) located in the ciliary body. This is formed by the two long posterior ciliary arteries and the seven anterior ciliary arteries. The iris blood vessels pass radially in a corkscrew pattern toward the pupillary margin, causing the meridional striations of the ciliary portion of the iris. At the collarette they anastomose to form the incomplete minor vascular circle of the iris. The vessels have thick collagen adventitia and a thin muscularis layer. The endothelila cells of the veins have a perivascular sheath. They drain into the vortex veins. The endothelil cells of the capillaries are typically nonfenestrated with junctional complexes (zonulae occludentes) that prevent the passage of large molecules. This vascular endothelium, together with the tight junctions of the pigment epithelium of the ciliary body processes, forms the blood-aqueous barrier. The ciliary body vessels, like those of the choroid, are fenestrated.

Nerve supply. The iris is richly supplied with nerves from the short ciliary (cholinergic) and long ciliary (sensory, adrenergic) nerves. The nerves are partially medullated and have a thick neurilemma. The motor innervation of the dilatator pupillae muscle emerges from adrenergic nerves accompanying the long ciliary nerves. Additionally, the long ciliary nerves transmit sensory fibers from the iris. The sphincter pupillae muscle is innervated by cholinergic fibers from the Edinger-Westphal nucleus of the oculomotor nerve that synapse in the ciliary ganglion and are distributed with short ciliary nerves. The adrenergic nerve supply of iris arteries is carried by the short ciliary nerves.

6. The Choroid

The choroid is the posterior part of the uvea, the middle tunic of the eye. The uvea develops from the mesenchyme surrounding the two vesicles that bud off the embryonic forebrain at the end of the first month in humans, eventually becoming the eyes. At about that time, melanocyte precursors migrate into the uvea from the neural crest; these do not differentiate into pigmented melanocytes until 7-8 months of gestation. The mesenchyme that forms the choriocapillaris at about 2 months must be in contact with the developing retinal pigment epithelium (RPE) in order to differentiate. Therefore, the choroid derives from different cell lines than do the retina and RPE, which both derive from the neural ectoderm. The choroid is comprised of blood vessels, melanocytes, fibroblasts, resident immune-competent cells and supporting collagenous and elastic connective tissue. As one of the most highly vascularized tissues of the body, its main function has been traditionally viewed as supplying oxygen and nutrients to the outer retina, and, in species with avascular retinas, to the inner retina as well. Other likely functions include light absorption (in species with pigmented choroids), thermoregulation via heat dissipation, and modulation of intraocular pressure (IOP) via vasomotor control of blood flow. The choroid also plays an important role in the drainage of the aqueous humor from the anterior chamber, via the uveoscleral pathway. This pathway is responsible for approximately 35% of the drainage in humans, a higher percentage, between 40 and 60%, in non-human primates, and a much lower percentage in the cat (about 3%) and rabbit (3-8%) (Alm and Nilsson, 2009; Nickla and Wallman, 2010).

Histology of the Choroid

The choroid extends from the margins of the optic nerve to the pars plana, where it continues anteriorly, becoming the ciliary body. Its innermost layer is the complex 5-laminar structure of Bruch's membrane, and its outermost one is the suprachoroid outside of which is the suprachoroidal space between choroid and sclera.

Histologically, the choroid has variously been divided into 4 to 6 layers, depending on whether the vascular region is considered as 1 or 2 layers (Sattler's and Haller's), and whether the lamina fusca is considered to be of scleral or choroidal origin. It is most commonly described as five layers: starting from the retinal (inner) side, these are Bruch's membrane, the choroiocapillaris, the two vascular layers (Haller's and Sattler's), and the suprachoroidea (Hogan et al., 1971). In humans, the choroid is approximately 200 μm thick at birth and decreases to about 80 μm by age 90 (Ramrattan et al., 1994).

Choriocapillaris

The choriocapillaris is a highly anastomosed network of capillaries, forming a thin sheet apposed to Bruch's membrane. The fibrous basement membrane of the capillary endothelial cells forms the outermost layer of Bruch's membrane in humans. The choriocapillaris is about 10 μm thick at the fovea, where there is the greatest density of capillaries, thinning to about 7 μm in the periphery. The capillaries arise from the arterioles in Sattler's layer, each of which gives rise to a hexagonal (or lobular)-shaped domain of a single layer of capillaries, giving a patch-like structure to the choriocapillaris. The capillaries are fenestrated and, in humans, are relatively large in diameter (20-40 μm), although possessing passages narrow enough to hinder the flow of 9 μm spheres (Bill et al., 1983). Because of the large area of the choriocapillaris, the velocity of red blood cells here is only about 77% that of the velocity of red blood cells in the retinal capillaries (Wajer et al., 2000). The fenestrated capillaries are highly permeable to proteins, contributing to the high oncotic pressure in the extravascular stroma, which fosters the movement of fluids from the retina to the choroid. Adjacent to Sattler's layer at the outer choriocapillaris there is a fibrous layer which is attached to the outer fibrous layer of Bruch's membrane by columns of collagen fibers running between the capillaries; these columns (or "pillars") may function to keep the capillary diameters constant (at least in primates) (Krebs and Krebs, 1991). Finally, the innermost choroidal layer is Bruch's membrane, a 5-layered structure consisting of (from outer to inner): basement membrane of the choroiocapillaris, outer collagenous zone, elastic layer, inner collagenous zone, and basement membrane of .the retinal pigment epithelium.

Choroidal Vascular Layers and Suprachoroid

The vascular region of the choroid consists of the outer Haller's layer of large blood vessels and the inner Sattler's layer of medium and small arteries and arterioles that feed the capillary network, and veins. The stroma (extravascular tissue) contains collagen and elastic fibers, fibroblasts, non-vascular smooth muscle cells and numerous very large melanocytes that are closely apposed to the blood vessels. As in other types of connective tissue, there are numerous mast cells, macrophages, and lymphocytes.

The suprachoroid is a transitional zone between choroid and sclera containing elements of both -- collagen fibers, fibroblasts and melanocytes.

The lamina fusca is the outermost layer of the suprachoroid (Fig. 4A), approximately 30 μm thick, consisting of several layers of closely-apposed, flattened fusiform melanocytes and fibroblast-like cells, with interspersed bundles of myelinated axons (De Stefano and Mugnaini, 1997b). Some anatomists identify the lamina fusca as the innermost layer of the sclera (Forrester et al., 2002; Watson and Young, 2004) The fibroblast-like cells form sheaths, or plates, that are connected to one another by adhering and occluding junctions (Krebs and Krebs, 1988). These cells synthesize and secrete the usual extracellular matrix components elastin, collagens and proteoglycans. The function of the melanocytes, apart from providing pigmentation, is unknown. However, their membranes contain endothelin-B receptors, which may mediate the endothelin 1-induced influx of calcium ions (Hirose et al., 2007), the functional implications of which are also not known.the endothelin 1- induced influx of calcium ions (Hirose et al., 2007), the functional implications of which are also not known.

Choroidal Blood Flow: Nourishment of the Retina

Despite the conspicuousness of the retinal blood vessels, the major blood supply to the retina is the choroid. Because the photoreceptors are extremely metabolically active, especially in darkness, when the light-gated ion channels are open, and active transport of ions is required to maintain ion homeostasis, over 90% of the oxygen delivered to the retina is consumed by the photoreceptors. In darkness, ninety percent of the oxygen comes from the choroidal circulation (Linsenmeier et al., 1981; Bill et al., 1983; Linsenmeier and Braun, 1992). To obtain this high transport of oxygen from the choroid, despite the barriers of Bruch's membrane and the retinal pigment epithelium, requires a steep gradient of oxygen tension, which is maintained by the high blood flow in the choroid, probably the highest of any tissue in the body per unit tissue weight, ten-fold higher than the brain (Alm and Bill,

1973; Alm, 1992). Consequently, the oxygen tension in the choroid stays high, with an arterial/venous difference of only 3% versus 38% for the retinal circulation.

Torsional oscillations of the eye during saccadic eye movements facilitate the diffusion of oxygen and nutrients across the retina by bulk flow (Pettigrew et al., 1990), a mechanism aided by the liquid phase of the vitreous being adjacent to the retina.

In the retina, the capillaries are the continuous type (the walls have no fenestrations), constituting the blood-ocular barrier, and are impermeable to even small molecular weight molecules such as glucose and amino acids, which require special transport systems to move them across the endothelium. The choroidal circulation is crucial in supplying nutrients as well as oxygen because the capillaries of the choroid are fenestrated, with especially large pores. These fenestrations have a high permeability not only to glucose but to low molecular weight substances such as albumen and myoglobulin. It was estimated that more than 50% of molecules the size of glucose or amino acids can pass through the fenestrations into the extracellular tissue, creating a very high glucose concentration there, thereby facilitating transport across the RPE to the retina (Bill et al., 1980). The high protein permeability of the choriocapillaris also allows the establishment of a high oncotic pressure, presumably contributing to movement of fluid out of the retina through the stroma and suprachoroid, and out the sclera (Bill, 1962; Marmor et al., 1980).

Choroid in High Myopia (Mrejen and Spaid, 2013)

Chorioretinal Atrophy in High Myopia

In many developed countries, a major cause of vision loss is high myopia, which is often defined as 6 or more diopters spherical equivalent myopic correction. High myopia is associated with excessive and progressive elongation of the globe and results in a variety of fundus changes that lead to visual impairment, including lacquer cracks in Bruch's membrane, CNV, and chorioretinal atrophy (Curtin et al, 1977; Hirata and Negi, 1998; Hotchkiss and Fine, 1981; Kitaguchi et al, 2007; Klein and Curtin, 1975; Lai et al, 2008; Morgan, 2003; Okabe et al, 1982). Myopic chorioretinal atrophy is a common and serious problem, and yet the mechanisms and pathologic course are not well understood. If retinal stretching was the main mechanism for visual impairment in highly myopic eyes, we would expect the visual function to be well correlated with the amount of myopia; clinically, however, visual function in highly myopic patients tends to be more correlated with age than degree of myopia (Saw et al, 2005; Vongphanit et al, 2002). Okabe et al analyzed three eyes with chorioretinal atrophy and pathologic myopia enucleated for various reasons: herpetic keratitis and secondary glaucoma, intraocular hemorrhage, and painful filamentous keratitis (Okabe et al, 1982). One eye had -20 D of myopia and the amount of myopia was not defined for the two other eyes. Histopathological observations showed the choroid was thin with vessels present in some areas but completely absent in others (Okabe et al, 1982). They hypothesized that the choriocapillaris was obstructed and disappeared earlier than the other choroidal vessels and that the choriocapillaris obstruction occurs in a lobulated fashion (Okabe et al, 1982). The associated diseases in these eyes may have affected their choroidal ultrastructure. There are no data on the ultrastructural modifications present at the early stages of high myopia. Animal models of myopia show decreased choriocapillaris density and diameter (Hirata and Negi, 1998). The photoreceptor packing density is decreased in high myopes (Chui et al, 2008). Both photoreceptors and choriocapillaris are rarefied as compared with emmetropic eyes.

Angiographic studies of the choroid with ICG reveals that the choroidal vasculature is altered in highly myopic eyes (Moriyama et al, 2007; Quaranta et al, 1996). A color Doppler ultrasonographic study found that the choroidal circulation was decreased in highly myopic eyes.1 As the choroid supplies oxygen and nutrition to the retinal pigment epithelial cells and the outer retina, compromised choroidal circulation may account, in part, for the retinal dysfunction and vision loss that is seen in high myopia.

Biometric Choroidal Changes in Highly Myopic Eyes and Clinical Significance

The choroid of highly myopic patients is significantly thinner than the choroid of non-myopic eyes (Fujiwara et al, 2009; Ikuno and Tano, 2009). A group of 18 patients (31 eyes), with a mean age of 51.7 years and a mean refractive error of -15.5 D was evaluated with regular SD-OCT. The mean subfoveal CT was 100.5 mm, thinner than in emmetropic eyes, and the eyes underwent further thinning with increasing age and posterior staphyloma height.94 The authors defined staphyloma height as the sum of four vertical measurements on SD-OCT foveal scans: the distance from the RPE line beneath the fovea to the nasal, temporal, superior, and inferior edges of the OCT image (Ikuno and Tano, 2009). They do not mention how the presence, shape, and exact location of the posterior staphyloma were determined. The posterior pole of any eye, whether it is myopic or not, is not a flat structure, and as such it should have some "height" as it is defined by this SD-OCT method of measurement. The height measured in this study is a reflection of the global curvature of the eye itself and does not necessarily imply any outpouching, as is required to define a posterior staphyloma. Conventional SD-OCT allows a relatively good visualization of the choroidal /sceral interface in highly myopic eyes because of the dramatic choroidal thinning (Ikuno and Tano, 2009). Ikuno et al reported that the choroidal/scleral interface is generally undetectable in eyes with a CT greater than 300 mm with regular SD-OCT (Ikuno and tano, 2009). This probably also depends on other factors, such as the degree of pigmentation of the RPE and choroid. Another group of 31 patients (55 eyes) with a mean age of 59.7 years and a mean refractive error of -11.9 D was evaluated with EDI-OCT. The mean subfoveal CT was 93.2 mm, and was negatively correlated with age ($p = 0.006$) and refractive error ($p < 0.001$) (Fujiwara et al, 2009). Eyes with a history of choroidal neovascularization also had a thinner choroid ($p = 0.013$), but the patients in this study were treated with photodynamic therapy, which may have damaged the choroid.55 In this EDI OCT study, subfoveal CT was found to decrease by 12.7 mm for each decade of life and by 8.7 mm for each diopter of myopia.55 The quantification of choroidal biometric changes may be useful for monitoring the progression and for estimating the relative risks for future development of the disease. A large proportion of patients with high myopia develop some visual deficit, and even modestly reduced visual acuities to the 20/30 or 20/40 level can have a significant impact on their quality of life (Nishida et al, 2012). The visual deficit developed in highly myopic eyes increases with age and amount of myopia. Nishida et al evaluated predictive factors for visual acuity using EDI-OCT in 145 highly myopic eyes with no macular pathology (Nishida et al, 2012). They evaluated subfoveal CT, foveal thickness, outer nuclear layer thickness, and inner segment to RPE aggregate thickness. The mean subfoveal CT was 158.6 mm. The subfoveal CT was inversely correlated with visual acuity and was also the only significant predictive factor of visual acuity in the pooled data (Nishida et al, 2012).

Imaging the Highly Myopic Disk

Intrachoroidal Cavitation

In 2003, Freund et al recognized peripapillary detachment in pathologic myopia (Freund et al, 2003). They reported an elevated, wellcircumscribed, dome-shaped, yellow-orange lesion inferior to theoptic disk along the inferior margin of the myopic conus. Toronzo and Gaudric renamed this anomaly intrachoroidal cavitation based on OCT analysis: a large intrachoroidal hyporeflective space with a flat RPE (Toranzo et al, 2005), a finding present in 4.9% of 632 highly myopic eyes in a Japanese study (Shimada et al, 2006). Some authors postulated that intrachoroidal cavitation is another cause of visual field defects in high myopia (Shimada et al, 2006), along with primary open-angle glaucoma, normal tension glaucoma, tilted disk syndromes, myopic conus, and macular atrophy. Wei et al, using Stratus-OCT, identified direct communication between the intrachoroidal cavity and the vitreous space in 6 out of 13 cases and hypothesized that liquid vitreous might be the source of the disruption of the choroid and fluid accumulation (Wei et al, 2009). EDI-OCT allowed identifying intrachoroidal cavitation that had been unrecognized clinically (Park et al, 2012). Spaide et al (Spaide et al, 1996) evaluated 16 eyes of 13 patients with peripapillary intrachoroidal cavitation using mainly SS-OCT and in one eye EDI-OCT and volume rendering. The patients had a mean age of 50.3 years and a mean refractive error of 12.5 D. All had a tilted disk with myopic conus. In all of the eyes, the sclera was bowed posteriorly focally below the region of the intrachoroidal cavitation, whereas the curvature of the RPE line overlying the lesion was not modified. Therefore there was no internal elevation of the lesion. There was full thickness defect in the retina, RPE, and inner choroid at the inferior border of the conus in only four eyes, indicating a direct communication between the vitreous cavity and the intrachoroidal cavity. They proposed that the primary cause of intrachoroidal cavitation formation was the posterior bowing of the sclera in the region of the conus that extended around the nerve to involve the choroid secondarily. In more exaggerated cases the posterior deflection of the sclera could allow fluid to enter through a full thickness defect in the overlying retina-RPE-Bruch's membrane at the border of the conus (Spaide et al, 2012).

7. The Ciliary Body

The ciliary body is a ring of tissue about 6 mm wide that extends from the scleral spur to the ora serrata of the retina.

Structure. It is divided into uveal and epithelial portions. The uveal portion is adjacent to the sclera and includes the suprachoroid (lamina fusca), the ciliary muscles, the blood vessel layer, and the lamina basalis choroideae (lamina vitrea). The epithelial portion is adjacent to the posterior chamber and includes the pars pana (orbiculus ciliaris) and the pars plicata (corona ciliaris) or ciliary processes.

Uveal portion. The ciliary muscle is the most prominent structure in the uveal portion of the ciliary body. It is composed of three groups of smooth muscle: (1) the longitudinal fibers (Brücke muscle), which are the outermost, parallel the surface of the overlying sclera, and constitute the main bulk of the muscle; (2) the radial fibers that originate from the anterior portion of the longitudinal fibers and run obliquely to become continuous with circular fibers;

and (3) the circular fibers (Müller muscle) that are the innermost portion of the ciliary muscle and parallel the lens equator.

Contraction of the circular fibers relaxes the lens zonule, which allows a greater curvature of the lens (accommodation). Parasympathetic (cholinergic) motor innervation originates in the Ediger-Westphal nucleus of the oculomotor (N III) nerve. Efferent visceral motor fibers pass from the inferior division of N III to synapse in the ciliary ganglion. Postganglionic fibers in 6 to 20 short ciliary nerves innervate the ciliary muscle and sphincter pupillae muscle. Contraction of the longitudinal portion of the ciliary muscle may retract the scleral pur and enlarge the canal of Schlemm.

The scleral surface of the ciliary body is the suprachoroid (lamina fusca). The vessel layer is composed mainly of the major arterial circle of the iris, its tributaries, and veins. There is no choriocapillaris. At the anterior termination of the choroid, Bruch membrane divides. The elastic layer derived from choroid disappears, but the inner cuticular layer that originates from the retinal pigment epithelium continues forward to the iris root as the basement membrane of the pigmented epithelium of the ciliary body.

Epithelial portion. The epithelial portion of the ciliary body is divided into the pars plana (orbiculus ciliaris) and the pars plicata (corona ciliaris). The pars plana is about 4 mm wide and extends anteriorly from the ora serrata ofv the retina. The pars plicata forms the most anterior 2 mm of the ciliary body.

It is formed of 60 to 70 folds, the ciliary processes, each of which is about 0.8 mm high and 1.0 mm wide. Each ciliary process consists of a finger of tissue covered with an outer layer og nonpigmeneted epithelium that covers a layer of pigmented epithelium surrounding a central vascular core.

The nonpigmented epithelium constitutes the anterior continuation of the sensory retina. Its basement membrane is continuous with the internal limiting membrane of the retina and is located on the posterior chamber side of the cell. The basement membrane of the pigmented epithelium is on the side of the cell nearest the sclera. Aqueous humor and hyaluronic acid are secreted through the apices of the nonpigmented epithelial cells of the ciliary processes. These cells have prominent Golgi complexes comparable to those of other secreting glandular cells. The apices of the cells of the pigmented epithelium and nonpigmented epithelium are in apposition, and the posterior aqueous humor secreted must pass between the cells of the nonpigmented epithelium to reach the posterior chamber.

The posterior margin of the pars plana portion of the ciliary body has a scalloped edge that corresponds to the retinal ora serrata. Each retinal tooth corresponds to a valley of the ciliary body. In this region the sensory retina abruptly changes into a single layer of elongated nonpigmented epithelium of the ciliary body. Surgical instruments may be introduced into the vitreous cavity and into the crystalline lens through the pars plana.

Blood supply. The blood supply of the ciliary body is mainly from the major arterial circle of the iris formed by the two long ciliary arteries and the penetrating branches of the seven anterior ciliary arteries.

Nerve supply. The motor nerve supply to the ciliary muscle is freom the oculomotor nerve by postganglionic parasympathetic fibers that synapse in the ciliary ganglion and are distributed by the short ciliary nerves. These nerves also carry thze sympathetic nerve supply of the uveal blood vessels.

Chambers of the Eye

The eye contains three chambers: the anterior chamber, the posterior chamber, and the vitreous cavity.

Anterior chamber. The anterior chamber is bounded anteriorly by the cornea, posteriorly by the front surface of the iris and lens, and peripherally by the the anterior chamber angle. The anterior chamber is deepest in its central portion (3 mm) and shallowest at the peripheral insertion of the iris. In humans, its volume is approximately 0.20 ml (Newell, 1986).

Posterior chamber. The posterior chamber (frontispiece) is bounded anteriorly by the iris, peripherally by the ciliary processes, and posteriorly by the anterior lens capsule and its zonule. Its volume in adults is about 0.06 ml. Aqueous humor is secreted by the nonpigmented epithelium of the ciliary processes into the posterior chamber and flows through the pupil into the anterior chamber (Newell, 1986).

8. The Retina

Embryologically part of the central nervous system (Bach and Seefelder, 1914; Dejean et al, 1958; Mann, 1964; Duke-Elder, 1963; Cook et al, 2003), the retina develops from invagination of the optic vesicle to form an outer layer, the retinal pigment epithelium, and an inner layer, the sensory retina. Moreover, an estimated 80% of all sensory information in humans is thought to be of retinal origin (Sharma and Ehinger, 2003), indicating the importance of retinal function for the ability to interact with the outside world.

The retina is the light-sensitive tissue that lines the inside of the eye. The retina functions in a manner similar to film in a camera. The optical elements within the eye focus an image onto the retina of the eye, initiating a series of chemical and electrical events within the retina. Nerve fibers within the retina send electrical signals to the brain, which then interprets these signals as visual images (Jakobiec, 1982).

The retina is the innermost layer of the eye. It lines the entire posterior portion of the eye with the exception of the area of the optic nerve and extends anteriorly to end 360 degrees circumferentially at the ora serrata.

The total area of the retina is approximately 1,100 mm^2. The circumferential diameter at the equator of the adult eye averages 69 mm. The retinal distance circumferentially passing posteriorly from a point on the ora serrata to a point on the ora serrata 180 degrees away is approximately 50 mm. The average healthy retina is 250 μm thick immediately adjacent to the temporal margin of the optic nerve.

The retina thickens to approximately 400 μm in the macular area around the fovea and thins to 150 μm in the fovea. This difference in thickness in the central and noncentral portions of the macula can be appreciated when the eye is examined with an ophthalmoscope. The retina thins as it approaches the equatorial region of the eye and further thins to 80 μm at the ora serrata.

Retinal nerve fibers exit the eye through the optic nerve, located nasally and on the same plane as the anatomical center of the retina. There is no retinal tissue overlying the optic nerve head. The optic nerve head or optic disc is oval in shape and measures approximately 1.75 mm. vertically and 1.5 mm horizontally. The center of the optic disc is located 4.5 mm to 5 mm nasal to the anatomical center of the retina.

The center of the retina provides the greatest resolving power of the eye. This area, responsible for central vision, is known as the macula. The center of the macula is called the fovea.

The inner surface of the retina is adjacent to the vitreous of the eye. The outermost layer of the retina, the retinal pigment epithelium, is tightly attached to the choroid.

Assuming that the ocular media (cornea, anterior chamber, lens, and vitreous) are not cloudy, the living retina can be examined using a direct or indirect ophthalmoscope or a retinal lens at the slit lamp. In addition, the retina may be photographed using a retinal camera. The arterioles and venules of the retina are the only blood vessels whose wall can be directly examined in the living human without an incision.

The retina, with the exception of the blood vessels coursing through it, is transparent to the examiner up to its outer layer, the retinal pigment epithelium. The transparent portion of the retina is known as the neurosensory retina. The examiner sees the neurosensory retina against the background orange color of the melanin containing retinal pigment epithelium and blood-filled choroidal layer of the eye.

The neuroretina is tightly attached to the underlying retinal pigment only at the margins of the optic nerve and at the ora serrata. There is a potential space between the neurosensory retina and the retinal pigment epithelium. In a retinal detachment, this space fills with fluid and detaches the neurosensory retina from the underlying retinal pigment epithelium.

The living retina may be imaged using fluorescein angiography, polarimetry, or optical coherence tomography.

The inner layer is stratified into many layers, but the pigment epithelium is only one layer thick. The layers of the retina nearest the choroid are designated as the outer layers and those nearest the vitreous humor as the inner layers. The retina extends from the optic nerve posteriorly to its scalloped margin (the ora serrata) anteriorly, where it continues as the epithelium of the ciliary body.

The major cellular components of the retina are the retinal pigment epithelium (RPE) cell, the photoreceptor cells, the interneurons, the ganglion cells, and the glial cells. Vascular cells are described in greater detail later.

The retina consists of millions of cells packed together in a tightly knit network spread over the surface of the back of the eye. These cells can be divided into a three basic cell types, photoreceptor cells, neuronal cells, and glial cells (Sterling, 1999).

Photoreceptor Cells

Photoreceptor cells consist principally of cones and rods. Cones function best under illuminated conditions and provide color vision. Rods function primarily in dim light and provide black-and-white vision. Each human retina contains approximately 120 million rods and 6 million cone photoreceptors.

Each rod or cone cell contains photoreceptor elements and an axon. Cones have a projection called a pedicle at the termination of the axon, which contacts a dendrite. Rods have a similar projection called a spherule. There are three types of cones, varying in specific sensitivity to different wavelengths (colors) of light.

Each photoreceptor portion of a rod or cone is anatomically divided into an outer segment and an inner segment. In a rod, the outer segment contains the pigment rhodopsin within free floating discs. These discs are stacked within a sleeve, similar to a roll of coins. Iodopsin pigment is contained within cones in folded layers inside a continuous outer membrane. The photoreceptor inner segment contains the cell nucleus and other subcellular structures.

The central retina is cone dominated and the peripheral retina is rod dominated. The highest density of cones is at the center of the fovea. There are no rods in the center of the fovea. At the center of the macula is the fovea, a pit where the cones are smallest and arranged in a mosaic to provide highest and most efficient optical density.

There is a third class of photoreceptors within the retina (in addition to the rods and cones). These are the much rarer intrinsically photosensitive retinal ganglion cells, which are stimulated by light even when all rods and cones are blocked. The photosensitive ganglion cells contain the pigment melanopsin. Alteration in this pigment by light is involved in non – image-forming responses to light, such as synchronization of circadian rhythms to the light-dark cycle, contributing to regulation of pupil size and influencing release of melatonin from the pineal gland.

Retinal Pigment Epithelium

Like the sensory components of the neuroretina, the RPE cell is of neuroectodermal embryonic origin (Bach and Seefelder, 1914; Dejean et al, 1958; Mann, 1964; Duke-Elder, 1963; Cook et al, 2003; Seefelder, 1930; Wolfensberger, 1998). The retinal pigment epithelium is a single layer of cells that extends to the optic berve margin posteriorly and to the ora serrata anteriorly, where it fuses with the anterior continuation of the sensory retina and continues forward as pigmeneted ciliary epithelium. Each adult human retina contains about 3.5 million RPE cells (Panda-Jonas et al, 1996) whose diameters vary fourfold between 14 mm in the central retina and 60 mm in the peripheral retina (Boulton et al, 2001). The density of RPE cells is greater in the fovea (5,000 cells/mm^2) than in the periphery (2,000 cells/mm2) (La Cour, 2003). In the central retina, where RPE cells are most tightly packed, they take the shape of regular hexagonal tiles that form a single layer of cuboidal epithelium. Tight junctions between adjacent RPE cells form the outer blood-retina barrier, an important physiologic barrier to the free flow of molecules between the leaky choriocapillaris and the photoreceptors of the neuroretina (Schnaudigel, 1913; Cunha-Vaz, 1913; Cunha-Vaz, 2004; Davson, 1990; Thumann et al, 2006; Strauss, 2005; Kanski and Milewski, 2002).

Cellular polarity and the abundance of mitochondria, endoplasmatic reticulum, and free ribosomes all indicate a very high level of metabolic activity in the RPE cell (Thumann et al, 2006; Strauss, 2005; Burke, 1998). Infoldings of the basal and apical surfaces greatly increase the RPE surface area, facilitating active transport across its cell surface with both the choriocapillaris and the photoreceptor layer (Kincaid and Green, 1999; La Cour, 2003; Strauss, 2005; Hughes et al, 1998; Marmor, 1999; Newmani, 2000). Though normally nondividing cells, the RPE can proliferate in response to a variety of pathological conditions. Melanin renders the RPE dark brown to black. It is synthesized from tyrosine via the tyrosinase pathway (Dowling, 2000). Pigmentation of the RPE is a rapid process that begins at about 35 days gestation and is complete within approximately 1 week (Kincaid, 1997). RPE cells show no or little racial variation in melanin pigmentation. Another pigment, lipofuscin, accumulates as an end-product of outer photoreceptor segment degradation in the

RPE and in Bruch's membrane. Though lipofuscin is a pigment of aging, small amounts of it can already be detected in the RPE of children (Marmor, 1999).

The cells of the retinal pigment epithelium contain varying amounts of melanin, which, on ophthalmoscopic examinantionn, give a granular appearance to the fundus (the pigment is of neural ectoderm origin and not of neural crest origin). In the region underlying the central sensory retina, the cells are slender and tall, but they are more cuboidal and irregular in the periphery. Their basement membrane is firmly attached to the cuticular portion of the Bruch membrane. The villous projections of the apices surround the outer segments of rods and cones in an interphotoreceptor matrix without specialized attachments.

Pigment epithelial cells are generally hexagonal, in flat section individual cells may have four to eight sides. The cells fit together like cobblestones in a regular arrangement. In cross-section, the pigment epithelial celles are divided into thirds, consisting of a base, a body, and an apex.

The base is adjacent to the cuticular portion of the Bruch membrane. It contains prominent infoldings of the basal plasma membrane, many mitonchondia, and little or no pigment. The cell nucleus and assorted organelles and lipofuscin occupy the body. The apex is topped with microvilli that enmesh the outer segments of rods and cones embedded in glycosaminoglycans. The apical cytoplasm contains ovoid pigment granules and partially digested outer segment disks (phagosomes). The lateral surfaces of adjacent cells at the apices (but not the microvilli) are bound together by terminal bars that are composed of a basilar portion (zonula adherens) and an apical portion (ronula occludens). There is no intercellular space at the level of these junctions, and together with the nonfenestrated retinal blood vessels they constitute the blood-retina barrier. After 30 years of age, lipofuscin is prominent in the pigment epithelium underlying the central retina.

Sensory Retina

The sensory retina (pars optica retinae) develops from the inner wall of the secondary optic vesicle. It consists of a layer of photoreceptor cells whose axons synapse with cells that modulate their response. These modular cells in turn synapse with cells that transmit spike discharges to the brain. The rods and cones, the light-sensitive cells of the retina, correspond to the sensory endings elsewhere in the nervous system. The glial sytem of Müller cells provide mechanical support of the retina.

Photoreceptor Cell

The photoreceptor cell may be divided into the following: (1) an outer segment, which is embedded in the microvilli of the retinal pigment epithelium cells; (2) a cilium, a tubular structure that connects the outer and inner segments; (3) an inner segment composed of an ellipsoid and a myoid; (4) the outer rod (cone) fiber connecting the inner segment to the cell body; (5) the cell body that contains the nucleus; and (6) the inner rod (or cone) fiber that terminates in a specialized synaptic ending.

The outer segment consists of a dense vertical stack of 700 flattened sacs or disks. The outer segment is surrounded by a plasma membrane that is continuous with the disks. The outer segment is surrounded by a plasma membrane that is continuous with the disks of cones but separate from rod disks. The space within each sac is occupied by the visual pigments.

Most (111 to 130 million) outer segments in humans consist of cylindrical disks (rods) containing the photopigment rhodopsin. Other outer segments (6.3 to 6.8 million) have a conical shape (cones) with the apex pointing outward and containing three different photopigments responsible for color vision. The outer tip of the rod is surrounded by the microvilli of the retinal pigment epithelium and the extracellular space containing glycosaminoglycans. Outside of the fovea centralis, the tapered portion of the cone does not reach the retinal pigment epithelium, and the microvilli of the retinal pigment epithelium are lengthened to reach the cone outer segment. In the foveal region, cones are more slender and resemble the cylindrical structure of rods.

The outer segment is connected to the inner segment by the cilium. The connecting cilium contains nine pairs of microtubules but lacks the central pair seen in mobile cilia. This structure transmits cellular components from the inner segment and cell nucleus to the disks and their plasma membrane.

The inner segment is divided into a refractile outer ellipsoid and a nonrefractile, basophilic inner myoid. The ellipsoid contains mitochondria grouped around the base of the cilium. The myoid portion (contractile in some amphibian) of the inner segment contains free and membrane-bound ribosomes, Golgi complexes, and a variety of vesicles and vacuoles. The division into ellipsoid and myoid portions is more distinct in rods than in cones.

The photoreceptors are the sensors of the visual system that convert the capture of photons into a nerve signal in a process called phototransduction (Levin, 2003). The human retina contains approximately four to five million cones and 77–107 million rods (Levin, 2003; Tessier-Lavigne, 2000; Wurtz and Kandel, 2000). Only cones are found in the foveola, whereas rods predominate outside the foveola in the remaining fovea and all of the peripheral retina. Among the three cone photoreceptors, red cones (63% or 2.9 million) are more common than green (32% or 1.4 million) and blue cones (5% or 0.2 million) (Oyster, 1999). Each photoreceptor consists of an outer segment (photopigment), inner segment (mitochondria, endoplasmatic reticulum), a nucleus, an inner fiber (analogous to an axon), and the synaptic terminal (Roof and Makino, 2000). The outer segment contains the photon-capturing photopigment. Opsin is a transmembranous protein that anchors the photopigment in the plasma membrane. In the outer segments, the plasma membrane is stacked into hundreds of flat discs, thereby increasing the density of retinal-opsin photopigment per photoreceptor cell. The discs in cones are deep invaginations of the outer segment membrane, while in rods, the discs are separate from the outer segment (except at the base). Shed discs are phagocytosed by the RPE. A nonmotile cilium connects the outer and inner segments. The inner segment contains the cellular machinery necessary to meet the high metabolic requirements of the photoreceptor cells. Its outer portion (the ellipsoid) is packed with mitochondria that produce ATP by oxidative phosphorylation, while the inner portion (the myoid) contains smooth and rough endoplasmic reticulum for synthetic activity as well as microtubules for intracellular transport. The photoreceptor nucleus contains all non-mitochondrial DNA. The inner fiber is the axon of the photoreceptor cell and transmits the photoreceptor cell signals to the outer plexiform layer (OPL) via its synaptic terminals. Due to the absence of inner nuclear layer cells in the foveola, foveolar inner fibers have to travel to the OPL in the surrounding macula to make synaptic contact. The synaptic neurotransmitter of the photoreceptor cell is glutamate, which is released in response to depolarization. The photoreceptor is most depolarized in darkness, whereas phototransduction results in gradated hyperpolarization. The terminal endings of the photoreceptors interact with neighboring photoreceptors and interneurons (horizontal and bipolar cells) and play a critical physiological role in the transmission and early processing of visual information in the retina.

Interneurons in the inner nuclear retinal layer connect the photoreceptor layer with the ganglion cell layer. These interneurons consist of the bipolar, horizontal, amacrine, and interplexiform cells, which form complex neuroretinal circuitries in the outer and inner plexiform layers (IPLs) that process the photoreceptor signal and transmit this information to the ganglion cell layer. In the simplest case, the photoreceptor cell is directly connected to a ganglion cell via a bipolar cell. *Bipolar cells* receive input from either rods or cones (Sharma and Ehinger, 2003; Radius and Anderson, 1979; Minckler, 1980). Cone bipolar cells may make contact with as few as one cone, while rod bipolar cells may receive input from up to 70 rods. Depending on their response to glutamate, bipolar cells are classified as being hyperpolarizing (OFF-center) or depolarizing (ON-center). Photoreceptors also interact with *horizontal cells* in the OPL (Ogden, 1983). Three types of horizontal cells have been described in the human retina (Fitzgibbon and Taylor, 1996; Fitzgibbon, 1997). *Amacrine cells* are mainly found in the inner nuclear layer, although some are seen in the ganglion cell layer and the IPL as well (Provis and Penfold, 2005). There are as many as 30 different types of amacrine cells, though the functional significance of each of these is not fully understood (Wurtz and Kandel, 2000). Amacrine cells are classified according to the size of their horizontal dendritic fields and the sublaminar level(s) within the IPL in which they synapse. The dendritic fields of amacrine cells vary between less than 100 mm (narrow-field) and greater than 500 mm (large-field) (Fitzgibbon and Taylor, 1996). Similarly, amacrine cells are uni-, bi-, or multistratified, creating connections both within and between the different strata of the IPL. Examples of different amacrine cell types are the narrow-field, multistratified AII amacrine cell that is involved in scotopic vision, and the wide-field starburst amacrine cell that is involved in motion detection (Wurtz and kandel, 2000). Another interneuron in the inner nuclear layer – the *interplexiform cell* – has processes extending into the inner and outer plexifom layers. Thus, on their way to the ganglion cell, visual signals are transmitted and modified by bipolar, horizontal, amacrine, and interplexiform cells as part of the visual processing within the retina (Ogden, 1983).

Ganglion Cells

Finally, the ganglion cells are responsible for transmitting visual information from the retina to the brain. The ganglion perikarya are located in the ganglion cell layer, while their dendrites make contact with bipolar and amacrine cells in the IPL. Up to 20 different ganglion cell types have been described in the human retina – the two best known types are the midget and the parasol cells, which make up about 80% of ganglion cell population (Wurtz and Kandel, 2000). The *midget ganglion cell* (also known as P or b cell) receives input from midget bipolar cells at a ratio of up to one-to-one in the fovea. It is a small cell with a relatively small dendritic arbor. The *parasol ganglion cell* (M or a cell) has a much more extensive dendritic arbor that resembles an opened umbrella in histological preparations of the retina. Midget and parasol cells project to the parvocellular and magnocellular layers of the lateral geniculate nucleus (LGN), respectively (Callaway, 2005; Davson, 1990). Because of the anatomic distance between the retina and the brain, the ganglion axons require effective mechanisms for transport of metabolites and organelles away from (anterograde) and back to (retrograde) the ganglion cell nucleus. Axonal transport occurs at slow (<10 mm/ day), high (hundreds of mm/day), or intermediate velocities. Most transport is slow and anterograde. An example of fast anterograde transport involves the transfer of vesicles containing neurotransmitter to the axonal synapses. Axon transport is an active process that requires adenosine triphosphate (ATP), which is supplied by the mitochondria in the axon. Interference with anterograde transport at the lamina cribrosa results in pathologic disc swelling.

Glial Cells

Four glial cell types are found in the retina: Müller cells, astrocytes, microglia, and occasionally, oligodendrocytes. *Müller cells* are the main glial cells of the retina (Newman, 2000; Oyster, 1999; Harris et al, 2001; Saint-Geniez and D'Amore, 2004). Their perikarya are located in the inner nuclear layer with cell processes that span the entire neuroretina (Newman, 2000). The proximal extensions of Müller cells expand and flatten to form so-called *endfeet* whose basal lamina forms the *inner limiting membrane* (Cioffi et al,2003). Distally, Müller's extensions give rise to the *outer limiting membrane* by forming a series of junctional complexes. Lateral extensions of Müller cells surround the retinal neurons. Müller cell processes also cover retinal blood vessels. Müller cells play a crucial role in maintaining the local environment that allows the visual process to function optimally. *Astrocytes* are thought to derive from stem cells in the optic nerve and are found in the superficial layers of the neuroretina where they surround ganglion cells, nerve fibers, and superficial retinal blood vessels (Provis, 2001). *Microglia* enter the retina from the circulation (Provis, 2001). They are phagocytic and part of the reticuloendothelial system. They are usually found in small numbers in the nerve fiber layer, but are mobile and can reach any part of the retina. *Oligodendrocytes* give rise to the myelin sheath in the peripheral nervous system. Though normally unmyelinated, retinal nerve fibers occasionally are seen to be myelinated, indicating that oligodendrocytes can reach the retina in certain conditions.

The retina is the neurosensory component of the eye. Its outer part is supplied by a vascular layer, the choroid, and protected by a tough outer layer, the sclera. The cellular elements of the retina are arranged and adapted to meet the functional requirements of the different regions of the retina.

Each of the microscopic layers of the retina has a name and contains various structures (Kolb et al, 1995).

Beginning with the innermost layer (closest to the vitreous) and proceeding outwards towards the choroid and sclera, these layers are as follows:

1. The inner limiting membrane
2. The nerve fiber layer
3. The ganglion cells layer
4. The inner plexiform layer
5. The inner nuclear layer
6. The outer plexiform layer
7. The outer nuclear layer
8. The outer limiting membrane
9. The rod and cone layer
10. The retinal pigment epithelium

Retinal Pigment Epithelium

Each eye contains about 3.5 million RPE cells (Panda-Jonas et al, 1996), which are held together by junctional complexes to form a continuous epithelial monolayer. The tight junctions (zonulae occludentes) between these RPE cells separate the choriocapillaris from the photoreceptors of the outer retina, thus creating the outer blood-retina barrier, a selective barrier between the outer retina and its choroidal blood supply (Schnaudigel, 1913; Cunha-Vaz, 1979; Cunha-Vaz, 2004; Davson, 1990; Thumann et al, 2006 Strauss, 2005; Kanski and Milewski, 2002). This barrier helps to control the extracellular milieu and maintain the function of the outer retina. During embryogenesis, the central neuroectoderm of the optic vesicle invaginates to form the inner leaf of the optic cup and becomes the sensory retina. The peripheral neuroectoderm of the optic vesicle forms the pigmented outer leaf of the optic cup and differentiates into the retinal pigment epithelium. As a result of this invagination, the neuroretina and the retinal pigment epithelium become apposed, being only separated by a potential subretinal space, which can fill with fluid and give rise to a retinal detachment.

Photoreceptor Layer

Rods and cones are tightly stacked together into a single pallisading layer of photoreceptors (Levin, 2003; Tessier-Lavigne, 2000; Roof and Makino, 2000; Curcio et al, 1987; Olver and McCartney, 1989; Olver et al, 1990;). This thin, subcellular stratum is the only light- sensitive part of the neuroretina and the site of phototransduction. All other layers of the neuroretina collectively serve to process and transmit these nerve signals.

External Limiting Membrane

This is not a true membrane, but created by junctional complexes between adjacent Müller cells as well as between Müller and photoreceptor cells. The subretinal space is a potential space lying between the outer blood retina barrier and the external limiting membrane (Alm et al, 1973; Alm and Bill, 1973).

Outer Nuclear Layer

The outer nuclear layer contains the nuclei of the photoreceptor cells and is thickest in the foveolar area. The human retina contains approximately four to five million cones and 77–107 million rods (Levin, 2003; Tessier-Lavigne, 2000; Wurtz and Kandel, 2000). Only cones are found in the foveola, whereas rods predominate outside the foveola throughout the remaining retina. The maximum rod density is found in the “rod ring” about 4.5 mm, or 20–25°, from the foveola (Sharma and Ehinger, 2003). The absence of rods from the foveola (“rod-free zone”) accounts for the physiological central scotoma that is experienced under extreme scotopic conditions.

Outer Plexiform Layer

In the OPL, photoreceptor cells of the outer nuclear layer form connections with the bipolar and horizontal cells of the inner nuclear layers. This is an important initial processing step in the retina: Individual cone photoreceptor signals are connected in such a way that they give rise to concentric receptive fields with an antagonistic center-surround organization. These signals are then transmitted to the next layer of processing, the IPL, by bipolar cells (Dowling, 2000; Zhu et al, 2000). The OPL has two components: the axons of the photoreceptor, bipolar and horizontal cells and their synaptic connections. The axons of the photoreceptor cells transmit the photosignal to the OPL and form a specialized structure, Henle’s fiber layer, in the central retina. The terminals of the photoreceptor cells – the rod spherules and cone pedicles – form the synapses between the photoreceptor, bipolar and horizontal cells (Wurtz and Kandel, 2000; Ogden, 1983).

Inner Nuclear Layer

This layer harbors the nuclei of not less than five different types of cells: the horizontal, the bipolar, the amacrine, the interplexiform, and the Müller cells. The horizontal cells are located along the outer limit of the inner nuclear layer facing the OPL, whereas the amacrine faces the IPL. The nuclei of the bipolar, interplexiform, and Müller cells take up intermediate positions (Newman, 2000; Wurtz and Kandel, 2000; Ogden, 1983).

Inner Plexiform Layer

The IPL is the second retinal processing layer with networks between bipolar, amacrine, and ganglion cells. The IPL shows sublayering into six lamina. This enables the parallel representation and processing of the photoreceptor input through specific interactions between the bipolar, amacrine, and ganglion cells in each of the six lamina of the IPL (Zhu et al, 2000).

Ganglion Cell Layer

This layer contains about 1.2 million ganglion cells as well as a number of other cell types, including "displaced" amacrine cells, astrocytes, enthothelial cells, and pericytes (Levin, 2003; Provis, 2001; Anderson and Quigley, 1992). The thickness of the ganglion cell layer is greatest in the perifoveal macula consisting of between eight and ten rows of nuclei (60–80 μm), decreases to a single row outside the macula (10–20 μm), and is absent from the foveola itself (Sharma and Ehinger, 2003; Kincaid and Green, 1999). The small midget and the larger parasol cells make up 80% of the ganglion cell layer and behave as either ON or OFF cells depending on the location of their dendrites in the ON or OFF-regions of the IPL. The ON-OFF center-surround organization of receptive fields that was first created in the OPL is thus maintained at the ganglion cell level (Tessier-Lavigne, 2000; Wurtz and Kandel, 2000; Zhu et al, 2000).

Nerve Fiber Layer

Ganglionic axons travel towards the optic nerve head within the nerve fiber layer. Thin and difficult to discern in the far periphery, the nerve fiber layer becomes thicker towards the disc as a result of the convergence of all retinal ganglion axon fibers on the optic disc. The axons are accompanied by astrocytes in the nerve fiber layer and are separated into small bundles by the cellular processes of Müller cells and the internal limiting membrane (Radius and Anderson, 1979). The exact cross-sectional ordering of the axonal fibers of the peripheral and central ganglion cells in the retina remains controversial (Minckler, 1980; Ogden, 1983; Fitzgibbon and Taylor, 1996; Fitzgibbon, 1997). Temporal to the disc lies the macula, which has the highest density of ganglion cells. Axons from the macula project straight to the disc, forming the papillomacular "bundle." The remaining axons of the temporal retina reach the optic disc only by arcing around the papillomacular bundle. As a result, all temporal ganglion cell axons originating from outside the macula are compressed into the superotemporal and inferotemporal sectors of the optic nerve, above and below the temporal entry of the papillomacular bundle fibers. The superior and inferior nerve fibers are therefore much thicker (almost 200 μm) compared to the papillomacular bundle (65 μm) and easier to see on clinical examination, especially in red-free light. Nasally, axons enter the nasal half of the optic disc more or less straight. In addition, ganglion axon fibers do not cross the horizontal meridian (the horizontal raphe).

Inner Limiting Membrane and Vitreoretinal Interface

The innermost processes of the Müller cell enlarge and flatten on the vitreal side to form the inner limiting membrane. Vitreous collagen fibrils insert into this membrane of the retina, so rendering the retina vulnerable to vitreoretinal traction forces (Cioffi et al, 2003).

The Fovea

Though the posterior pole (the anatomic macula) makes up less than 4% of the entire retina, it accounts for all central and most photopic vision (Provis and Penfold, 2005). Because of its special histological organization, the posterior pole is subdivided into four concentric regions: the perifovea, the parafovea, the foveal slope, and the foveola (Provis and Penfold, 2005). The *perifovea* is the outermost region of the anatomic macula that borders the peripheral retina. It is rich in retinal blood vessels and has a high rod–cone ratio of 33–130:1, an increased cone density compared with the peripheral retina, and a ganglion cell layer that is greater than a single cell layer in thickness. The *parafovea* is located between the fovea and the perifovea. It contains less retinal vessels, has a reduced rod: cone ratio of 4:1, and has the highest density of ganglion cells. The fovea contains the *foveola*, a flat central depression in the fovea and the site of maximum visual acuity. The foveola is surrounded by the *foveal slope* or clivus. Importantly, the clivus marks the switch from vascular to avascular retina (the FAZ) and from rod-dominated to cone-dominated retina (Provis and Penfold, 2005). The foveola itself is created in two opposing tissue migrations: the slow peripheral displacement of the inner nuclear and ganglion cells, while red and green cone photoreceptors in the surrounding outer retina migrate towards the foveola (Hendrickson, 1993; Hendrickson, 1994). As a result of these migrations, the fovea thins and forms a central depression, the foveola. The foveola is populated by cone photoreceptors and Müller cells only. Rods are excluded from the foveolar depression, so are blue cones, all ganglion and inner retinal cells, blood vessels, and other glial cells (Provis and Penfold, 2005; Newell, 1996). The human rodfree zone constricts from 2.00 mm^2 at 22 fetal weeks to less than 0.40 mm2 at 45 months (Hendrickson, 1993). As a result of this concentration, the highest density of cone photoreceptors in the adult human retina is produced, varying between 100,000 and 324,000 cones/mm2 (Tessier-Lavigne, 2000). In the adult, the rod-free zone is 350 mm in diameter, or 1° of visual angle (Tessier-Lavigne, 2000). In this most tightly packed foveolar region, the foveolar cones are compressed to about 1–1.5 μm and elongated to 70 μm (Davson, 1990). The inner fibers of the foveolar cone remain in contact with the bipolar and horizontal cells during their peripheral displacement and become considerably elongated. The radial arrangement of these axonal fibers in the clivus gives rise to Henle's layer. While the absence of retinal vessels in the FAZ removes a source of optical impediment, it also means that the central fovea is entirely dependent on blood supply from the choriocapillaris. Ganglion axons from the temporal retina do not cross the fovea, but arc around the fovea. The density of cones falls rapidly from an average peak of 199,000 cells/mm^2 in the foveola to about 20,000/mm^2 at the edge of the fovea and about 5,000/mm^2 outside the fovea. The functional consequence of this extreme specialization of foveal organization is that, though maximal central visual acuity can be generated in a very small area of the entire retina under photopic conditions, visual acuity is already halved at 1° eccentricity, quartered at 5° eccentricity, and is brought to less than 10% outside the temporal arcades, while the rod-free foveola is functionally blind under extreme scotopic conditions (Oyster, 1999)

Blood Supply of the Retina

Apart from the foveolar avascular zone (FAZ) and the extreme retinal periphery, which are thin enough to be supplied by diffusion from the choroidal circulation, the remaining human retina is too thick to be supplied by either the retinal or the choroidal circulation alone. The reason for this dual dependence is that diffusion time increases by the square of the distance. It has been calculated that it takes a glucose molecule 50 ms to diffuse 10 mm, but 100 times longer (5 s) to reach 100 mm (Oyster, 1999). The choroidal circulation thus supplies the outer retina, whereas the inner retina is supplied by the retinal circulation (Harris et al, 2001; Saint-Geniez and D'Amore, 2004; Provis, 2001). The oxygen tension is lowest in the watershed area between the two circulations (Cioffi et al, 2003).

Topographic Organization of the Retina

The adult *posterior pole* (anatomic macula or area centralis) is about 4.5–6 mm in diameter, centered on the fovea, and located between the superior and inferior temporal arcades. The *macula* (anatomic fovea centralis) is located approximately 3 mm temporal to the optic disc and is about 1.5 mm, or one disc size, in diameter (Kincaid and Green, 1999). The center of the macula lies just below the horizontal meridian (Williams and Wilkinson, 1992), a relationship that is used to study rotation during incyclo and excyclotorsion. The presence of xanthophyll, a yellow carotenoid pigment, gives the region its name – the macula lutea. The most central part of the macula, the *fovea* (anatomic foveola), is formed by a central, circa 0.35 mmwide depression and represents the retinal region of greatest visual acuity (Oyster, 1999). Clinically, it is recognized by the foveal reflex, blunting or loss of which may indicate early macular disease. The foveola is demarcated by a sloping wall, the clivus, which contributes to the annular light reflex that is seen in children and young adults. The foveola has the highest density of cone photoreceptors (199,000/mm2), which are narrowed and elongated in this location to maximize light detection further (Curcio et al, 1990). The long axons of the foveal cones form Henle's layer as they radiate out of the central depression. The fovea develops by an opposing process of outward displacement of the cells of the inner nuclear and ganglion cell layers, while the cone photoreceptors migrate toward the center (Hendrickson, 1993; Hendrickson, 1994; Provis et al, 1998). Rod photoreceptors are excluded from the foveal outer retina ("rod-free zone"). As a result, the foveola contains only cone photoreceptors and some Müller cells. The central 500 mm of the fovea contains no retinal capillaries (the *foveal avascular zone (FAZ)*), making the fovea dependent on blood supply from the choriocapillaris. The exact extent of the FAZ can be delineated with accuracy only by fluorescein angiography. Retinal blood vessels from the temporal retina do not cross the central fovea but arc around it. The *peripheral retina* comprises the remaining retina outside the temporal retinal arteries. Anatomically, the peripheral retina possesses only one layer of ganglion cells. The ampullae of the vortex veins lie just posterior to the equator, while the long posterior ciliary arteries and nerves mark the horizontal meridian. The *ora serrata* delineates the anterior termination of the sensory retina and the beginning of the pars plana of the ciliary body. At this junction, the sensory retina is reduced to a single cell layer which, anteriorly, becomes the nonpigmented ciliary epithelium whereas the retinal pigment epithelium (RPE) is replaced by pigmented ciliary epithelium. Junctional complexes between the pigmented and nonpigmented ciliary epithelia abolish the potential subretinal space that exists between the RPE and the neuroretina, making the pars plana a relatively safe site for surgical access to the posterior segment.

9. The Vitreous

Vitreous cavity. The vitreous cavity is the largest cavity of the eye. It is bounded anteriorly by the lens, zonule, and ciliary body and posteriorly by the retina and optic nerve. It has a volume of 4.5 ml.

The Vitreous Humor

The vitreous humor is a transparent gel structure composed of a random network of uniformly thin collagen fibrils suspended in a highly dilute solution of salts, protein, and hyaluronic acid. Its main component is water (98.5% to 99.7%). In young adults it is about 80% gel and 20% liquid vitreous humor that contains hyaluronic acid but no fibrils. With aging, the volume of liquid vitreous increases to about 50%.

The vitreous is shaped like a sphere with a segment removed anteriorly to provide a saucer-shaped depression forv the lens (lenticular fossa). In the region of depression, the vitreous humor is condensed and described clinically as the anterior hyaloid face. The vgitreous humor adheres firmly to the peripheral retina and to the ciliary epithelium in the region of the pars plana (vitreous base) and to the margin of the optic disc. Sometimes it is strongly attached to retinal blood vessels. The anterior hyaloid may be loosely attached to the posterior capsule of the lens (Weigert hyaloideocapsular ligament).

In the healthy young eye, the vitreous humor is in contact with the entire retina and is attached to the internal limiting lamina of the retina by scattered collagenous filaments. YThese attachments may cause retinal tears by traction if the vitreous humor degenerates and collapses.

The vitreous humor may be divided into two portions: a cortical portion, which circumscribes the entire vitreous body adjacent to the lens and retina, and a central portion. The vitreous base is a 2 mm band of vitreous that straddles both the ora serrata and pars plana to which it is attached by many fibrils. At the periphery of the optic disc, fibrils extend between the vitreous and the footplates of Müller cells. Embryologically, the vitreous is divided into primary (mesenchymal, canal of Cloquet), secondary (most of the adult vitreous), and tertiary (the lens zonule) parts.

The central vitreous has a less dense structure with fewer fibrils than the vitreous of the cortex. The vitreous cortex contains a few cells called "hyalocytes", which are vbelieved to be phagocytes, connective tissdue cells of the macrophage type.

Macroscopic Morphology

In an emmetropic adult human eye the vitreous is approximately 16.5 mm in axial length with a depression anteriorly just behind the lens (patellar fossa). The hyaloideocapsular ligament of Weiger is the annular region (1 – 2 mm in width and 8 – 9 mm in diameter) where the vitreous is attached to the posterior aspect of the lens. Erggelet's or Berger's space is at the center of the hyaloideocapsular ligament. The canal of Cloquet arises from this space and courses posteriorly through the central vitreous, which is the former site of the hyaloid artery in the embryonic vitreous. 16 The former lumen of the artery is an area devoid of collagen fi brils and surrounded by multifenestrated sheaths that were previously the basal laminae of the hyaloid artery wall (Sebag, 1989). Posteriorly, Cloquet's canal opens into a funnel-shaped region anterior to the optic disc, known as the area of Martegiani. Within the adult human vitreous fine, parallel fibers course in an anteroposterior direction, are continuous, and do not branch. The fibers arise from the vitreous base, where they insert anterior and posterior to the ora serrata. Various concepts are used to explain the connection between the peripheral anterior vitreous fibers and the retina and pars plana (Sebag, 1989), but all agree that the pathophysiology of retinal tears is vitreous traction upon foci of strong adhesion at the vitreoretinal interface in these locations. As the central fibers near the vitreous cortex course posteriorly, they are circumferential with the vitreous cortex, while central fibers "undulate" in a confi guration parallel to Cloquet's canal. Ultrastructural studies demonstrate that collagen, organized in bundles of packed, parallel fi brils, is the only microscopic structure that corresponds to these fibers (Seabag and Balazs, 1989). It is hypothesized that visible vitreous fi bers form when hyaluronan molecules no longer separate the microscopic collagen fibrils, which results in the aggregation of collagen fibrils into bundles from which hyaluronan molecules are excluded (Sebag and Balazs, 1989; Sebag, 1989; Sebag, 1987). The areas adjacent to these large fibers have a low density of collagen fibrils and a relatively high concentration of hyaluronan molecules. Composed primarily of "liquid vitreous," these areas scatter very little incident light and, when prominent, constitute "lacunae" seen in aging.

Microscopic Morphology

The vitreous cortex is defined as the peripheral "shell" of the vitreous that courses forward and inward from the anterior vitreous base, the "anterior vitreous cortex," and posteriorly from the posterior border of the vitreous base, the "posterior vitreous cortex." The posterior vitreous cortex is 100 – 110 mm thick and consists of densely packed collagen fibrils (Sebag, 1989; Sebag, 1994). Although no direct connections exist between the posterior vitreous and the retina, the posterior vitreous cortex is adherent to the internal limiting lamina of the retina, which is actually the basal lamina of retinal Müller cells. The exact nature of the adhesion between the posterior vitreous cortex and the internal limiting lamina is not known, but it most probably results from the action of various extracellular matrix molecules (Sebag, 1991). A hole in the prepapillary vitreous cortex can sometimes be visualized clinically when the posterior vitreous is detached from the retina. If peripapillary glial tissue is torn away during posterior vitreous detachment and remains attached to the vitreous cortex about the prepapillary hole, it is referred to as Vogt's or Weiss' ring. Vitreous can extrude through the prepapillary hole in the vitreous cortex but does so to a lesser extent than through the premacular vitreous cortex. Various vitreomaculopathies can result (Sebag, 1992). Other mechanisms, particularly tangential vitreomacular traction (Gass, 1995), are implicated in the pathogenesis of macular holes. Embedded within the posterior vitreous cortex are hyalocytes. These mononuclear cells are spread widely apart in a single layer situated 20 – 50 μ m from the internal limiting membrane of the retina. The highest density of hyalocytes is in the vitreous base, followed next by the posterior pole, with the lowest density at the equator. Hyalocytes are oval or spindle shaped, 10 – 15 μ m in diameter, and contain a lobulated nucleus, a well-developed Golgi complex, smooth and rough endoplasmic reticula, many large lysosomal granules (periodic acid-Schiff positive), and phagosomes . Balazs (Balazs, 1984) pointed out that hyalocytes are located in the region of highest hyaluronan concentration and suggested that these cells are responsible for hyaluronan synthesis. Hyalocyte capacity to synthesize collagen was fi rst demonstrated by Newsome *et al.* (Newsome, 1976) Thus, in a similar fashion to the chondrocyte metabolism in the joint, hyalocytes may be responsible for vitreous collagen synthesis at some point(s) during life. The phagocytic capacity of hyalocytes is consistent with the presence of pinocytic vesicles and phagosomes and the presence of surface receptors that bind immunoglobulin G and complement (Sebag, 1994). It is intriguing to consider that hyalocytes are among the fi rst cells to be exposed to any migratory or mitogenic stimuli during various disease states, particularly proliferative vitreoretinopathy. Therefore, the role of these cells must be considered when the pathophysiology of all proliferative disorders at the vitreoretinal interface is considered, including premacular membrane formation. The basal laminae about the vitreous are composed of type IV collagen closely associated with glycoproteins (Sebag, 1994). At the pars plana, the basal lamina has a true lamina densa. The basal lamina posterior to the ora serrata is the internal limiting lamina of the retina. The layer immediately adjacent to the Müller cell is a lamina rara, which is 0.03 – 0.06 mm thick. The lamina densa is thinnest at the fovea (0.01 – 0.02 mm) and disc (0.07 – 0.1 mm). It is thicker elsewhere in the posterior pole (0.5 – 3.2 mm) than at the equator or vitreous base (Sebag, 1989; Sebag, 1994). The anterior surface of the internal limiting lamina (vitreous side) is normally smooth, whereas the posterior aspect is irregular, as it fi lls the spaces created by the irregular surface of the subjacent retinal glial cells. This feature is most marked at the posterior pole, whereas in the periphery both the anterior and posterior aspects of the internal limiting lamina are smooth. The signifi cance, if any, of this topographic variation is not known. At the rim of the optic disc the retinal internal limiting lamina ceases, although the basal lamina continues as the “inner limiting membrane of Elschnig.” Heergaard et al, 1988) This membrane is 50 mm thick and is believed to be the basal lamina of the astroglia in the papilla. At the central-most portion of the optic disc the membrane thins to 20 mm, follows the irregularities of the underlying cells of the optic nerve head, and is composed only of glycosaminoglycans with no collagen (Heergaard et al, 1988). This structure is known as the “central meniscus of Kuhnt.” The thinness and chemical composition of these structures may account for, among other phenomena, the frequency with which abnormal cell proliferation arises from or near the optic disc in proliferative diabetic retinopathy and premacular membranes with macular pucker. The vitreous is known to be most fi rmly attached at the vitreous base, disc, and macula and over retinal blood vessels. The posterior aspect (retinal side) of the internal limiting lamina demonstrates irregular thickening the farther posteriorly from the ora serrata (Sebag, 1989; Sebag, 1994). So-called attachment plaques between the Müller cells and the internal limiting lamina have been described in the basal and equatorial regions of the fundus but not in the posterior pole, except for the fovea (Sebag, 1989; Sebag, 1994). It has been hypothesized that these develop in response to vitreous traction upon the retina. The thick internal limiting lamina in the posterior pole dampens the effects of this traction, except at the fovea, where the internal limiting lamina is thin. The thinness of the internal limiting lamina and the purported presence of attachment plaques at the central macula could explain the predisposition of this region to changes induced by traction. An unusual vitreoretinal interface overlies retinal blood vessels. Physiologically, this may provide a shock-absorbing function to dampen arterial pulsations. However, pathologically, this structural arrangement could also account for the proliferative and hemorrhagic events upon retinal blood vessels that are associated with vitreous traction.

The Visual Pathways

Visual stimuli originating in the retina pass to the brain in the optic nerve. Fibers originating from the retina nasal to a vertical line through the foveola decussate in the optic chiasm and join axons from the contralateral temporal retina in the optic tract. They synapse in the lateral geniculate body, and axons from the lateral geniculate body pass in the optic radiation to the visual cortex in the occipital lobe.

Visual Nerve

The Optic Nerve

The optic nerve is a portion of a white fiber tract of the central nervous system that consists of axons of retinal ganglion cells. The optic nerve (the second cranial nerve) is actually part of the central nervous system, extending directly from the brain into the orbit). Like the rest of the central nervous system, the optic nerve is invested within a dural sheath and leptomeninges, surrounded by cerebrospinal fluid, and in part, is covered with myelin. However, only the anterior part of this heavilybmyelinated tract is termed the optic nerve. It extends from the optic disk at a level with the retina within the eye to the optic chiasm, where, in normal humans, half of the fibers decussate to the opposite side of the brain in the optic chiasm. Thereafter, crossed nasal fiber and uncrossed temporal fibers constitute the optic tract.

The optic nerve is is about 50 mm long and extends from the eye to the optic chiasm. It is often described as consisting of four portions (divided into four portions): (1) intraocular, about 1 mm; (2) orbital, about 30 mm (24-30 mm); (6) intracanalicular, about 4 to 10 mm; (4) intracranial, about 10 mm.

Optic Disc (Opti Nerve Head)

The intraocular portion of the optic nerve includes the opti disk and the portion of the optic nerve within the posterior scleral foramen. The optic disk is located about 3 mm nasal to and about 0.8 mm above the foveola. It is composed of axons of ganglion cells. The choroid and all layers of the retina, except the nerve fiber layer, terminate at the optic disk margin. Because the photosensitive rods and cones are absent, this area is blind (the blind spot of Mariotte in visual field testing). The optic nerve head is 1 mm deep in the anetroposterior direction and 1.5 mm (horizontally) by 1.8 mm (vertically) in diameterat the level of the retina (Jonas et al, 1988). The retinal ganglion axons make an orthogonal turn from the nerve fiber layer and pass through one of 200-300 holes that perforate the lamina cribosa, the collagenous support of the optic disc (Anderson, 1969) These axons must pass from an area of higher tissue pressure (intraocular compartiment) to a zone of lower pressure (retrobulbar space). The collagen plates and specialized glial tissue maintain the pressure differential. The arterial supply shifts from the central retinal artery to branches of the ophthalmic artery. The axons become myelinated immediately at the posterior end of the optic nerve head.

The optic nerve exits from the eye through the posterior scleral foramen bridged with the lamina cribosa that is formed by fibrous tissue fromnthe sclera, elastic tissue of the choroid and Bruch membrane, and astroglia derived from the septal system of the nerve. Posterior to the optic disk the nerve fibers are myelinated, whereas anterior to the optic disk they are normally not myelinated. The portion of the optic nerve visible within the eye is about 1.5 mm in diameter.

The retinal nerve fiber layer and the optic nerve head (ONH) are biological structures, are not uniform in appearance, and show a remarkable variation within the normal population.

The normal measurements of the ONH with respect to ethnic background and the measurement technique have been reported (Samarawickrama, 2012). Optic nerve head parameters have shown a high inter-individual variability in the normal population.

A previous study using 107 freshly enucleated unfixed white human donor eyes revealed a minimal disk diameter of 1.67 ± 0.72mm (mean±standard deviation) and a maximal diameter of 1.92 ± 0.32 mm with a mean disk area of 2.59 0.±72 mm2 (minimum 0.68 mm2, maximum 4.42 mm^2) (Jonas et al, 1988). Clinical studies showed a similar inter-individual variation in disk measurement. For subjects of European descent, reported mean values for the vertical optic disk diameter were 1.76 to 1.87 mm in small-sample-size studies (Ewen et al, 2006; Jonas et al, 2003; Neubauer et al, 2006; Thomas et al, 2005).

Mean optic disk areas determined by planimetry ranged between 2.29 mm^2 and 3.09 mm^2.(Arvind et al, 2008; Budde et al, 2000; Jonas et al, 2006; Jonas et al, 2003; Lempert, 2008; Monteiro, 2006; Ramakrishnan et al,2005; Rudnicka et al, 2001; Soubrane and Bressler, 2001; Thomas et al, 2005; Xu et al,2008; Xu et al, 2007), a mean vertical cup diameter of 1.06 ± 0.23 mm from the Vellore Eye Study,79,163 0.75 ± 0.29 mm in 62 Americans31 and 0.061 inches (1.53 mm) with a standard error of 0.0004 from the Beaver Dam Eye Study.44 Optic cup area showed means varying between 0.53 mm^2 and 1.40 mm^2 (Samarawickrama, 2012). Recent reports have quoted mean vertical cup-to-disk diameter ratios varying from 0.3 to 0.5 (Samarawickrama, 2012) and mean cup-to-disk area ratios have varied from 0.14 to 0.37 (Samarawickrama, 2012).

Reports based on Heidelberg Retinal Tomography (HRT) have documented mean optic disk areas of between 1.79 mm2 and 2.67 mm2 in normal populations (Samarawickrama, 2012) and mean optic cup areas have varied between 0.32 mm2 and 0.95 mm2 in different populations (Samarawickrama, 2012) Mean cup-to-disk area ratio has been reported to lie between 0.19 to 0.37 (Samarawickrama, 2012). Data on mean vertical disk and cup diameter derived by HRT; reported a mean vertical disk and cup diameter of 1.65 ± 0.20 mm and 0.81 ±0.29 mm, respectively, from a sample of 62 Indian subjects.163 Vertical cup-to-disk ratio, reported in a range from 0.26 to 0.48 (Samarawickrama, 2012) with one report in a sample of subjects of predominantly African descent having a mean vertical cup-to-disk ratio of 0.59 ±0.10.175.

Recent reports using OCT have documented mean optic disk area in various normal populations between 1.60 mm^2 and 2.63 mm^2, (Samarawickrama, 2012) mean optic cup area between 0.34 mm2 and 0.93 mm2 (Samarawickrama, 2012) and mean cup-to-disk area ratios between 0.16 and 0.45 (Samarawickrama, 2012). One report, sampling a population predominantly of Africa ancestry, reported a larger mean optic cup area (1.35 ± 0.66 mm2) resulting in a larger mean cup-to-disk area ratio (0.49 ± 0.17) than in other populations. 175 Only one study, the Sydney Myopia Study, documented ONH parameters in a childhood population-based sample, with a mean optic disk area of 2.34 ±0.41 mm2, mean optic cup area of 0.46 ± 0.32 mm2, resulting in a mean cup-to-disk area ratio of 0.21 ± 0.14 (Samarawickrama, 2012).

Vertical optic disk diameter, documented in six reports, varied between 1.7 mm and 2.04 mm.23,106,119,149,176 Mean optic cup diameters were only described in two reports, measuring 0.73 ± 0.28 mm in a sample of 2,054 children106 and 0.93 ± 0.34 mm in a sample of 150 adult Indian subjects.23 Mean vertical cup-to-disk ratio was reported in quite a few reports and varied in adults between 0.34 and 0.55 (),5,18,23,30,39,65,80,96,104,106,122, 128,149,176,181 with one report in persons of African descent as high as 0.65 ± 0.13,175 while a report in children predominantly aged 12 years measured it as 0.39 ± 0.14.106 Recently, publications based on spectral-domain OCT have shown a mean disk area between 1.83 mm2 and 2.39 mm2, a mean cup area between 0.57 mm2 and 0.71 mm2, and a mean vertical cup-to-disk ratio between 0.48 and 0.50, similar to results published for time-domain OCT (Chang et al, 2009; Chen et al, 2008; Leung et al, 2010; Mwanza et al,2011).

Ethnic Variations in Normal Optic Nerve Head Parameters

Normal ONH parameters vary considerably between ethnicities (Samarawickrama, 2012). A rule of thumb may be that the closer to the equator that the patient's ancestors come from, the larger the optic disk. African Americans may have on average the largest optic disks, followed by Indians, Chinese, and then Europeans. Interestingly, the central corneal thickness follows a reverse direction with the highest corneal thickness measurements found in white patients, followed by Chinese, and the thinnest corneas in Indians and Sub-Saharan Africans (Samarawickrama, 2012).

Normal optic nerve parameters for white patients have been extensively reported (El Dairi et al, 2009; Girkin et al,2004; Harizman et al, 2006; Hawker et al, 2005; Hermann et al, 2004; ; Ikram et al, 2002; Jonas et al, 1995; Kamppeter et al, 2006; Medeiros et al, 2005; Melberg et al, 1995; Paunescu et al, 2004; Racette et al, 2005; Rekic et al, 2007; Reus and Lemij, 2005; Savini et al, 2005; van Koolwijk et al, 2007; Wang et al, 2007; Wollstein et al, 2005Zangwill et al, 2004), with a mean disk area ranging from 1.65-2.34 mm^2, mean cup area from 0.12-0.70mm^2, and mean cup-to-disk area ratio from 0.16-0.55 mm. Normal parameters for those of African descent have a mean optic disk area ranging between 1.84 mm^2 and 2.50 mm^2, mean cup area between 0.57 mm^2 and 0.95 mm^2, and mean cup-todisk area ratio between 0.23 mm and 0.49 mm (Deleon-Ortega et al, 2007; El Dairi et al, 2009; Girkin et al, 2004; Harizman et al,2006; Racette et al, 2005; Vessani et al, 2009; Zangwill et al, 2004). It appears that those of Indian descent generally had larger optic disk parameters than those of Asian descent, though similar optic cup parameters, when measured by both HRT and OCT. Normal parameters for Asian patients include a mean disk area range from 1.97-2.67 mm^2, mean cup area from 0.47-0.93 mm^2, and mean cup-to-disk area ratio from 0.20-0.37 mm (Abe et al, 2009; Chen and Huang, 2005;Choi et al, 2005; He et al, 2008; Itai et al, 2003; Kunimatsu et al, 2005; Leung et al, 2007; Leung et al, 2007; Liu et al, 2000; Min et al, 2005; Nagai-Kusuhara et al, 2008; Ruangvaravate and Neungton, 2008; Saito et al, 2008; Tong et al, 2007; Uchida et al, 2005; Xu et al, 2008). Normal parameters for Indian patients include a mean disk area ranging from 2.24-2.93 mm^2, mean cup area from 0.60--0.98 mm^2, and mean cup-to-disk area ratio from 0.25-0.73 mm (Agarwal et al, 2003; Arvind et al,2008; Dacosta et al, 2008; Jonas et al, 2003; Ramakrishnan et al, 2005; Sihota et al, 2008; Thomas et al, 2005). For Latinos, normal parameters include amean disk area ranging from1.95-2.56mm^2, mean cup area from0.74-0.93mm^2, and mean cup-todisk area ratio from 0.29-0.32 mm (Anton et al,2007; de la Rosa, 2007; Monteiro, 2006; Olmedo et al, 2005; Shine and Coates, 2005). Normal parameters for other populations including Turkish, Italian, German, Greek, and Swiss include a mean disk area ranging from 1.90-3.09 mm^2, mean cup area from 0.32-0.65 mm^2, and mean cup-to-disk area ratio from 0.14-0.34 mm (Budde et al, 2000; Cankaya et al, 2008; Deleon-Ortega et al, 2007; Durukan et al, 1980; Gherghel et al, 2000; Sampaolesi and Sampaolesi, 2001; Tekeli et al, 2008; Topouzis et al, 2006; Uysal et al, 2007).

Peripapillary Atrophy (Samarawickrama, 2012)

Peripapillary atrophy (PPA) is a clinical finding associated with chorioretinal thinning, photoreceptor loss, and disruption of the retinal pigmented epithelium.103 PPA surrounds the ONH and has been differentiated into a peripheral ''alpha'' zone and a central ''beta'' zone (Jonas et al, 1989; Rensch and Jonas, 2008). Alpha PPA is characterized by an irregular hypo- or hyperpigmentation adjacent to the retinal margin. Beta PPA is characterized as the unconcealed view of the sclera and sometimes the choroidal vessels, associated with thinning of chorioretinal tissue (Rensch and Jonas, 2008). Both alpha and beta PPA have been found to increase with age at a rate of approximately 0.21mm^2 per decade, and both are significantly correlated with optic disk size (Wang et al,2008). Many automated disk assessment modalities rely on retinal pigmentation to define the disk margin, and this may be under- or over-estimated in the presence of PPA (Kunimatsu et al, 2008; Lai et al, 2003; Na et al,2010). Size and shape of both zones of PPA can be assessed by simple ophthalmoscopy, and they can be measured by planimetry of optic disk photographs or by manually interactive measurements on confocal laser scanning images of the ONH (Kono, 1999). Because the beta zone with its histologic features of a loss of retinal pigment epithelium cells and photoreceptors and a thinning of the choroid can be imaged by confocal laser scanning tomography, the spectral-domain OCT devices may in future be able to give some measurements of PPA (Lee et al,2011; Nonaka et al,2011; Park et al,2010).

Influence of Aging on the Optic Nerve Head

Aging leads to a loss of retinal cells at a rate of about 0.3% per year of life, as shown for retinal photoreceptors and retinal pigment epithelium cells (Panda Jonas et al,1995; Panda Jonas et al, 1996) as well as for the number of retinal ganglion cell axons or optic nerve axons (Dolman et al, 1980; Jonas et al, 1990). Out of an original population of about 1.4 million axons at birth, white patients lose about 5,000 per year of life. It has also been suggested that there is a decrease in cup-to-disk ratio and neuroretinal rim area as age increased in studies based on Asian populations (kashiwagi et al, 2000; Kee et al, 1997); this was not found to be statistically significant, however. Healey et al (Healey et al, 1997) reported in a population based study that both optic disk diameter and cup-todisk ratio increased with increasing in age (0.001 mm and 0.001, respectively, for every 1 year increase in age; $p < 0.001$) and neural rim width decreased by 0.001 mm for every year increase in age ($p < 0.001$). See et al (Rensch and Jonas, 2008) found in a longitudinal study over 7 years that the neuroretinal rim decreased by 0.07% per year in normal patients. Previous cross-sectional studies found that older persons had thinner retinal nerve fiber layers compared to younger persons (Bowd et al, 2002; Sung et al, 2009).

In contrast, a longitudinal study conducted over 13 years in adults by Moya et al (Moya et al, 1999) found no significant change in optic nerve appearance or rim/disk area with age (p50.95), which differs from the findings by both See et al and Healey et al. (Healey et al, 1997) Taken together, it appears that the ONH is relatively stable in adulthood.

In summary, in normal adult populations HRT measures the mean optic disk area as between 1.79 mm^2 and 2.67 mm^2; planimetry reports it as between 2.29 mm^2 and 3.09 mm^2; OCT reports a mean between 1.60 mm^2 and 2.63 mm^2. Many studies have shown that persons of African descent tend to have larger optic disks, optic cups, and cup-to-disk ratios compared to white persons. Studies in adults indicate that the ONH is constantly changing, with a general loss of axons with increasing age (Samarawickrama, 2012).

Optic Nerve

The retinal ganglion axon fibers travel within the nerve fiber layer to converge on the optic disc while obeying strict retinotopic organization. The adult optic nerve head is typically elliptical in shape, having a slightly greater mean vertical (1.9 mm) than mean horizontal (1.7–1.8 mm) diameter (Levin, 2003), though its size and shape can vary greatly even in healthy eyes (Levin, 2003; Anderson and Quigley, 1992; Wilson et al, 2006; Tsai et al, 1995; Kanski and Nischal, 1999). In children, the optic disc and optic nerve achieve 75% of their adult size around term and 95% before the end of the first postnatal year (Jonas and Garway-Heath, 2000). The retinal axons leave the retinal plane to enter the optic nerve head at an angle of about 90° taking up position in a specific order: central RCG axons are located in the inner part of the optic nerve rim whilst peripheral RCG axons are found in the outer layers of the optic disc rim. The central part of the optic nerve head that contains no retinal fibers and appears optically empty forms the optic cup. The relationship between disc and cup size (the cupdisc ratio) can vary widely in healthy eyes (Kanski and Nischal, 1999). All retinal ganglion axons pass through the optic nerve head, which consists of three parts: the preliminary portion (between the lamina cribrosa and the vitreous), the lamina cribrosa, and the postlaminar portion. Surrounded by astrocytes in the prelaminar portion, the axon bundles stream through the foramina of the lamina cribrosa, which is made of condensations of scleral collagen, to enter the postlaminar portion where oligodendrocytes and connective tissue become part of the glial structure. A number of histological structures delineate the prelaminar optic nerve head from the vitreous (*internal limiting membrane of Elschnig* with the *central meniscus of Kuhnt*), the retina (*intermediary tissue of Kuhnt*), and the choroid (*border tissue of Jacoby*). In the oligodendrocyte-containing postlaminar portion, the axon fibers become myelinated and the optic nerve ensheathed by the meninges. After passing through the optic nerve disc, the retinal axons travel in the intraorbital (about 30 mm), the intracanalicular (5–12 mm), and the intracranial portions of the optic nerve (8–19 mm). At the optic chiasma, the nasal fibers decussate to join the temporal fibers of the contralateral optic nerve to form the optic tract, which projects to the LGN, the pretectal nuclei, the superior colliculus, the hypothalamus, and possibly other brain structures (Levin, 2003). The blood circulation of the optic nerve head is Primarily by the *circle of Zinn and Haller* and the peripapillary choroid of the posterior ciliary artery circulation (Levin, 2003; Anderson and Quigley, 1992; Hayreh, 1995). The central retinal artery circulation makes significant contributions only to the superficial optic nerve fiber layer (not the prelaminar portion of the optic nerve head) and the posterior portion of the optic nerve head. Thus, the posterior ciliary artery circulation supplies both the outer retina via the choriocapillaris and most of the optic nerve head. However, unlike the fenestrated capillaries of the choriocapillaris, the capillaries of the optic nerve head are nonfenestrated with tight junctions. In addition, the optic nerve head vessels are capable of autoregulation unlike the choriocapillaris. Even though the optic nerve head circulation is derived from the posterior ciliary circulation, its blood-retina barrier function and capability to autoregulate resemble more the retinal than the choroidal circulation (Anderson and Quigley, 1992). Because all retinal ganglion cell axons and all retinal blood vessels have to pass through the optic disc, relatively small lesions at the optic disc and in the optic nerve can have devastating clinical effects (Brown, 1999; Rimmer ett al, 1993). Pathology affecting these ganglionic axons along their anatomic course between the retina and the brain gives rise to characteristic visual field defects (Fekrat and Finkelstein, 1990; Anderson and Patella, 1999) and patterns of neural rim loss and pallor (Tsai et al, 1995; Kline et al, 2004; Miller and Newman, 1999; Glaser, 1999; Liu et al, 2001) that help to localize lesions clinically.

Intraorbital Optic Nerve

The orbital portion of the optic nerve has a S-shaped curve to permit movements of the eye. It is sheathed with a dense outer dura mater, a middle arachnoid mater, and an innermost, a middle arachnoid mater, and an innermost pia mater. These extend from the optic foramen to the globe, where the dura mater and arachnoid sheaths blend into the sclera. Near the globe the long and short ciliary arteries and nerves are arranged about its circumference. The central retinal artery and vein penetrate the optic nerve 12 mm behind the globe. At the apex of the orbit, the optic nerve is surrounded by the tendinous origin of the recti muscles, the ligament of Zinn.

Intracanalicular Optic Nerve

In its intracanalicular portion, the optic nerve passes through the optic foramen together with the ophthalmic artery and the sympathetic nerves accompany this artery. At the anterior margin of the optic foramen the dura mater covering the nerve divides so that one portion continues as the periosteum of the orbit and the other continues as the dural sheath of the optic nerve. Within the optic canal, the dura mater is adherent to bone, arachnoid, and pia mater so that the nerve is firmly fixed.

Intracranial Optic Nerve

The intracranial portion of the optic nerve passes medially to form the chiasm. Once past the hard fold of dura above the intracranial opening of the canal, the intracranial optic nerve runs for 12-16 mm to reach the optic chiasm. The intracranial optic nerve is now about 4.5 nmm in average diameter.

Structure

The optic nerve contains between 1.1 and 1.3 million afferent axonsthat derive from retinal ganglion cells and profect to the eight primary visual nuclei (Fredericks et al, 1988; Sadun, 1986; Sadun et al, 1986; Sadun et al, 1986(2-5)) of ganglion cells subserving vision,,pupillary reflex, and ocular movements. Axons from ganglion cells of the fovea centralis may provide up to 90% of the axons of the optic nerve.

References

Abe H, Shirakashi M, Tsutsumi T, et al. Laser scanning tomography of optic discs of the normal Japanese population in a population-based setting. *Ophthalmology.* 2009;116:223-230

Agarwal HC, Gulati V, Sihota R. The normal optic nerve head on Heidelberg Retina Tomograph II. *Indian J Ophthalmol* 2003;51:25-33.

Alm A, Bill A. Ocular and optic nerve blood flow at normal and increased intraocular pressure in monkeys (Macaca iris): A study with radioactively labelled microspheres including flow determination in brain and some other tissues. *Exp Eye Res* 1973;15:15-29.

Alm A, Bill A. Ocular and optic nerve blood flow at normal and increased intraocular pressure in monkeys. *Exp. Eye Res* 1973;15:15–29.

Alm, A., Bill, A., Young, FA: The effects of pilocarpine and neostigmine on the blood flow through the anterior uvea in monkeys: a study with radioactively labelled microspheres. *Exp. Eye Res* 1973; 15, 31.

Amann J, Holley GP, Lee SB, Edelhauser HF. Increased endothelial cell density in the paracentral and peripheral regions of the human cornea. *Am J Ophthalmol.* 2003;135: 584-590.

American Academy of Ophthalmology (AAO), Basic and Clinical Science Course. Section 11: Lens and Cataract, 2010-2011.

Anderson D, Braverman S. Reevaluation of the optic disc vasculature. *Am J Ophthalmol* 1976; 82:165-174.

Anderson D, Hoyt W, Hogan M. The fine structure of the astroglia in the human optic nerve and optic nerve head. *Trans Am Ophthalmol Soc* 1967;65:275-305.

Anderson D, Hoyt W. Ultrastructure of the intraorbital portion of human and monkey optic nerve. *Arch Ophthalmol* 1969; 82:506-530.

Anderson D. Ultrastructure of the human and monkey lamina cribrosa and optic nerve head. *Arch Ophthalmol* 1969;82:800-814.

Anderson D. Ultrastructure of the optic nerve head. *Arch Ophthalmol* 1970;83:63-73.

Anderson, D.R., Patella, V.M.: *Automated Static Perimetry*, 2nd edn. Mosby, St. Louis 1999

Anderson, D.R., Quigley, H.A.: The optic nerve. In: Hart Jr., W.M. (ed.) Adler's Physiology of the Eye, 9th edn, pp. 616–639. Mosby, St. Louis 1992

Anton A, Moreno-Montanes J, Blazquez F, et al. Usefulness of optical coherence tomography parameters of the optic disc and the retinal nerve fiber layer to differentiate glaucomatous, ocular hypertensive, and normal eyes. *J Glaucoma.* 2007;16:1-8

Apt L. An anatomic reevaluation of rectus muscle insertions. *Trans Am Ophthalmol Soc* 1988;78:365.

Arvind H, George R, Raju P, et al. Neural rim characteristics of healthy South Indians: the Chennai Glaucoma Study. *Invest Ophthalmol Vis Sci.* 2008;49:3457-3464

Bach, L., Seefelder, R.: Atlas zur Entwicklungsgeschichte des menschlichen Auges. Verlag von Wilhelm Engelmann, Leipzig 1914

Balazs E A . The vitreous. In: Davson H, ed. *The Eye*, Vol la .London: Academic Press ; 1984.: 533 – 89.

Beebe DC, Coats JM. The lens organizes the anterior segment: specification of neural crest cell differentiation in the avian eye. *Dev Biol* 2000; 220:424–431. Available at:http://www.sciencedirect.com/science?_obZMImg&_imagekeyZB6WDG-45K169G1K1&_cdiZ6766&_userZ10&_piiZS0012160600996386&_originZsearch&_coverDateZ04%2F15%2F2000&_skZ997799997&viewZc&wchpZdGLzVtb-zSkWA&md5Zb03e6a3a34ab49b6ae0cfdeb15674485& ieZ/sdarticle.pdf. Accessed November 23, 2010

Bill A, Sperber G, Ujiie K. Physiology of the choroidal vascular bed. *Int. Ophthalmol* 1983;6:101–107.

Bill A, Tornqvist P, Alm A. The permeability of the intraocular blood vessels. *Trans. Ophthal. Soc.* UK 1980;100:332–336.

Boote C, Dennis S, Newton RH, Puri H, Meek KM. Collagen fibrils appear more closely packed in the prepupillary cornea: optical and biomechanical implications. *Invest Ophthalmol Vis Sci* 2003; 44:2941–2948. Available at: http://www.iovs.org/content/44/7/2941.full.pdf. Accessed November 24, 2010

Boulton, M., Dayhaw-Barker, P.: The role of the retinal epithelium: topographical variation and ageing changes. *Eye* 2001; 15, 384-389 .

Bourne WM, Nelson LR, Hodge DO. Central corneal endothelial cell changes over a ten-year period. *Invest Ophthalmol Vis Sci* 1997; 38:779–782. Available at: http://www.iovs.org /content/ 38/3/779.full.pdf. Accessed November 23, 2010

Bron AJ, Tripathi RC, Tripathi BJ. Wolff's Anatomy of the Eye and Orbit, 8th ed. London: *Chapman & Hall*, 1997

Brown NP, Bron AJ: Lens Disorders. Clinical Manual of Cataract Diagnosis. *Oxford: Butterworth-Heinemann Ltd*, 1996

Brown, G.C.: Arterial occlusive disease. In: Regillo, C.D., Brown, G.C., Flynn, H.W. (eds.) *Vitreoretinal Disease*, pp. 97–115. Thieme, New York, Stuttgart 1999

Budde WM, Jonas JB, Martus P, et al. Influence of optic disc size on neuroretinal rim shape in healthy eyes. *J Glaucoma*. 2000;9:357-362

Burke, J.M.: Determinants of retinal pigment epithelial cell phenotype and polarity. In: Marmor, M.F., Wolfensberger, T.J. (eds.) *The Retinal Pigment Epithelium*, pp. 86–102. Oxford University, Oxford 1998

Callaway, E.M.: Structure and function of parallel pathways in the primate early visual system. *J. Physiol* 2005; 566, 13-19.

Cameron JD. Corneal reaction to injury. In: Krachmer JH, Mannis MJ, Holland EJ, eds, Cornea, 2nd ed. Philadelphia, PA, Elsevier *Mosby*, 2005; 115-133

Cankaya AB, Elgin U, Batman A, et al. Relationship between central corneal thickness and parameters of optic nerve head topography in healthy subjects. *Eur J Ophthalmol.* 2008;18:32-38

Chang RT, Knight OJ, Feuer WJ, et al. Sensitivity and specificity of time-domain versus spectral-domain optical coherence tomography in diagnosing early to moderate glaucoma. *Ophthalmology*. 2009;116:2294-2299

Chen HY, Huang ML. Discrimination between normal and glaucomatous eyes using Stratus optical coherence tomography in Taiwan Chinese subjects. *Graefes Arch Clin Exp Ophthalmol*. 2005;243:894-902

Chen TC, Zeng A, Sun W, et al. Spectral domain optical coherence tomography and glaucoma. *Int Ophthalmol. Clin*. 2008;48:29-45.

Choi MG, Han M, Kim YI, et al. Comparison of glaucomatous parameters in normal, ocular hypertensive and glaucomatous eyes using optical coherence tomography 3000. *Korean J Ophthalmol*. 2005;19:40-46.

Cioffi, G.A., Granstam, E., Alm, A.: Ocular circulation (Chapter 33). In: Kaufman, P.L., Alm, A. (eds.) Adler's Physiology of the Eye, 10th edn, pp. 747–784. *Mosby*, St Louis 2003.

Cogan DG, Kuwabara T. Arcus senilis: its pathology and histochemistry. *Arch Ophthalmol*. 1959;61:553–560.

Cogan DG, Kuwabara T. Focal senile translucency of the sclera. *Arch Ophthalmol*. 1959;62:604-610.

Cook, C., Sulik, K.K., Wright, K.W.: Embryology. In: Wright, K.W., Spiegel, P.H. (eds.) *Pediatric Ophthalmology and Strabismus*, 2nd ed, 2003; pp. 3–38. Springer, Berlin.

Cunha-Vaz, J.G.: The blood-ocular barriers. *Surv. Ophthalmol.* 1979; 23, 279–296.

Cunha-Vaz, J.G.: The blood-retinal barriers system. Basic concepts and clinical evaluation. Review. *Exp. Eye Res* 2004 78, 715-721.

Curcio, C.A., Sloan, K.R., Kalina, R.E., Hendrickson, A.E.: Human photoreceptor topography. *J. Comp. Neurol* 1990; 292, 497-523 .

Curcio, C.A., Sloan, K.R., Packer, O., Hendrickson, A.E., Kalina, R.E.: Distribution of cones in human and monkey retina: individual variability and radial asymmetry. *Science* 1987; 236, 579-582.

Dacosta S, Bilal S, Rajendran B, et al. Optic disc topography of normal Indian eyes: an assessment using optical coherence tomography. *Indian J Ophthalmol*. 2008;56:99-102

Davson, H.: Retinal structure and organization (chapter 5). In: Davson, H. (ed.) *Physiology of the Eye*, 5th edn, pp. 205–218. MacMillan, London 1990

Davson, H.: The aqueous humour and the intraocular pressure (chapter 1). In: Davson, H. (ed.) *Physiology of the Eye,* 5th edn, pp. 3–95. MacMillan, London 1990.

de la Rosa MG, Gonzalez-Hernandez M, Lozano-Lopez V, et al. Optic disc tomography and perimetry in controls, glaucoma suspects, and early and established glaucomas. *Optom Vis Sci*. 2007;84:33-41.

De Stefano M, Mugnaini E. Fine structure of the choroidal coat of the avian eye: lymphatic vessels. *Invest. Ophthalmol. Vis. Sci* 1997b;38:1241–1260

Dejean, C.H., Hervouët, F.R., Leplat, G.: L'embryologie de l'oeil et sa tératologie. Société Française d'Ophtalmologie. Paris: Masson. *Libraire de l'Académie de Médicine*,1958 pp. 1-728.

Deleon-Ortega J, Carroll KE, Arthur SN, et al. Correlations between retinal nerve fiber layer and visual field in eyes with nonarteritic anterior ischemic optic neuropathy. *Am J Ophthalmol*. 2007;143:288-294

Derek W. DelMont DW, Kim T. Anatomy and physiology of the cornea. *J Cataract Refract Surg* 2011; 37:588-598

Dolman CL, McCormick AQ, Drance SM. Aging of the optic nerve. *Arch Ophthalmol.* 1980;98:2053-2058.

Dowling, J.E.: Retinal neurophysiology. In: Albert, D.A., Jakobiec, F.A. (eds.) *Principles and Practice of Ophthalmology*, 2nd edn, pp. 1713–1729. Saunders, Philadelphia 2000.

Duke-Elder S, Wybar K: The eye. In Duke-Elder S (ed): *The Anatomy of the Visual System*, Vol II. St. Louis: CV Mosby, 1961:75–386

Duke-Elder, S., Cook, C.: Normal and abnormal development. Part 1. Embryology. In: Duke-Elder, S. (ed.) *System of Ophthalmology*,1963 vol 3, pp. 190–201. Henry Kimpton, London 1963

Durmus M, Karadag R, Erdurmus M, et al. Assessment of cup-to-disc ratio with slit-lamp funduscopy, Heidelberg Retina Tomography II, and stereoscopic photos. *Eur J Ophthalmol.* 2009;19:55-60

Durukan AH, Yucel I, Akar Y, et al. Assessment of optic nerve head topographic parameters with a confocal scanning laser ophthalmoscope. *Clin Experiment Ophthalmol.* 2004;32:259-264

Edelhauser HF. The balance between corneal transparency and edema. The Proctor lecture. *Invest Ophthalmol Vis Sci.* 2006; 47:1755-1767.

El Dairi MA, Asrani SG, Enyedi LB, et al. Optical coherence tomography in the eyes of normal children. *Arch Ophthalmol.* 2009;127:50-58

Ewen A, Lee KE, Klein BE, et al. Comparability of cup and disk diameters measured from nonstereoscopic digital and stereoscopic film images. *Am J Ophthalmol.* 2006;141: 1126-1128

Farjo A, McDermott M, Soong HK. Corneal anatomy, physiology, and wound healing. In: Yanoff M, Duker JS, eds, *Ophthalmology*, 3rd ed. St. Louis, MO, Mosby, 2008; 203–208

Fekrat, S., Finkelstein, D.: Venous occlusive disease. In: Regillo, C.D., Brown, G.C., Flynn, H.W. (eds.) Vitreoretinal Disease, pp. 117–132. Thieme, New York, Stuttgart 1999

Ferreras A, Pablo LE, Larrosa JM, et al. Discriminating between normal and glaucoma-damaged eyes with the Heidelberg Retina Tomograph 3. *Ophthalmology.* 2008; 115:775-781

Ferreras A, Pajarin AB, Polo V, et al. Diagnostic ability of Heidelberg Retina Tomograph 3 classifications: glaucoma probability score versus Moorfields regression analysis. *Ophthalmology.* 2007;114:1981-1987

Fini ME, Stramer BM. How the cornea heals; cornea-specific repair mechanisms affecting surgical outcomes. *Cornea* 2005; 24 (suppl 1):S2–S11.

Fitzgibbon, T., Taylor, S.F.: Retinotopy of the human retinal nerve fibre layer and optic nerve head. *J. Comp. Neurol* 1996; 375, 238–251.

Fitzgibbon, T.: The human fetal retinal nerve fiber layer and optic nerve head: a DiI and DiA tracing study. *Vis. Neurosci* 1997; 14, 433-447.

Folberg R. Chapter 1. The eye. In: Spencer WH, ed. Ophthalmic Pathology. An Atlas and Textbook. 4th ed. Philadelphia, PA: W. B. Saunders, Co.; 1996:1–37.

Forrester J, Dick A, McMenamin P, Lee W. Anatomy of the eye and orbit. In: Forrester JV, Dick AD, McMenamin P, Lee WR, eds. *The eye: Basic sciences in practice*. London: WB Saunders; 1996:1-86.'

Fredericks CA, Giolli RA, Blanks RH, Sadun AA. The human accessory optic system. *Brain Res* 1988;454:116-122.

Fredericks CA, Giolli RA, Blanks RH, Sadun AA. The human accessory optic system. *Brain Res* 1988;454:116-122.

Gass J D M . Reappraisal of biomicroscopic classifi cation of stages of development of a macular hole . *Am J Ophthalmol* . 1995 ; 119 : 752 – 9 .

Geroski DH, Matsuda M, Yee RW, Edelhauser HF. Pump function of the human corneal endothelium; effects of age and cornea guttata. *Ophthalmology* 1985; 92:759-763; discussion by J Sugar, 763

Gherghel D, Orgul S, Prunte C, et al. Interocular differences in optic disc topographic parameters in normal subjects. *Curr Eye Res*. 2000;20:276-282

Gipson IK, Joyce NC. Anatomy and cell biology of the cornea, superficial limbus, and conjunctiva. In: Albert DM, Jakobiec FA, eds, Principles and Practice of Ophthalmology, 3rd ed. Philadelphia, PA, Saunders, 2008; 423-420

Gipson IK, Yankauckas M, Spurr-Michaud SJ, Tisdale AS, Rinehart W. Characteristics of a glycoprotein in the ocular surface glycocalyx. *Invest Ophthalmol Vis Sci* 1992; 33:218-227. Available at: http://www.iovs.org/content/33/1/218.full.pdf. Accessed November 24, 2010

Girkin CA, McGwin G Jr, Long C, et al. Subjective and objective optic nerve assessment in African Americans and whites. *Invest Ophthalmol Vis Sci*. 2004;45:2272-2278

Glaser, J.S.: Topical diagnosis: prechiasmal visual pathways. In: Glaser, J.S. (ed.) *Neuro-Ophthalmology*, 3rd edn, pp. 95–198. Lippincott Williams&Wilkins, Philadelphia 1999.

Grossniklaus HE, Nickerson JM, Edelhauser HF, Bergman LA, Berglin L. Anatomic alterations in aging and age-related diseases of the eye. *Invest Ophthalmol Vis Sci* 2013;54(14):ORSF23-7.doi:10.1167/iovs.13-12711. Review

Hall ER, Klein BE, Knudtson MD, et al. Age-related macular degeneration and optic disk cupping: the Beaver Dam Eye Study. *Am J Ophthalmol*. 2006;141:494-497

Hanna C, Bicknell DS, O'Brien JE. Cell turnover in the adult human eye. *Arch Ophthalmol* 1961; 65:695-698

Hanson S, Krishnan SK, Phillips J. Observer experience and cup:disc ratio assessment. *Optom Vis Sci*. 2001;78:701-75

Harizman N, Oliveira C, Chiang A, et al. The ISNT rule and differentiation of normal from glaucomatous eyes. *Arch Ophthalmol*. 2006;124:1579-1583

Harris, A., Gingaman, D.P., Ciulla, T.A., Martin, B.J.: Retinal and choroidal blood flow in health and disease. In: Ryan, S.J. (ed.) The Retina, 3rd edn, pp. 68–88. Mosby, St Louis 2001

Hawker MJ, Ainsworth G, Vernon SA, et al. Observer agreement using the Heidelberg retina tomograph: the Bridlington Eye Assessment Project. *J Glaucoma*. 2008;17: 280-286

Hawker MJ, Vernon SA, Ainsworth G, et al. Asymmetry in optic disc morphometry as measured by Heidelberg retina tomography in a normal elderly population: the Bridlington Eye Assessment Project. *Invest Ophthalmol Vis Sci*. 2005;46:4153-4158

Hawker MJ, Vernon SA, Ainsworth G. Specificity of the Heidelberg Retina Tomograph's diagnostic algorithms in a normal elderly population: the Bridlington Eye Assessment Project. *Ophthalmology*. 2006;113:778-785

Hawker MJ, Vernon SA, Tattersall CL, et al. Linear regression modeling of rim area to discriminate between normal and glaucomatous optic nerve heads: the Bridlington Eye Assessment Project. *J Glaucoma* 2007;16:345-351.

Hayreh S, Vrabec F. The structure of the head of the optic nerve in the rhesus monkey. *Am J Ophthalmol* 1966; 61:136

Hayreh, S.S.: The optic nerve head circulation in health and disease. The 1994 Von Sallman Lecture. *Exp. Eye Res* 1995; 61, 259–272.

He M, Liu B, Huang W, et al. Heritability of optic disc and cup measured by the Heidelberg Retinal Tomography in Chinese: the Guangzhou twin eye study. *Invest Ophthalmol Vis Sci.* 2008;49:1350-1355

Healey PR, Mitchell P, Smith W, et al. The influence of age and intraocular pressure on the optic cup in a normal population. *J Glaucoma*. 1997;6:274-278

Helveston E, Merriam W, Ellis F, Schelhamer R, Gosling G. The trochlea: a study of the anatomy and physiology. *Ophthalmology* 1982;89:124-133.

Hendrickson, A.E.: Morphological development of the primate retina. In: Simons, K. (ed.) Early Visual Development, Normal and Abnormal, pp. 287–295. Oxford University, New York, Oxford 1993

Hendrickson, A.E.: Primate foveal development: A microcosm of current questions in neurobiology. Recent developments. *Invest. Ophthalmol. Vis. Sci* 1994; 35, 3129–3133.

Hermann MM, Garway-Heath DF, Jonescu-Cuypers CP, et al. Interobserver variability in confocal optic nerve analysis (HRT). *Int Ophthalmol*. 2005;26:143-149

Hermann MM, Theofylaktopoulos I, Bangard N, et al. Optic nerve head morphometry in healthy adults using confocal laser scanning tomography. *Br J Ophthalmol*. 2004;88:761-765

Hildebrand GD, Fielder AR. Anatomy and physiology of the retina. In, Reynolds J and Olitsky (eds), Pediatric Retina.DOI:10.1007:978-3-642-12041-1-2. Springer Verlag Berlin Heidelberg, 2011.

Hirata A, Negi A. Morphological changes of choriocapillaris in experimentally induced chick myopia. *Graefe's Arch Clin Exp Ophthalmol* 1998;236:132–137.

Hirose A, Azuma H, Tokoro T, Hirai K. Endothelin-B receptors on suprachoroidal melanocytes mediate and endothelin-1-induced increase in the intracellular calcium concentration of rabbit ocular suprachoroidal tissue. *Curr. Eye Res* 2007;32:585-591.

Hogan M, Alvarado J, Weddell J: Histology of the Human Eye—An Atlas and Textbook. Philadelphia: WB Saunders, 1971

Hogan, M.J., Alvarado, J.A., Weddell, J.E.: Retina. In: Histology of the Human Eye. An Atlas and Textbook, pp. 393–521. Saunders: Philadelphia 1971

Hogan, MJ.; Alvarado, JA.; Weddell, JE. Histology of the Human Eye. Saunders Company; Philadelphia: 1971.

Hrynchak P, Hutchings N, Jones D, et al. A comparison of cup-to-disc ratio evaluation in normal subjects using stereo biomicroscopy and digital imaging of the optic nerve head. *Ophthalmic Physiol Opt.* 2003;23:51-59

Hughes, B.A., Gallemore, R.P., Miller, S.S.: Transport mechanisms in the retinal pigment epithelium. In: Marmor, M.F., Wolfensberger, T.J. (eds.) The Retinal Pigment Epithelium, pp. 103–134. Oxford University, Oxford 1998

Ikram MK, Borger PH, Assink JJ, et al. Comparing ophthalmoscopy, slide viewing, and semiautomated systems in optic disc morphometry. *Ophthalmology*. 2002;109:486-493

Iliev ME, Meyenberg A, Garweg JG. Morphometric assessment of normal, suspect and glaucomatous optic discs with Stratus OCT and HRT II. *Eye*. 2006;20:1288-1299

Itai N, Tanito M, Chihara E. Comparison of optic disc topography measured by retinal thickness analyzer with measurement by Heidelberg Retina Tomograph II. *Jpn J Ophthalmol.* 2003;47:214-220

Jakobiec FA. *Ocular Anatomy, Embryology, and Teratology*. Philadelphia, PA: Harper & Row Publishers, Inc; 1982.

Jester JV, Moller-Pedersen T, Huang J, Sax CM, Kays WT, Cavangh HD, Petroll WM, Piatigorsky J. The cellular basis of corneal transparency: evidence for 'corneal crystallins'. *J Cell Sci* 1999; 112:613–622. Available at: http://jcs.biologists.org/cgi/reprint/112/5/613. Accessed November 23, 2010

Johnson DH, Bourne WM, Campbell RJ. The ultrastructure of Descemet's membrane. I. Change with age in normal corneas. *Arch Ophthalmol.* 1982;100:1942-1947.

Jonas JB, Gusek GC, Guggenmoos-Holzmann I, et al. Size of the optic nerve scleral canal and comparison with intravital determination of optic disc dimensions. *Graefes Arch Clin Exp Ophthalmol.* 1988;226:213-215

Jonas JB, Muller Bergh JA, Schlotzer Schrehardt UM, et al. Histomorphometry of the human optic nerve. *Invest Ophthalmol Vis Sci.* 1990;31:736-744

Jonas JB, Nguyen XN, Gusek GC, et al. Parapapillary chorioretinal atrophy in normal and glaucoma eyes. I. Morphometric data. *Invest Ophthalmol Vis Sci.* 1989;30: 908-918

Jonas JB, Schmidt AM, Muller Bergh JA, et al. Optic nerve fiber count and diameter of the retrobulbar optic nerve in normal and glaucomatous eyes. *Graefes Arch Clin Exp Ophthalmol.* 1995;233:421-424

Jonas JB, Stroux A, Martus P, et al. Keratometry, optic disc dimensions, and degree and progression of glaucomatous optic nerve damage. *J Glaucoma.* 2006;15:206-212

Jonas JB, Thomas R, George R, Berenshtein E, Muliyil J. Optic disc morphology in south India: the Vellore Eye Study. *Br J Ophthalmol* 2003;87:189

Jonas JB, Thomas R, George R, et al. Optic disc morphology in south India: the Vellore Eye Study. *Br J Ophthalmol.* 2003;87:189-196

Jonas, J., Garway-Heath, T.: Primary glaucomas: optic disc features. In: Hitchings, R.A. (ed.) *Glaucoma*, pp. 29–38. BMJ books, London 2000.

Kaimbo DK, Kayembe D. Orbital measurements in Zairian children. Inner canthal, outer orbital, inert-pupillary distances and proptosis. [Artcle in French]. *J Fr Ophtalmol* 1994; 17:496-500.

Kamppeter BA, Schubert KV, Budde WM, et al. Optical coherence tomography of the optic nerve head: interindividual reproducibility. *J Glaucoma.* 2006;15:248-254

Kanski, J.J., Milewski, S.A.. Introduction. In: Kanski, J.J., Milewski, S.A. (eds.) Diseases of the Macula, pp. 1–18. Mosby, St Louis 2002

Kanski, J.J., Nischal, K.K.: The optic disc. In: Ophthalmology. Clinical Signs and Differential Diagnosis, pp. 247–285. Mosby: St Louis 1999

Kashiwagi K, Tamura M, Abe K, et al. The influence of age, gender, refractive error, and optic disc size on the optic disc configuration in Japanese normal eyes. *Acta Ophthalmol Scand.* 2000;78:200-203

Kim JS, Ishikawa H, Gabriele ML, Wollstein G, Bilonick, et al. Retinal nerve fiber layer thickness measurement comparability between time domain optical coherence tomography (OCT) and spectral domain OCT. *Invest Ophthalmol Vis Sci.* 2010;51:896-902

Kincaid, M.C., Green, W.R.: Anatomy of the vitrous, retina and choroid. In: Regillo, C.D., Brown, G.C., Flynn, H.W. (eds.) Vitreoretinal Disease, pp. 11–24. Thieme, New York, Stuttgart 1999

Kincaid, M.C., Green, W.R.: Anatomy of the vitrous, retina and choroid. In: Regillo, C.D., Brown, G.C., Flynn, H.W. (eds.) Vitreoretinal Disease, pp. 11–24. Thieme, New York, Stuttgart 1999

Kincaid, M.C.: Pathology of the retina. In: Sassani, J.W. (ed.) Ophthalmic Pathology with Clinical Correlations, pp. 269–291. Lippincott-Raven, Philadelphia 1997

Kline, L.B., Bajandas, F.J.: Visual fields. In: Kline, L.B., Bajandas, F.J. (eds.) Neurophthalmology. Review Manual, 5th edn, pp. 1–45. Slack, Thorofare 2004

Kolb H, Fernandez E, Nelson R. *The Organization of the Retina and Visual System*. Salt Lake City, UT: National Library of Medicine, National Institutes of Health; 1995.

Kono Y, Jonas JB, Zangwill L, et al. Agreement of measurement of parapapillary atrophy with confocal scanning laser ophthalmoscopy and planimetry of photographs. *J Glaucoma*. 1999;8:105-110

Krebs W, Krebs IP. Ultrastructural evidence for lymphatic capillaries in the primate retina. *Arch Ophthal* 1988;106:1615-1616.

Krebs, W.; Krebs, I. Primate Retina and Choroid: Atlas of Fine Structure in Man and Monkey. Springer-Verlag; New York: 1991.

Kunimatsu S, Tomidokoro A, Saito H, et al. Performance of GDx VCC in eyes with peripapillary atrophy: comparison of three circle sizes. *Eye*. 2008;22:173-178

Kunimatsu S, Tomita G, Araie M, et al. Frequency doubling technology and scanning laser tomography in eyes with generalized enlargement of optic disc cupping. *J Glaucoma*. 2005;14:280-287

Kuszak JR, Brown HG. Embryology and anatomy of the lens. In: Albert DM, Jakobiec FA, eds. Principles and practice of ophthalmology. Basic sciences. Philadelphia: WB Saunders; 1994:82-96.

La Cour, M.: The retinal pigment epithelium. In: Kaufman, P.L., Alm, A. (eds.) Adler's Physiology of the Eye, 10th edn, pp. 348–357. Mosby, St Louis 2003.

Lai E, Wollstein G, Price LL, et al. Optical coherence tomography disc assessment in optic nerves with peripapillary atrophy. *Ophthalmic Surg Lasers Imaging*. 2003;34: 498-504

Lee EJ, Kim TW, Weinreb RN, et al. beta-Zone parapapillary atrophy and the rate of retinal nerve fiber layer thinning in glaucoma. *Invest Ophthalmol Vis Sci*. 2011;52:4422-4427

Lempert P. Optic disc area and retinal area in amblyopia. *Semin Ophthalmol*. 2008;23:302-306

Lenzi GL, Fieschi C. Superior orbital fissure syndrome: a review of 130 cases. *Eur Neurol* 1977;16:23-30.

Leung CK, Cheng AC, Chong KK, et al. Optic disc measurements in myopia with optical coherence tomography and confocal scanning laser ophthalmoscopy. *Invest Ophthalmol Vis Sci*. 2007;48:3178-3183

Leung CK, Medeiros FA, Zangwill LM, et al. American Chinese glaucoma imaging study: a comparison of the optic disc and retinal nerve fiber layer in detecting glaucomatous damage. *Invest Ophthalmol Vis Sci*. 2007;48:2644-2652

Leung CK, Ye C,Weinreb RN, et al. Retinal nerve fiber layer imaging with spectral-domain optical coherence tomography a study on diagnostic agreement with Heidelberg Retinal Tomograph. *Ophthalmology*. 2010;117:267-274

Levin, L.A.: Optic nerve. In: Kaufman, P.L., Alm, A. (eds.) Adler's Physiology of the Eye, 10th edn, pp. 603–638. Mosby, St Louis 2003.

Levin, L.A.: Optic nerve. In: Kaufman, P.L., Alm, A. (eds.) Adler's Physiology of the Eye, 10th edn, pp. 603–638. Mosby, St Louis 2003

Li W, Hayashida Y, Chen Y-T, Tseng SCG. Niche regulation of corneal epithelial stem cells at the limbus. *Cell Res* 2007; 17:26–36. Available at: http://www.nature.com/cr/journal /v17/ n1/pdf/7310137a.pdf. Accessed December 1, 2010

Linsenmeier RA, Braun RD. Oxygen distribution and consumption in the cat retina during normoxia and hypoxia. *J. Gen. Physiol* 1992;99:177–197.

Linsenmeier RA, Goldstick TK, Blum RS, Enroth-Cugell C. Estimation of retinal oxygen transients from measurments made in the vitreous humor. *Exp. Eye Res* 1981;32:369-379.

Liu X, Ling Y, Zheng X, et al. Study on stereometric parameters of optic nerve head of normal, big-cupped disk and glaucomatous eyes using Heidelberg retina tomograph. *Yan Ke Xue Bao.* 2000;16:163-167

Liu, G.T., Volpe, N.J., Galetta, S.L.: Vision loss: retinal disorders of neuro-ophthalmic interest. In: Liu, G.T., Volpe, N.J., Galetta, S.L. (eds.) Neuro-Opthalmology. Diagnosis and Management, pp. 58–102. Saunders, Philadelphia 2001.

Mallajosyula S. Surgical atlas of orbital diseases. Jaypee Brothers Medical Publishers (P) Ld, New Delhi, 2009 pp 3-22.

Mann, I.: The Development of the Human Eye, 3rd edn. British Medical Association, Tavistock Square, London 1964.

Marmor MF, Abdul-Rahim AS, Cohen SD. the effect of metabolic inhibitors on retinal adhesion and subretinal fluid reabsorbtion. *Invest. Ophthalmol. Vis. Sci* 1980;19:893-903.

Marmor, M.F.: Retinal and retinal pigment epithelial physiology. In: Regillo, C.D., Brown, G.C., Flynn, H.W. (eds.) Vitreoretinal Disease, pp. 25–38. Thieme, New York, Stuttgart 1999

Maurice D. Cornea and sclera. In Davson H (ed). Physiology of the Eye, 2nd ed. Boston: Little, Brown and Co, 1969:6,14,15

Maurice DM. The transparency of the corneal stroma [letter]. *Vision Res* 1970; 10:107-108

McBrien N, Sahebjada S, Arumugam B, Chow A, Jobling AI, Gentle A. Role of M4 receptor antagonist in control of myopic eye growth. *Invest. Ophthalmol. Vis. Sci.* 2009 E-Abstract #3850.

McCaa CS. The Eye and Visual Nervous System: Anatomy, Physiology and Toxicology. *Environmental Health Perspectives* 1982;44: 1-8.

Medeiros FA, Zangwill LM, Bowd C, et al. Agreement between stereophotographic and confocal scanning laser ophthalmoscopy measurements of cup/disc ratio: effect on a predictive model for glaucoma development. *J Glaucoma.* 2007;16:209-214

Medeiros FA, ZangwillLM, Bowd C, et al. Evaluation of retinal nerve fiber layer, optic nerve head, and macular thickness measurements for glaucoma detection using optical coherence tomography. *Am J Ophthalmol.* 2005;139:44-55.

Meek KM, Boote C. The organization of collagen in the corneal stroma. *Exp Eye Res* 2004; 78:503-512.

Melberg NS, Williams DF, Balles MW, et al. Vitrectomy for vitreomacular traction syndrome with macular detachment. *Retina.* 1995;15:192-197

Migliori ME, Gladstone GJ. Determination of the normal range of exophthamometric values for black and white adults. *Am J Ophthalmol* 1984;98(4):438-442.

Miller, N.R., Newman, N.J.: Anatomy and physiology of the retina and optic nerve: Distinguishing retinal from optic nerve disease (chapter 2). Anomalies of the optic disc (chapter 3). Topical diagnosis of acquired optic nerve disorders (chapter 4). In: Miller, N.R., Newman, N.J. (eds.) Walsh and Hoyt's Clinical Neuro-Ophthalmology. The essentials, 5th edn, pp. 59–166. Williams & Wilkins, Baltimore 1999

Min KH, Seong GJ, Hong YJ, et al. Optic nerve head topographic measurements and retinal nerve fiber layer thickness in physiologic large cups. *Korean J Ophthalmol.* 2005;19:189-194

Minckler, D.S.: The organization of nerve fiber bundles in the primate optic nerve head. *Arch. Ophthalmol* 1980; 98, 1630– 1636 .

Monteiro ML. Anterior ischemic optic neuropathy: a comparison of the optic disc area of patients with the arteritic and non-arteritic forms of the disease and that of normal controls. *Arq Bras Oftalmol.* 2006;69:805-810

Mrejen S R, Spaide RF. Optical coherence tomography imaging of the choroid and beyond.. *Surv Ophthalmol* 2013;58:387-429.

Müller LJ, Pels E, Vrensen GFJM. The specific architecture of the anterior stroma accounts for maintenance of corneal curvature. *Br J Ophthalmol* 2001; 85:437–443. Available at: http://www.ncbi.nlm.nih.gov/pmc/articles/PMC1723934/pdf/v085p00437.pdf. Accessed November 24, 2010

Mwanza JC,Oakley JD, Budenz DL, et al. Ability of Cirrus HDOCT optic nerve head parameters to discriminate normal from glaucomatous eyes. *Ophthalmology.* 2011;118:241-248.

Na JH, Moon BG, Sung KR, et al. Characterization of peripapillary atrophy using spectral domain optical coherence tomography. *Korean J Ophthalmol* 2010;24:353-359.

Nagai-Kusuhara A, Nakamura M, Tatsumi Y, et al. Disagreement between Heidelberg Retina Tomograph and optical coherence tomography in assessing optic nerve head configuration of eyes with band atrophy and normal eyes. *Br J Ophthalmol* 2008;92:1382-1386

Neubauer AS, Krieglstein TR, Chryssafis C, et al. Comparison of optical coherence tomography and fundus photography for measuring the optic disc size. *Ophthalmic Physiol Opt.* 2006;26:13-18.

Newell FW. Ophthalmology. Principles and concepts. Sixth edition. The C.V. Mosby Company, St Louis, 1986.

Newell, F.: Anatomy and embryology. In: Newell, F. (ed.) Ophthalmology. Principles and Concepts, 8th edn, pp. 3–73. St. Mosby, Louis 1996.

Newman, E.A.: Müller cells and the retinal pigment epithelium. In: Albert, D.A., Jakobiec, F.A. (eds.) Principles and Practice of Ophthalmology, 2nd edn, pp. 1763–1785. Saunders, Philadelphia 2000

Nickla DL, Wallman J. The multifunctional choroid. *Prog Retin Eye Res.* 2010 March ; 29(2): 144–168. doi:10.1016/j.preteyeres.2009.12.002.

Ogden, T.E.: Nerve fiber layer of the macaque retina: retinotopic organization. *Invest. Ophthalmol. Vis. Sci* 1983; 24, 85-98.

Oliveira-Soto L, Efron N. Morphology of corneal nerves using confocal microscopy. *Cornea* 2001; 20:374-384

Olmedo M, Cadarso-Suarez C, Gomez-Ulla F, et al. Reproducibility of optic nerve head measurements obtained by optical coherence tomography. *Eur J Ophthalmol.* 2005; 15:486—492

Olver, J.M., McCartney, A.C.E.: Orbital and ocular microvascular corrosion casting in man. *Eye* 1989;3, 588–596.

Olver, J.M., Spalton, D.J., McCartney, A.C.E.: Microvascular study of the retrolaminar optic nerve in man: The possible significance on anterior ischaemic optic neuropathy. *Eye* 1990;4, 7–24 .

Oyster, C.: Blood supply and drainage (Chapter 6). In: Oyster, C. (ed.) The Human Eye – Structure and Function, pp. 247–289. Sinauer Associates, Sunderland, Massachusetts 1999

Oyster, C.: Retinal III: regional variation and spatial organization (Chapter 15). In: Oyster, C. (ed.) The Human Eye – Structure and Function, pp. 649–700. Sinauer Associates, Sunderland, Massachusetts 1999

Oyster, C.: Retinal III: regional variation and spatial organization (Chapter 15). In: Oyster, C. (ed.) The Human Eye – Structure and Function, pp. 649–700. Sinauer Associates, Sunderland, Massachusetts 1999.

Panda Jonas S, Jonas JB, Jakobczyk Zmija M. Retinal photoreceptor density decreases with age. *Ophthalmology.* 1995;102:1853-1859.

Panda Jonas S, Jonas JB, Jakobczyk Zmija M. Retinal pigment epithelial cell count, distribution, and correlations in normal human eyes. *Am J Ophthalmol.* 1996;121:181-189

Panda-Jonas, S., Jonas, J.B., Jakobczk-Zmija, M.: Retinal pigment epithelial cell count, distribution and correlations in normal human eyes. *Am. J. Ophthalmol* 1996; 121, 181–189.

Park DJJ, Karesh J. Topographic anatomy of the eye: an overview.Chapter 1.Tasman W and Jaeger EA, editors. In Duane's Ophthalmology on CD Rom, Philadelphia: Lippincott Williams & Wilkins, 2006 edition.

Park SC, De Moraes CG, Tello C, et al. In vivo microstructural anatomy of beta-zone parapapillary atrophy in glaucoma. *Invest Ophthalmol Vis Sci.* 2010;51:6408-6413.

Paunescu LA, Schuman JS, Price LL, et al. Reproducibility of nerve fiber thickness, macular thickness, and optic nerve head measurements using StratusOCT. *Invest Ophthalmol Vis Sci.* 2004;45:1716-1724

Pettigrew JD, Wallman J, Wildsoet C. Saccadic oscillations facilitate ocular perfusion from the avian pecten. *Nature* 1990;343:362-363.

Phelps Brown N, Bron AJ. Lns structure . In: Phelps Brown N, Bron AJ, Phelps Brown NA, eds. Lens disorders: aclinical manual of cataract diagnosis. *Oxford Butterworth-Heinemann*,1996:32-47.

Polse KA, Brand RJ, Cohen SR, Guillon M. Hypoxic effects on corneal morphology and function. *Invest Ophthalmol Vis Sci* 1990; 31:1542–1554. Available at: http://www.iovs.org/content/ 31/8/1542.full.pdf. Accessed November 23, 2010

Provis, J.M., Diaz, C.M., Dreher, B.: Ontogeny of the primate fovea: a central issue in retinal development. *Prog. Neurobiol* 1998; 54, 549-580.

Provis, J.M., Penfold, P.L., Cornish, E.E., Sandercoe, T.M., Madigan, M.C.: Anatomy and development of the macula: specialisation and the vulnerability to macular degeneration. *Clin. Exp. Optometry* 2005; 88, 269-281.

Provis, J.M.: Development of the primate retinal vasculature. *Prog. Ret. Eye Res* 2001; 20, 799-821.

Racette L, Boden C, Kleinhandler SL, et al. Differences in visual function and optic nerve structure between healthy eyes of blacks and whites. *Arch Ophthalmol.* 2005;123: 1547-1553.

Radius, R.H., Anderson, D.R.: The histology of retinal nerve fiber layer bundles and bundle defects. *Arch. Ophthalmol* 1979; 97, 948-950.

Ramakrishnan R, Kader MA, Budde WM. Optic disc morphometry with optical coherence tomography: comparison with planimetry of fundus photographs and influence of parapapillary atrophy and pigmentary conus. *Indian J Ophthalmol.* 2005;53:187-191

Ramrattan RS, van der Schaft TL, Mooy CM, de Bruijn WC, Mulder PGH, de Jong P. Morphometric analysis of Bruch's membrane, the choriocapillaris and the choroid in aging. Invest. *Ophthalmol. Vis. Sci* 1994;35:2857-2864.

Ramratten RS, van der Schaft TL, Mooy CM, et al. Morphometric analysis of Bruch's membrane, the choriocapillaris, and the choroid in aging. *Invest Ophthalmol Vis Sci.* 1994;35: 2857-2864.

Rekic A, Breznik M, Cvenkel B. Çomparison of optic nerve head topography in healthy adults using a Heidelberg retina tomograph and retinal thickness analyzer. *Int Ophthalmol.* 2007;27:1-9

Rensch F, Jonas JB. Direct microperimetry of alpha zone and beta zone parapapillary atrophy. *Br J Ophthalmol.* 2008;92:1617-1619

Reus NJ, Lemij HG. Relationships between standard automated perimetry, HRT confocal scanning laser ophthalmoscopy, and GDx VCC scanning laser polarimetry. *Invest Ophthalmol Vis Sci.* 2005;46:4182-4188

Rimmer, S., Keating, C., Chou, T., Farb, M.D., Christenson, P.D., Foos, R.Y., Bateman, J.B.: Growth of the human optic disk and nerve during gestation, childhood, and early adulthood. *Am. J. Ophthalmol* 1993; 116, 748–753.

Roof, D.J., Makino, C.L.: The structure and function of retinal photoreceptors. In: Albert, D.A., Jakobiec, F.A. (eds.) Principles and Practice of Ophthalmology, 2nd edn, pp. 1624–1673. Saunders, Philadelphia 2000.

Rotchford AP, Johnson GJ. Glaucoma in Zulus: a population- based cross-sectional survey in a rural district in South Africa. *Arch Ophthalmol.* 2002;120:471-478

Ruangvaravate N, Neungton C. Normative data of optic nerve head in Thai population by laser scanning tomography: Siriraj study. *J Med Assoc Thai.* 2008;91:859-863

Rudnicka AR, Frost C, Owen CG, et al. Nonlinear behavior of certain optic nerve head parameters and their determinants in normal subjects. *Ophthalmology.* 2001;108: 2358-2368

Rüfer F, Schröder A, Erb C. White-to-white corneal diameter; normal values in healthy humans obtained with the Orbscan II topography system. *Cornea* 2005; 24:259-261.

Rutin U. Fundus appearance in the normal eye. I. The choroid. *Am J Ophthalmol* 1967;64:821-839.

Sacks J. The shape of the trochlea. *Arch Ophthalmol* 1984;102:932.

Sadun AA, Johnson BM, Smith LEH. Neuroanatomy of the human visual system: Part II. Retinal projections to the superior colliculus and pulvinar. *Neuroophthalmology* 1986;363-370.

Sadun AA, Johnson BM, Smith LEH. Neuroanatomy of the human visual system: Part II. Retinal projections to the superior colliculus and pulvinar. *Neuroophthalmology* 1986;363-370.

Sadun AA, Johnson BM., Schaecter J. Neuroanatomy of the human visual system: Part III. Three retinal projections to the hypothalamus. *Neuroophthalmology* 1986;6:371-379.

Sadun AA, Johnson BM., Schaecter J. Neuroanatomy of the human visual system: Part III. Three retinal projections to the hypothalamus. *Neuroophthalmology* 1986;6:371-379.

Sadun AA. Neuroanatomy of the human visual system: Part I. Retinal projections to the LGN and pretectum as demonstrated with a new stain. *Neuroophthalmology* 1986;6:353-361.

Saint-Geniez, M., D'Amore, P.A.: Development and pathology of the hyaloid, choroidal and retinal vasculature. *Int. J. Dev. Biol* 2004; 48, 1045–1058.

Saito H, Tomidokoro A, Tomita G, et al. Optic disc and peripapillary morphology in unilateral nonarteritic anterior ischemic optic neuropathy and age- and refractionmatched normals. *Ophthalmology.* 2008;115:1585-1590.

Samarawickrama C, Hong T, Jost B. Jonas JB, Mitchell P. Measurement of Normal Optic Nerve Head Parameters. *Surv Ophthalmol* 2012; 57:317-336.

Sampaolesi R, Sampaolesi JR. Large optic nerve heads: megalopapilla or megalodiscs. *Int Ophthalmol.* 2001;23: 251-257

Sarks SH. New vessel formation beneath the retinal pigment epithelium in senile eyes. *Br J Ophthalmol.* 1973;57:951-965.

Saude T. The internalocular media. In: Ocular anatomy and physiology, Oxford: *Blackwell Scientific*; 1993:36-52.

Savini G, Espana EM, Acosta AC, et al. Agreement between optical coherence tomography and digital stereophotography in vertical cup-to-disc ratio measurement. *Graefes Arch Clin Exp Ophthalmol.* 2009;247:377-383

Savini G, Zanini M, Carelli V, et al. Correlation between retinal nerve fibre layer thickness and optic nerve head size: an optical coherence tomography study. *Br J Ophthalmol.* 2005;89:489-492

Schnaudigel, O.: Die Vitalfärbung mit Trypanblau am Auge. Albrecht von Graefes Arch. *Ophthalmol* 1913; 86, 93–97.

Sealand JH. The lens capsule and zonulae. Acta Ophthalmol 1992; 70:7-12.

Sebag J , Balazs E A. Morphology and ultrastructure of human vitreous fibers . *Invest Ophthalmol Vis Sci.* 1989; 30: 187 – 91.

Sebag J . Age-related changes in human vitreous structure. *Graefes Arch Clin Exp Ophthalmol.* 1987; 225: 89 – 93 .

Sebag J . Age-related diff erences in the human vitreoretinal interface. *Arch Ophthalmol.* 1991; 109: 966 – 71.

Sebag J . Anatomy and pathology of the vitreo-retinal interface. *Eye.* 1992; 6: 541 52.

Sebag J . Letter to the editor. *Arch Ophthalmol.* 1991; 109: 1059 – 60 .

Sebag J . Surgical anatomy of vitreous and the vitreoretinal interface. In: Tasman W, Jaeger E , eds. Clinical ophthalmology, Vol 6 Philadelphia: JB Lippincott; 1994: 1 – 36.

Sebag J . The Vitreous-Structure, Function, and Pathobiology. New York: Springer-Verlag; 1989.

Sebag J. The Vitreous: structure, function, and pathobiology. New York: Springer-Verlag, 1989

Seefelder, R.: Die Entwicklung des menschlichen Auges. In: Schieck, F., Brückner, A. (eds.) Kurzes Handbuch der Ophthalmologie, pp. 476–518. Springer, Berlin 1930.

Sharma, R.K., Ehinger, B.E.J.: Development and structure of the retina. In: Kaufman, P.L., Alm, A. (eds.) Adler's Physiology of the Eye, 10th edn, 2003 pp. 319–347. Mosby, St Louis 2003.

Sharma, R.K., Ehinger, B.E.J.: Development and structure of the retina. In: Kaufman, P.L., Alm, A. (eds.) Adler's Physiology of the Eye, 10th edn, pp. 319–347. Mosby, St Louis 2003

Shine NP, Coates H. Systemic ototoxicity: a review. *East Afr Med J.* 2005;82:536-539.

Sihota R, Srinivasan G, Dada T, et al. Is the ISNT rule violated in early primary open-angle glaucoma—a scanning laser tomography study. *Eye.* 2008;22:819-824.

Simon G, Ren Q. Biomechanical behavior of the cornea and its response to radial keratotomy. *J Refract Corneal Surg* 1994; 10:343–351; comments by RK Maloney, ST Feldman, K Buzard, G Simon, Q Ren, 351-356

Snell RS, Lemp MA. The eyeball. Clinical anatomy of the eye. Oxford: Blackwell Scientific; 1989:119-194.

Soubrane G, Bressler NM. Treatment of subfoveal choroidal neovascularisation in age related macular degeneration: focus on clinical application of verteporfin photodynamic therapy. *Br J Ophthalmol.* 2001;85:483-495

Spencer WH. Chapter 3. Cornea. In: Spencer WH, ed. Ophthalmic Pathology. An Atlas and Textbook. 4th ed. Philadelphia, PA: W. B. Saunders, Co.; 1996:157–333.

Spencer WH. Chapter 4. Sclera. In: Spencer WH, ed. Ophthalmic Pathology. An Atlas and Textbook. 4th ed. Philadelphia, PA: W. B. Saunders, Co.; 1996:334–371.

Spencer WH. Chapter 8. Vitreous. In: Spencer WH, ed. Ophthalmic Pathology. An Atlas and Textbook. 4th ed. Philadelphia, PA: W. B. Saunders, Co.; 1996:623-666.

Sterling P. Deciphering the retina's wiring diagram. *Nat Neurosci.* Oct 1999;2(10):851-853.

Stevenson TC. Intrascleral nerve loops: a clinical study of frequency and treatment. *Am J Ophthalmol* 1963; 55:935

Stiemke MM, Edelhauser HF, Geroski DH. The developing corneal endothelium: correlation of morphology, hydration and Na/K ATPase pump site density. *Curr Eye Res* 1991; 10: 145–156

Strauss, O.: The retinal pigment epithelium in visual function. *Physiol. Rev* 2005; 85, 845–881

Streeten BW, Eshaghian J. Human posterior subcapsular cataract: a gross and flat preparation study. *Arch Ophthalmol.* 1978;96:1653-1658.

Tekeli O, Turacli ME, Atmaca LS, et al. Evaluation of the optic nerve head with the heidelberg retina tomograph in diabetes mellitus. *Ophthalmologica.* 2008;222:168-172

Tessier-Lavigne, M.: Visual processing by the retina. In: Kandel, E.R., Schwartz, J.H., Jessell, T.M. (eds.) Principles of Neural Science, 4th edn, pp. 507–522. McGraw-Hill, New York 2000

Thomas R, George R, Muliyil J, et al. Correlation of confocal laser scanning tomography with planimetric photographic measurements of the optic disc in a normal South Indian population: the Vellore Eye Study. *Indian J Ophthalmol.* 2005;53:289-294

Thumann, G., Hoffmann, S., Hinton, D.R.: Cell biology of the retinal pigment epithelium. In: Ryan, S.J. (ed). Retina, 4th (ed), pp. 137–152. Elsevier-Mosby, St. Louis 2006

Tong L, Chan YH, Gazzard G, et al. Heidelberg retinal tomography of optic disc and nerve fiber layer in Singapore children: variations with disc tilt and refractive error. *Invest Ophthalmol Vis Sci.* 2007;48:4939-4944

Topouzis F, Coleman AL, Harris A, et al. Association of blood pressure status with the optic disk structure in nonglaucoma subjects: the Thessaloniki eye study. *Am J Ophthalmol.* 2006;142:60-67

Tripathi RC, Tripathi BJ. Functional anatomy of the anterior chamber angle. In Duane TD, Jaeger EA (eds): Biomedical Foundations of Ophthalmology. Philadelphia: Lippincott, 1982

Tripathi RC, Tripathi BJ. Human trabecular endothelium, corneal endothelium, keratocytes, and scleral fibroblasts in primary cell culture. A comparative study of growth characteristics, morphology, and phagocytic activity by light and scanning electron microscopy. *Exp Eye Res* 1982;35:611

Tsai, C.S., Zangwill, L., Gonzalez, C., Irak, I., Garden, V., Hoffman, R., Weinreb, R.N.: Ethnic differences in optic nerve head topography. *J. Glaucoma* 1995; 4(4), 248-257.

Uchida H, Yamamoto T, Araie M, et al. Topographic characteristics of the optic nerve head measured with scanning laser tomography in normal Japanese subjects. *Jpn J Ophthalmol.* 2005;49:469-476.

Uysal Y, Bayer A, Erdurman C, et al. Sensitivity and specificity of Heidelberg Retinal Tomography II parameters in detecting early and moderate glaucomatous damage: effect of disc size. *Clin Experiment Ophthalmol.* 2007;35:113-118

Van Heynigen R. What happens to the human lens in cataract. *Sci Am.* 1976;233:70-81.

van Koolwijk LM, Despriet DD, van Duijn CM, et al. Genetic contributions to glaucoma: heritability of intraocular pressure, retinal nerve fiber layer thickness, and optic disc morphology. *Invest Ophthalmol Vis Sci.* 2007;48:3669-3676

Vannas S, Teir H. Observations on structure and age changes in the human sclera. *Acta Ophthalmol* 1960; 38:268

Vessani RM,Moritz R, Batis L, et al.Comparison of quantitative imaging devices and subjective optic nerve head assessment by general ophthalmologists to differentiate normal from glaucomatous eyes. *J Glaucoma.* 2009;18:253-261

Wajer SD, Taomoto M, McLeod DS, McCally RL, Nishiwaki H, Fabry RL, Lutty GA. Velocity measurements of normal and sickle cell red blood cells in the rat retinal and choroidal vasculatures. *Microvasc. Res* 2000;60:281-293.

Wang XY, Huynh SC, Burlutsky G, et al. Reproducibility of and effect of magnification on optical coherence tomography measurements in children. *Am J Ophthalmol.* 2007; 143:484-488

Wang Y, Xu L, Zhang L, et al. Peripapillary atrophy in elderly Chinese in rural and urban Beijing. *Eye.* 2008;22:261-266

Watsky MA, McDermott ML, Edelhauser HF. In vitro corneal endothelial permeability in rabbit and human: the effects of age, cataract surgery and diabetes. *Exp Eye Res* 1989; 49. 751-767

Watson PG, Young RD. Scleral structure, organization and disease. A review. *Exp. Eye Res* 2004;78:609-623.

Weale RA. A Biography of the Eye: Development, Growth Age. London: H.K. Lewis, 1982

Whikehart DRA, Parikh CH, Vaughn A, Mishler K, Edelhauser HF. Evidence suggesting the existence of stem cells for the human corneal endothelium. *Mol Vis.* 2005;11:816-824.

Whitnall S: The Anatomy of the Human Orbit and Accessory Organs of Vision. London: Oxford University Press, 1932

Wiley L, SundarRaj N, Sun T-T, Thoft RA. Regional heterogeneity in human corneal and limbal epithelia: an immunohistochemical evaluation. *Invest Ophthalmol Vis Sci* 1991; 32:594-602. Available at: http://www.iovs.org/content/32/3/594.full.pdf. Accessed November 24, 2010

Williams KK, Noe RL, Grossniklaus HE, Drews-Botsch C, Edelhauser HF. Correlation of histologic corneal endothelial cell counts with specular microscopic cell density. *Arch Ophthalmol.* 1992;110:1146-1149.

Williams, T.D., Wilkinson, J.M.: Position of the fovea centralis with respect to the optic nerve head. *Optom. Vis. Sci* 1992; 69, 369-377.

Wilson, C., Theodorou, M., Cocker, K.D., Fielder, A.: The temporal retinal blood vessels and preterm birth. *Br. J. Ophthalmol.* 2006;90(6), 702–704.

Wolfensberger, T.J.: The historical discovery of the retinal pigment epithelium. In: Marmor, M.F., Wolfensberger, T.J. (eds.) The Retinal Pigment Epithelium, pp. 13–22. Oxford University, Oxford 1998

Wollstein G, Ishikawa H, Wang J, et al. Comparison of three optical coherence tomography scanning areas for detection of glaucomatous damage.*Am J Ophthalmol.* 2005;139:39-43

Wurtz, R.H., Kandel, E.R.: Central visual pathways. In: Kandel, E.R., Schwartz, J.H., Jessell, T.M. (eds.) Principles of Neural Science, 4th edn, pp. 523–547. McGraw-Hill, New York 2000

Xu J, Ishikawa H, Wollstein G, et al. Automated assessment of the optic nerve head on stereo disc photographs. *Invest Ophthalmol Vis Sci.* 2008;49:2512-2517

Xu L, Wang Y, Yang H, et al. Size of the neuroretinal rim and optic cup and their correlations with ocular and general parameters in adult Chinese: the Beijing eye study. *Br J Ophthalmol.* 2007;91:1616-1619

Yee RW, Matsuda M, Schultz RO, Edelhauser HF. Changes in the normal corneal endothelial cellular pattern as a function of age. *Curr Eye Res* 1985; 4:671-678

Yeh S, Foroozan R. Orbital apex syndrome. *Curr Opin Ophthalmol* 2004;15:490-498.

Zangwill LM, Weinreb RN, Berry CC, et al. Racial differences in optic disc topography: baseline results from the confocal scanning laser ophthalmoscopy ancillary study to the ocular hypertension treatment study. *Arch Ophthalmol.* 2004;122:22-28

Zhu, M., Madigan, M.C., Van Driel, D., Maslim, J., Billson, F., Provis, J.M., Penfold, P.L.: The human hyaloid system: cell death and vascular regression. *Exp. Eye Res* 2000; 70, 767-776.

Chapter IV

Geometrical Optics

Abstract

This chapter presents the theory of geometrical optics with the application of theory to clinical practice. Geometrical optics deals with the formation of image by rays of optical instruments (like lenses, prisms and mirrors) and the various pathways light travels as it moves from an object, through an optical system, and, ultimately, arrives at the image.

An important aspect of geometrical optics is the ability to predict image position and size theoretically (given the object position and lens power) without going to the trouble of doing the experiment. Physical optics deals with the nature of light itself (*e.g.*, electromagnetic waves and photons).

Image properties depend primarily on the routes light travels rather than on the nature of light per se. The refracting lane is an ideal laboratory for demonstrating the principles of geometrical optics (Thall, 2006).

1. Definitions

The word *lens* may refer to a single piece of glass (or other material) or to a combination of individual lenses assembled to function as a unit. *Element* refers specifically to an individual lens.

A common photographic lens consisting of six individual elements. A rotationally symmetric optical system has an axis of symmetry called the *optical axis*). Most optical systems consist of several lenses symmetrically arranged along a common axis. Rotating the system about the axis does not alter the imaging characteristics. Rotationally asymmetric systems do not have an axis.

A *vertex* is any intersection of the axis with a lens surface. At the vertex, the axis is normal (*i.e.*, perpendicular) to the lens surface. The vertices are the intersections of the lens surfaces with the axis. The axis is perpendicular to the lens surfaces at the vertices.

Objects

An object may be luminous or nonluminous. A *luminous object* or *source* produces light and is visible in otherwise total darkness. Every point on a luminous object (e.g., candle flame) radiates light in all directions. *Nonluminous objects* do not produce light and are visible only when illuminated by a source. When light strikes a point on a nonluminous object, it is *diffusely reflected* or scattered in all directions (diffuse reflection).

Diffuse reflection should not be confused with *specular reflection.* In specular reflection, light (the incident light) symmetrically rebounds in a single direction (e.g., mirrors) instead of scattering in many directions (objects). From the standpoint of geometrical optics, the most important characteristic of an object, whether luminous or nonluminous, is that every point of the object radiates light in all directions (diffuse reflection).

A *point source* occupies no volume (*i.e.,* a point in the mathematical sense) and radiates light in all directions. Point sources do not exist, but conceptually, objects are simply a collection of point sources. Every object point is a point source radiating in all directions. Point sources simplify the analysis of optical systems by making it possible to deal with one object point at a time.

The Stigmatic Image

The word *stigmatic* derives from the Greek "stigma," meaning stylus or point, and emphasizes the point-to-point nature of the stigmatic image.

Each point on a screen (*e.g.,* piece of paper) placed near an object receives light from many object points, and no image appears. An appropriate lens placed between screen and object redirects light so that each point on the screen receives light from a single object point, thereby producing an image. Without the lens, light from a single object point distributes over the entire screen, mixing with light from every other object point. With the lens, however, light from a single object point falls on a single screen point and does not mix with light from any other object point. The lens redirects light so that each point on the screen receives light from only one object point. An image is produced. The image is defined as a point or extended source that the pencil/beam of rays go to.

The one-to-one correspondence between object and image points is the essential feature of the *stigmatic image.* Imaging is a two-step process. In the first step, an object distributes light in all directions. This is an important step. If an object radiates light in only one direction, then it will be visible from only one vantage point. It would be visible to only one observer. Scattering light makes objects visible from many directions simultaneously. Objects scatter in many directions and thus are visible to several observers simultaneously. Although beneficial, scattering necessitates a second step, the redirection of light by an optical system to produce an image.

The Ideal Image

Besides stigmatism, there are other desirable image properties. The image of a flat object that is normal to the axis should, likewise, be flat and normal to the axis. Some lenses produce stigmatic, but curved, images. The technical term for this is *field curvature.* Photographic film is usually flat. A photograph of a curved image taken with flat film is out of focus at the edges. Non-ideal optical systems may image planes perpendicular to the axis as curved surfaces. If this is a camera using a flat piece of film, the photograph will be blurry at the edges. The retina is curved, but the macula is flat. Only the macula is capable of high acuity, so field curvature is undesirable in the eye.

However, an enlarged image differs from the original object by only a scale factor. Distortion is a greater disruption of the image. No simple change in scale can make a distorted image resemble the object.

Field curvature and distortion are not always undesirable. Photographers use distortion for aesthetic effects. Panoramic cameras have field curvature but use curved film to compensate. Nevertheless, geometrical optics defines the *ideal image* as stigmatic and free of field curvature or distortion. The ideal image may be enlarged, reduced, or inverted with respect to the object.

Rays

A *ray* is an abstract representation of a light path. An arrow indicates the propagation direction. Rays represent paths, not the light moving along those paths. A ray gives no indication of the physical characteristics (*e.g.,* intensity, wavelength, and so forth) of the light traveling along the ray.

It may seem somewhat pedantic, but lenses bend light, not rays. When a ray strikes the surface of a lens or mirror, it does not deviate. The light moving along the ray changes direction and begins to move along a new ray. Rays continue straight through the surface of a mirror or a lens, but the light does not Technically, a ray never deviates. The ray extends as a straight line to infinity. Lenses (or mirrors) do not change the ray's direction. At the lens, the light traveling along the ray changes direction. The light stops moving along the object ray and begins moving along the image ray. Rays extend infinitely in both directions. Light travels over only a segment of the ray. The distinction between a ray and the light moving along a ray becomes important later when dealing with pupils and virtual images. For clarity, illustrations usually show only the portion of a ray over which light travels, but rays are straight and infinite in extent.

It must be noted that it is common practice and more economical to use statements such as "the lens bends the ray" instead of "the lens bends light traveling along the ray." Of course, the implication is that the light bends, not the ray.

Any ray that intersects the object point is an *object ray.* Similarly, *image rays* intersect the image point. Object rays represent light before it has entered the optical system, and image rays represent light after it emerges from the system. Every object ray entering an optical system gives rise to a unique image ray. Thus, every object ray is associated with a unique image ray, and vice versa.

An *ideal lens* is a rotationally symmetric optical system that produces an ideal image of any object. At this point the imaging properties of the lens are the main concern, and there is no need to worry about how many elements are in the lens or any other aspects of its construction. Consequently, ideal lenses are illustrated as "black boxes".

Objects are usually three-dimensional, but it is easier to describe optical properties using flat objects confined to planes. An *object plane* is normal to the axis and contains an object. Every point in an object plane is a potential object point or point source. Image planes are normal to the axis, and every point in the image plane is a potential image point.

Conjugate refers, in a rather general way, to the object-image relationship. Let O and O' be, respectively, an object point and its image. O is conjugate to O'. Similarly, O' is conjugate to O.

Collectively, O and O' constitute a pair of conjugate points.

Transverse magnification is the ratio of image height to object height. Two aspects of magnification are confusing. In common parlance, magnification implies enlargement, but in optics, magnification applies to any image whether larger or smaller than the object. Images are scale models of the object, and magnification is the scale factor. Magnification also indicates the image's orientation with respect to the object. A negative magnification indicates an inverted image. For example, a magnification of -2 means the image is inverted and twice the size of the object. A magnification of 0.5 indicates that the image is upright and half the size of the original.

Transverse magnification applies to linear dimension. Thus, a 1-inch-wide, 2-inch-high object magnified by a factor of two gives a 2-inch-wide, 4-inch-high image. Both the height and width change by a factor of two, increasing the image's area by a factor of four.

The ratio of the image size to the object size or image vergence to object vergence is called transverse or linear magnification. $M\,T = I/O = U/V = v/u$

2. Properties of Ideal Lenses

The ideal lens produces a one-to-one correspondence between object points and image points. Consequently, no two object points share the same image point. Thus, necessarily, the image of every object point has a different location in space.

This reasoning extends to every point on an object ray. Every point on an object ray has a unique image point, and the image ray associated with the object ray passes through all of these image points. The object ray and its associate image ray are conjugate. To summarize, light moving along an object ray enters an optical system, deviates, and emerges, traveling along an image ray. Every point on the object ray must have an image somewhere on the image ray.

From a clinical viewpoint, the most important property of ideal lenses deals with object and image planes. Associated with every object plane is a unique image plane. Every point in the object plane has an image somewhere in the associated image plane (*i.e.,* the object and image planes are conjugate). No two object planes share the same image plane; every object plane has an image plane in a different location. This property seems inconsistent with daily experience. To be seen clearly, the image must be on the retina. According to this property, only one object can have an image plane on the retina at any one time; despite this fact, everything in a scene seems to be in focus simultaneously.

How can the properties of imaging systems be reconciled with common experience? First, the impression that all objects in a scene are in focus simultaneously is not correct. We have a mistaken notion that everything is in focus simultaneously because we pay attention only to part of a scene at any one time. As we shift our attention, the eye keeps various objects in focus by varying accommodation. Nevertheless, many objects are simultaneously in focus despite being various distances from the observer. This is due to depth-of-focus.

In any case, image position changes as object position changes. Magnification also changes with object position. Image position also depends on lens power.

3. Infinite Conjugates and Focal Planes

As the distance between an object point and lens increases, the object rays tend to become parallel. It takes a little imagination, but rays from an infinitely distant object point are parallel. When the infinitely distant object point is on the optical axis, the object rays will be parallel to each other and parallel to the axis. If the distant object point is not on the axis, the object rays are still parallel to each other, but not parallel to the axis. The amount of divergence of the light is inversely proportional to the distance from the source. If the distance is expressed in meters, the vergence is in units of diopters: 1/Distance in Meters = Diopters.

Rays from an infinitely distant object point on the axis yield rays parallel to the axis. Rays from an infinitely distant object off axis yield rays parallel to each other but not parallel to the axis.

When the rays emerging from a lens are strongly convergent, the image is close to the lens. The less divergent the rays, the farther the image from the lens. If the image rays are parallel, the image point is at infinity. Image rays parallel to each other and also parallel to the axis give an infinitely distant image point on the axis. Image rays parallel to each other but not parallel to the axis give infinitely distant image points off-axis.

Objects that are not infinitely distant but far away give rays that are nearly parallel. Objects 20 feet (6 m) or more distant give rays so close to parallel that, for clinical purposes, they may be considered at infinity.

Object rays parallel to each other and to the axis produce image rays that converge at the *secondary focal point*. Because the object rays arose from an infinitely distant object point, the secondary focal point is the image of an on-axis object point at infinity. The *secondary focal plane* is normal to the axis through the secondary focal point. Off-axis points at infinity image at various points on the secondary focal plane.

An object point at the primary focal point produces image rays that are parallel to each other and the axis. Thus, the primary focal point's image is on-axis at infinity. The primary focal plane is normal to the axis through the primary focal point. Object points on the primary focal plane give image rays that are parallel to each other but not necessarily parallel to the axis.

4. Graphically Locating the Image

This section describes a means of locating the image using a graphical technique called *ray sketching*.

Image location partially depends on the properties of the lens. Thus, it is impossible to locate an image by any method without some specific information about the lens. In ray sketching, the *cardinal points* contain the lens information.

Consider an ideal lens. For every object plane there is a unique conjugate image plane and a unique magnification. There is one pair of conjugate planes that yields a magnification exactly equal to 1. In other words, an object located at P has an image in plane P', and the image has the same size and orientation as the original object. This specific pair of conjugate planes is called the *principal planes* or *planes of unit magnification.* The object plane P is the *primary principal plane,* and the image plane P' is the *secondary principal plane. The points of intersection of planes P and P' with the optical axis are, respectively, the primary and secondary principal points.*

The *nodal points* are another pair of useful landmarks located on the axis. An object ray passing through the primary nodal point is conjugate to an image ray passing through the secondary nodal point, and both rays make the same angle with the optical axis. There are no nodal planes associated with the nodal points.

The nodal point is the point in the eye where light entering or leaving the eye and passing through the nodal point, is undeviated. This allows similar triangles to be used to determine the retinal image size of an object in space. For example, to determine the retinal image size of a Snellen letter (viewed at 6 meters), the following formula would be used: Retinal image height/Snellen letter height = 17mm/6000mm.

Collectively, the principal, focal, and nodal points constitute the cardinal points of the optical system. All the information about the lens and its imaging properties is contained in the position of these points on the axis. Fundamentally, the only difference between two ideal imaging systems is the location of their cardinal points.

Ray Sketching

Starting with an ideal optical system, the task is to determine image location and size for a given object (Where is the image formed and what is the magnification?).

Step 1

Ignore the presence of the lenses because the locations of the cardinal points completely determine the properties of an ideal system. If necessary, redraw the object and optical system to scale using just the optical axis and cardinal points. Draw the principal planes through the principal points and normal to the axis.

Step 2

Pick some point on the object but not on the optical axis. Rays emanate from this point in all directions. In particular, one of these rays will be parallel to the optical axis. Draw the ray parallel to the axis from the object point to the primary principal plane.

Conceptually, this ray extends backward to infinity; in principle, this ray goes through the axial object point at infinity.

Step 3

The object ray drawn in step 2 goes through two important object points: 1) the axial object point at infinity and 2) a point on the primary principal plane (point M). The image ray must go through the images of these two object points. The image of M is M'. M' is a point on the secondary principal plane at the same height above the axis as point M because the principal planes are conjugate with a magnification of 1.

Thus, the image ray must go through M' and the secondary focal point. The image ray is drawn through these two points.

Step 4

Many other rays emanate from the object point, including one that goes through the primary image point F. Draw this ray and extend it to the principal plane.

Step 5

The ray drawn in step 5 must be conjugate to an image ray parallel to the axis (because the object ray goes through the primary focal point). The image ray must also pass through Q', the image of Q. Draw the second image ray through Q' and parallel to the axis.

Step 6

All the rays from the object point must intersect at the image point, so the two rays just drawn must also intersect at the image point. The intersection of the two image rays locates one image point.

The rest of the image is drawn normal to the axis (Draw the rest of the image perpendicular to the axis and through the image point. Because the drawing is to scale, the magnification can be found by measuring the object and image heights and taking the ratio.).

Step 7

Only two rays are necessary to locate the image, but it may help to draw a third ray from the object point to the primary nodal point N.

Step 8

The image ray conjugate to the object ray drawn in step 7 goes through the secondary nodal point and is parallel to the object ray. This ray should intersect the other two at the image point.

To summarize, rays emerge from an object point in all directions, and there is no easy way to determine the image rays associated with most of these object rays. However, for three special object rays, the conjugate image rays can be determined with the aid of the cardinal points. These three special object rays are: 1) the ray parallel to the axis, 2) the ray through the primary focal point F, and 3) the ray through the primary nodal point N. The intersection of the image rays conjugate to these object rays locates the image.

It is important to realize that ray sketching does not give the actual path of a ray within the lens itself. Ray sketching gives only the final image ray associated with a particular object ray.

With use of a different technique called *ray tracing,* it is possible to determine the exact path light follows. Ray tracing requires a detailed description of the optical system (not just the cardinal points) and considerable calculation. The strength of ray sketching is that it skips all the intermediate details and gives the correct result without calculation. The gain in simplicity comes at the expense of detailed information about the light path within the lens system itself.

5. Locating Images by Vergence

Light diverges from the object point and converges to the image point. Vergence is a quantitative measure of light's degree of convergence or divergence. When distance from an object point increases, divergence decreases. Similarly, as distance from the image point increases, convergence decreases. Thus, vergence is inversely proportional to distance from an object or image point. By convention, divergent light has a negative vergence, and convergent light has a positive vergence.

Vergence is a property of a ray, and every point on a ray has a different vergence. To give a concrete example, consider an object point 25 cm away from the primary principal plane of an ideal lens and 5 cm in front of the primary focal plane. When rays from the object point cross the primary focal plane, they have a vergence of -20.00 D. The vergence is negative because the light is divergent. The number 20.00 is the reciprocal of the distance in meters between the object point and focal plane (5 cm = 0.05 m, 1/0.05 = 20). The uppercase "D" is the standard abbreviation for *diopter.* The diopter is the standard unit of vergence used clinically. When the light reaches the primary principal plane, the vergence is -4.00 D. Again, the vergence is negative because the light is divergent. The number 4 is the reciprocal of the distance between the object point and principal plane (0.25 m).

Upon emerging from the lens, the light's vergence has changed. An ideal lens is simply a vergence changer. The power of the lens specifies the amount of vergence change the lens produces.

To give a second example, if the object point was 25 cm from the primary principal plane, then light (at the primary principal plane) would have a vergence of -4.00 D. The lens changes the vergence by + 5.00 D, giving light at the secondary principal plane a vergence of + 1.00 D. The image is 100 cm behind the secondary principal plane.

Vergence is the reciprocal of distance. Units of length, or distance, include inches, meters, centimeters, and so forth. Therefore, the units of vergence are reciprocal inches $(in)^{-1}$), reciprocal meters $(m)^{-1}$), reciprocal centimeters $(cm)^{-1}$), and so forth. Vergence is expressible in any of these inverse units. However, lens power and vergence add only when both are in the same units. To avoid confusion, it is universal clinical practice to use units of inverse meters for both vergence and lens power. The unit of diopter was created as a matter of convenience. By definition, one diopter equals one inverse meter.

It is conventional practice to round vergence to two decimal places, and the sign, whether positive or negative, should always be written. In most mathematical work, plus signs are redundant and not written, but the most common mistake in vergence calculations is inadvertently dropping a minus sign. Always writing the sign helps to prevent this.

Transverse magnification can be calculated by use of vergence. The ratio of object vergence to image vergence gives the transverse magnification.

Finally, note that parallel light rays neither converge nor diverge, and thus have a vergence of zero diopters. By convention, light from objects or images more than 20 feet away is so close to parallel that it is assigned a vergence of zero.

6. Virtual Images and Virtual Objects

Where is the image of an object 12.5 cm in front of a + 3.00 D lens? The object vergence is -8.00 D (at the lens), so the image vergence is -5.00 D. The negative vergence means that the image rays emerging from the lens are still divergent. Granted, the image rays are less divergent than the object rays (by three diopters in this case), but the image rays remain divergent. There is no real image, and this can be verified by use of a candle and trial lens.

Suppose a + 6.00 D lens is placed 5 cm behind the original + 3.00 D lens. The divergent light emerging from the first lens reaches the second lens, which does have enough power to converge light and form a real image. What is the location of the image formed by the second lens?

To answer this question, it is necessary to know the vergence of light incident on the second lens. Light has a vergence of -5.00 D when it emerges from the first lens, but the vergence changes as the light travels from the first lens to the second lens. The change in vergence produced simply by light moving from one place to another within the same medium is the *vergence change on transfer*. Because of the vergence change on transfer, it is necessary to determine the vergence of the light incident on the second lens.

Vergence is always related to the distance between an object or image point and some point of interest on the ray (such as the point where the ray meets the lens). Thus, to determine the vergence of the light incident on the second lens, the image rays emerging from the first lens must be associated with some image point. The image point is found by extending the divergent image rays backward until they meet at a common point. The image point is 20 cm in front of the first lens (found by taking the reciprocal of the vergence).

No light goes through this virtual image point. Light does not travel over the part of the image rays extended backward. The virtual image point is a mathematical construct; if a piece of paper is placed 20 cm in front of the first lens, no image will be observed. This mathematical construct is called virtual because it does not represent a real image. It is called an image because it is associated with the image rays emerging from the first lens.

The virtual image is 25 cm in front of the second lens. Thus, light incident on the second lens has a vergence of -4.00 D. Light emerging from the second lens has a vergence of + 2.00 D, giving an image 50 cm behind the second lens.

Next, consider an object far away from a + 2.00 D lens. The lens forms an image 50 cm behind itself. Where is the image if a + 6.00 D lens is placed 25 cm behind the first lens? Again, the vergence of the light incident on the second lens is the key issue. Light incident on a lens from a real object is always divergent. However, in this case, the light incident on the second lens is convergent. The convergent light is associated with an object point 50 cm behind the lens, but real objects are always in front of a lens. This example represents a virtual object. The virtual object is 25 cm behind the second lens, giving the incident light a vergence of + 4.00 D. Rays emerging from the second lens have a vergence of + 10.00 D, giving an image 10 cm behind the second lens.

It is often incorrectly stated that real images are always inverted and virtual images are erect. There is no inherent relationship between an image's orientation and its status as real or virtual. An image is real if the image rays are convergent, and virtual if the image rays are divergent. An object is real if the object rays are divergent, and virtual if the object rays are convergent.

7. Refractive Index

A *medium* is anything that light can travel through, such as glass, liquids, air, a vacuum, and even some metals. The speed of light varies in each medium. Light travels fastest in a vacuum and slower in any material medium.

Rather than deal directly with light's speed in a medium, it is usually more convenient to use *refractive index.* The refractive index of a medium is the ratio of light's speed in the vacuum to its speed in the medium. For example, the refractive index of spectacle crown glass is 1.523, indicating that light's speed in glass is about two-thirds its speed in a vacuum. Refractive index is always a number greater than or equal to 1. It is routine practice to use the lowercase letter “n” to indicate refractive index in formulas and equations.

Refractive index varies with wavelength. In general, the shorter the wavelength, the higher the refractive index. For instance, in spectacle crown glass, light of wavelength 656 nm (corresponding to red) has an index of 1.520, whereas light of wavelength 480 nm (corresponding to blue) has an index of 1.531. *Dispersion* is the variation of refractive index with wavelength. In the crown glass example, the dispersion is 0.011 (= 1.531 - 1.520). Each medium exhibits a different amount of dispersion, and not all media are dispersive. All wavelengths travel the same speed in a vacuum. The dispersion of air is so small that it can be ignored.

Refractive index is quite sensitive to chemical composition. It is easy to measure the refractive index difference between distilled water and physiologic saline. In the past, glycosuria was diagnosed by measuring urine refractive index. Manufacturers alter the optical properties of glass by adding small amounts of rare earth elements such as barium. Over 200 different types of optical glass with different indices (and dispersions) are commercially available.

Environmental factors such as temperature and atmospheric pressure can also influence refractive index, but the effects are usually small enough to be ignored. A notable exception is the index of silicone (20°C), which is strongly temperature dependent. Manufacturers should measure the power of silicone intraocular lenses at (or adjusted for) eye temperature (35°C) rather than at room temperature, or a clinically significant error in power may occur. Humidity can affect the refractive index of soft contact lenses by altering the water content.

8. Fermat's Principle, Refraction, and Reflection

Optical systems produce images by redirecting light. Fermat's principle governs the movement of light through an optical system. According to Fermat's principle, natural processes occur in extreme ways. Applied to light, Fermat's principle states that light travels from point A to point B along the path requiring the least time.

For instance, suppose light moves from A to B by reflection from a flat mirror. One path is shorter than any other; therefore, light moving along this path reaches B in the least time. Light moves from A to B only along this path. Of course, A is a point source and gives off light in all directions. Other rays from A reflect in different directions and do not reach B.

It is possible to show mathematically that for the shortest path the incident and reflected rays are always symmetric. Thus, the *law of* (specular) *reflection* follows from Fermat's principle. To state the law of reflection formally, it is necessary to define some additional terms. The *surface normal* is an imaginary line perpendicular to a surface at the point where a ray strikes the surface. There is a different surface normal at every point on a surface. The *angle of incidence* is the angle between the surface normal and the incident ray. The *angle of reflection* is the angle between the surface normal and the reflected ray. The law of reflection states that the incident ray, reflected ray, and surface normal lie in the same plane, and the angles of incidence and reflection are equal.

A flat mirror reflects a single ray from A to B. To produce a stigmatic image of A at B, all rays striking the mirror must pass through B. By Fermat's principle, this can happen only if every path from A to B has the same length. Bending the mirror equalizes the path lengths. The mirror's shape must be perfect, and it is not easy to fabricate such a mirror. If the shape is slightly off, some reflected rays will miss B but pass nearby.

Next, consider light traveling from an object point A in air (n_1 = 1) to some point B in glass (n_2 = 1.5). Because light moves relatively slowly in glass, light reaches B faster by other paths. Path 3 is the shortest in glass but the longest in air. The time saved by traveling a short distance in glass is more than offset by the extra distance in air, so path 3 is not the fastest. Path 2 is the fastest, representing the best compromise between air and glass.

The law of reflection, or Snell's law, is also mathematically derivable from Fermat's principle. Snell's law is easier to express as a formula than it is to express in words.

d=$n_1$sin (angle of incidence) $n_2$sin (angle of refraction)

As in the law of reflection, the incident ray, refracted ray, and surface normal lie in the same plane. Notice that when light moves from a lower refractive index to a higher index, it bends toward the surface normal. Conversely, light bends away from the surface normal when moving from a higher index to a lower index.

Just as in reflection, it is possible to bend the refracting surface to achieve a stigmatic image of A at point B. Again, all of the light from A must reach B simultaneously.

The laws of reflection and refraction are consequences of Fermat's principle, but there is an important distinction between the laws and the principle. When given a ray incident on a refracting surface, use Snell's law to determine the path of the refracted ray. When given two points separated by a refracting surface, use Fermat's principle to determine the path or paths light follows when moving between the two specified points. Similar reasoning applies to reflection.

An interesting phenomenon occurs when light moves from a higher index medium to a lower index medium. If the angle of incidence exceeds the *critical angle,* light does not pass into the lower index medium. Instead, light is reflected. This is called *total internal reflection* (TIR). The critical angle depends on the ratio of the refractive indices of the two media.

Optically, TIR is very useful. Many instruments for measuring refractive index use TIR. However, TIR can also cause problems. TIR makes it impossible to view the anterior chamber angle without a gonioscopy lens.

9. The Spherical Refracting Surface

Most lenses have spherical or plano (flat) surfaces. Some lenses have aspheric (anything not spherical) but rotationally symmetric surfaces, such as paraboloids, ellipsoids, and hyperboloids. Aspherics are uncommon in ophthalmology because they are usually costly to manufacture and unnecessary.

A spherical refracting surface does not produce a stigmatic image.

A small aperture can restrict rays so that only rays near the axis reach the image. With this restriction, the image becomes stigmatic. This is the paraxial approximation.

Paraxial means “near the axis.” To be paraxial, the ray must stay close to the axis over its entire path from object to image. Thus, the paraxial approximation is valid only for object (and image) points near the axis.

How far from the axis can a ray be and still qualify as paraxial? There is no definitive answer to this question. For very precise work, the rays may need to be quite close to the axis. For less demanding applications, rays can be farther from the axis.

Spherical refracting surfaces do not produce stigmatic images. However, under paraxial conditions, the spherical refracting surface becomes an ideal imaging system. It is legitimate to treat an optical system as ideal whenever the paraxial approximation is valid. The paraxial approximation is valid in most clinical situations.

10. The Paraxial Power of a Spherical Surface

A spherical surface of radius r (in meters) separating two media of index n_1 and n_2 has a paraxial power (in diopters) of:

$$Power = \frac{n_2 - n_1}{r}$$

Surfaces convex toward the higher index medium have positive power. Surfaces convex toward the lower index medium have negative power. Flat surfaces have zero power.

If the surface reflects instead of refracts, the power is:

$$Power = \frac{2}{r}$$

This formula is simpler because reflection does not involve refractive index. Concave reflecting surfaces have positive power. Convex reflecting surfaces have negative power. Flat surfaces have zero power. These equations relate the shape of a surface (the radius of curvature) to its optical function (the power). A spectacle prescription specifies power. The optician must grind a lens to the shape that produces the desired power. The optician uses these formulas to make the appropriate shape. These formulas apply only when the paraxial approximation is valid.

11. The Thin Lens Approximation

When light traverses a lens, its vergence changes at the front surface, as the light moves from the front to the back surface (called the *vergence change on transfer*), and at the back surface. The lens power is the sum of these three vergence changes. If paraxial conditions apply, it is easy to calculate the vergence change at each surface by using the equations. It is more difficult to calculate the vergence change on transfer. However, this is usually quite small, especially if the lens is thin. In the thin lens approximation, the vergence change on transfer is ignored and the lens power is calculated simply as the sum of the individual surface powers. How thin does a lens have to be to qualify as thin? Again, there is no definite answer to this; it depends on the accuracy demanded by the situation. Clinically, most lenses may be considered as thin. The principal planes of thin lenses overlap. This greatly simplifies vergence calculations in many situations.

12. Lens Shape and Fabrication

Two lenses with the same power may have quite different shapes. Despite the variety of shapes, positive lenses are always thicker in the center than at the edge, and vice versa for negative lenses.

Usually, spectacles are manufactured from semifinished blanks. The side of the blank that ultimately becomes the front surface of the spectacle lens is already polished to its final shape. If the spectacle is a bifocal, trifocal, or progressive add, the front surface contains the finished add power. The power of the distance portion of the front surface is the *base curve.* To fill a prescription, the optical lab selects a blank (with the appropriate add if necessary) and then grinds and polishes only the back surface of the blank. Finally, the lens is edged to fit the frame.

Spectacles are more cosmetically acceptable if the front surface has positive power. Even minus prescriptions usually have a weakly positive front surface. For instance, a -6.00 D spectacle usually has a + 2.00 D front (base curve) and a -8.00 D back. In the case of a negative prescription, the back surface must have extra minus power to overcome the positive power of the front surface. For high minus prescriptions, it is not possible to make the back surface strong enough, so both the front and back surfaces have minus power.

Semifinished blanks are available in a limited number of base curves. Sometimes a lab changes a patient's base curve when filling a new prescription, and this can cause problems, especially in older patients. Cylinder is ground on the back surface as minus cylinder regardless of how the prescription is written.

13. Thick Lenses

Occasionally, the thin lens approximation is not valid, and the lens must be treated as a thick lens. The principal planes of a thick lens do not overlap. The locations of the principal planes vary with lens shape even though the lens power does not change.

The principal planes are sometimes inside the lens. Earlier, it was stated that an object at the primary principal plane has an image at the secondary principal plane. This is true even when the principal planes are inside the lens. This can be demonstrated, but it is difficult to do so. Of course, when the principal planes are not inside the lens, it is easy to show that they are, indeed, planes of unit magnification.

In planoconvex or planoconcave lenses, one principal plane is always at the vertex of the curved surface. However, in general, the principal points do not coincide with the vertices. This is a problem because it makes it difficult to know exactly where the principal planes are located, and vergences are calculated from the principal planes, not the vertices.

To measure the power, the distances between the principal planes and the vertices must be taken into account.

The thin lens approximation greatly simplifies everything. The distance between the front and back vertices of a thin lens is zero. Both principal planes and both vertices overlap, and the lens is denoted by a single line.

14. Reduced Vergence

An object can be immersed in water, and images can form in the vitreous. For these situations, vergence calculations must be made by use of *reduced vergence.*

Reduced vergence is equal to the vergence multiplied by the refractive index. The term is confusing because, numerically, reduced vergence is larger than vergence. For example, light from an object 1 m from a thin lens has a vergence of -1.00 D at the lens. If the lens and object are submerged in water (n = 1.33), the reduced vergence is -1.33 D.

If the lens has a power of + 5.00 D when immersed in water, then the image rays have a reduced vergence of + 3.67 D, giving an image in water 36 cm (1.33/3.67) behind the lens.

15. Axial Magnification

Consider a three-dimensional object 25 cm long imaged by a + 5.00 D thin lens. The front of the object lies in an object plane 25 cm from the lens and has an image 1 m behind the lens. The back of the object lies in a plane 50 cm from the lens and has an image 33 cm behind the lens. The object has a length of only 25 cm, but the image has a length of 67 cm. The length of the image is magnified by a factor of 67/25, or 2.66. This is *axial magnification.*

In general, axial magnification may be defined for any two pairs of conjugate planes. Axial magnification usually varies for every different pair of object planes. In general, axial magnification is the distance between two image planes divided by the distance between the conjugate object planes.

16. A Focal Systems: Telescopes

Consider a system consisting of two thin lenses, + 2.00 D and + 10.00 D, separated by 60 cm. Parallel rays from a distant on-axis object point focus 50 cm behind the first lens and diverge again to become parallel rays after traversing the second lens.

This system does not produce a net change in vergence. Thus, the refractive power of this system is zero. This system has no focal points, no nodal points, and no principal points. This is an afocal system and cannot be analyzed in the same way as the previous examples.

Another confusing term in optics is the word power. This system has no refractive power. Nevertheless, it does make objects appear larger. The word *power* applied to afocal systems refers to its magnification, not to its refractive, or vergence changing, power. The power of the system is the refractive power of the second lens (+ 10.00 D) divided by the refractive power of the first lens (+ 2.00 D) and multiplied by -1. In this case, the power is -5.

Although the system has no cardinal points, it still produces images of objects. For every object plane there is a unique image plane. However, unlike focal systems, afocal systems have the same transverse magnification for every pair of conjugate planes. This transverse magnification is the reciprocal of the power. For this example, the transverse magnification is -0.2. Thus, the image of any object is inverted and one fifth the size of the object.

If the image is smaller than the object, why does it appear larger? The reason is that the axial magnification is the square of the power. In this example, the axial magnification is 25, which means that the image may be one fifth as large as the object but it is 25 times closer. The overall effect is that the image appears five times larger than the object.

The afocal system is called a *Keplerian* or *astronomical* telescope. The first lens is the *objective* and is a low-power plus lens. The second lens is the *eyepiece* or *ocular* and is a high-power plus lens. The lenses are separated by the sum of their focal lengths. The image is inverted, but prisms can reinvert the image. An alternate design also uses a low-power positive objective and a high-power negative ocular separated by the difference in focal lengths. The image is upright. This is the Galilean telescope.

The main application of afocal systems in ophthalmology is in low-vision work. Galilean telescopes are especially useful because they are shorter and give upright images, making them beneficial as spectacle-mounted visual aids. Keplerian telescopes with prisms give upright images, but the prisms add weight. They are better as hand-held visual aids and are especially useful for patients requiring high magnification.

Telescopes

Telescopes are afocal optical systems consisting of two lenses, separated in space, in air. There are two types of telescopic systems, Keplerian and Galilean.

a. Keplerian telescopes have a weak (+) objective lens and a strong (+) eyepiece lens.

The lenses are separated by the sum of their focal lengths. Keplerian (astronomical) telescopes form an inverted image so they require an erecting lens or prisms to make it a Terrestrial telescope.

b. Galilean telescopes has a weak (+) objective lens and a strong (-) eyepiece lens. The lenses are separated by the difference of their focal lengths. Galilean telescopes form an erect/upright image.

17. The Nonstigmatic Image

An image is never a perfect scale duplicate of the object, exact in every detail. A certain loss of detail is inherent in the imaging process. At best, an image is an imperfect facsimile of the original object.

The loss of detail occurs because images are not stigmatic. The stigmatic image is an idealization that cannot be achieved. Light from an object point does not come to a perfect point focus. Instead, light from a single object point is distributed over a small but definite area of the image. The light may spread over a region as small as a few microns in diameter or as large as 100 µm (0.1 mm) in diameter.

The failure to achieve a perfect stigmatic focus accounts for the loss of detail.

The fact that images are nonstigmatic has a small effect on image location and size, but usually this effect is insignificant. The methods based on stigmatic imaging that were developed to predict image location and size have sufficient accuracy for most clinical purposes. It is not necessary to rethink the entire analysis of optical systems.

However, although stigmatic imaging is an acceptable model for explaining some image characteristics, it is unacceptable for analyzing image quality. Stigmatic images are perfect down to the finest detail; real images are not. A different approach is necessary to analyze image quality.

18. Diffraction

Diffraction is a consequence of light's wave nature; it is not a "geometrical phenomenon." Snell's law and the other rules of geometrical optics do not take diffraction into account.

Diffraction causes a stigmatic image point to spread out into a round spot. This spot is called the Airy disk after the astronomer who described its characteristics. The larger the Airy disk, the greater the loss of detail. Basically, the size of the Airy disk is:

$$d = \frac{1.22\,(W)\,(\textit{focal length})}{A}$$

Where d = the diameter of the Airy disk, W = the wavelength of the light (about 0.55 μm), and A = the diameter of the aperture stop.

For a given lens, the diameter of the Airy disk increases as the aperture decreases. Consider two lenses identical in power, both producing (geometrically) stigmatic images, but one with a smaller diameter. The smaller-diameter lens gives a poorer image because of greater diffraction.

The smaller the lens diameter (maintaining the power constant), the greater the diffraction effects, the larger the airy disc, and the worse the image.

19. Aberrations

Even in the absence of diffraction it is impossible to achieve a stigmatic image in most cases. Every object point requires a differently shaped surface to produce a stigmatic image. An optical system can produce a stigmatic image of one or perhaps a few object points, but for most object points the image will not be stigmatic.

Ignoring diffraction, any deviation from ideal behavior is an *aberration.* Field curvature and distortion are two examples of aberrations, but the image is still stigmatic in these aberrations. In other aberrations, the image is nonstigmatic.

There are several different types of aberrations. Each type of aberration is unique in its behavior and optical characteristics.

Generally, decreasing the lens (or pupil) size decreases the aberration. Some aberrations improve dramatically with small decreases in lens diameter; others are barely affected or completely unaffected.

Pupil size plays an important role in image quality. If the pupil is small enough, diffraction is the major factor limiting image quality. If the pupil is large, aberrations limit image quality. The best pupil size is a compromise between aberrations and diffraction. The term diffraction-limited is often mistakenly used to imply a high-quality optical system, but this simply means that diffraction limits the optical quality. Any optical system can be made diffraction-limited by sufficiently reducing the aperture. Depending on pupil size, diffraction-limited systems may be inferior to systems limited by aberrations.

Chromatic aberration is a particularly important type of aberration. The refractive index of a material is different for every wavelength; as discussed earlier, this is called dispersion. The effect of this variation in index is that red light focuses behind blue light. The eye exhibits a large amount of chromatic aberration, but image processing by the brain prevents us from being conscious of it. It is easy to demonstrate chromatic aberration by means of the duochrome (or bichrome) technique used in refraction. Chromatic aberration of the eye results in green light being focused in front of the retina, yellow light at the retinal plane, and red light behind the retina. Therefore, when red is brighter, it indicates that more minus is needed to move the focus of red light further behind the retina. When green is brighter, more plus is needed to move the green light to focus further into the posterior chamber.

20. Image Quality

Loss of detail is inherent in the imaging process, but some optical systems preserve more detail than others. How can the performance of an optical system be gauged objectively and quantitatively?

It is fairly simple to assess the quality of a diffraction-limited system. The image of every object point is an identical Airy disk, and the size of the disk determines the amount of detail that is lost. The size of the Airy disk can be calculated from a formula, but it is better to evaluate an optical system by some bench test rather than rely on a calculation. In a resolution test, the United States Air Force resolution target is imaged by an optical system. Because of diffraction, the smaller line groups are blurry. The resolution is the smallest group of lines that appear as distinctly separate in the image.

The resolution test is quite analogous to a Snellen acuity. The results are expressed in terms of line pairs per millimeter rather than a Snellen fraction. One hundred line pairs per millimeter corresponds to 20/20.

As an optical test, resolution has some disadvantages. The test depends on a subjective judgment by an observer. It is not truly quantitative because there are only a limited number of line groups. It is impossible to pinpoint the resolution exactly because the true resolution falls somewhere between the groups on the target. Nevertheless, for a diffraction-limited system, resolution is a very useful test of optical performance.

However, in the presence of aberrations, resolution does not provide an adequate assessment of optical performance. Two systems can have identical resolutions and yet produce very different images. The *modulation transfer function* (MTF) provides a more complete evaluation of optical performance, but it is a more complicated test.

If a single pure tone is recorded, the frequency of the recording matches the frequency of the original, but the volume changes. The ratio of the recorded volume to the original volume is the response of the audio system to that particular frequency. If an audio system has different responses to different frequencies, the recorded sound will not match the original. However, if the audio system has the same response to all frequencies, the recorded sound will duplicate the original. A graph of response versus frequency (called a frequency response curve) can be constructed.

Images can be analyzed in the same way to find a pure tone in an optical equivalent. The optical analog of a pure tone is a *sine wave grating* (SWG). The frequency of the grating is determined by the horizontal peak-to-peak distance. The grating contrast is indicated by the difference in brightness between the brightest and darkest points and is analogous to the volume of a tone. One difference between sound and optics is that SWGs have an orientation--vertical, horizontal, or any oblique axis. Unlike the sine wave grating, which gradually changes from dark to light, the Ronchi ruling changes abruptly. In a sense, Snellen optotypes resemble Ronchi rulings more than sine wave gratings.

Just as sound is a mixture of pure frequencies, images are a mixture of SWGs. The image of a single SWG has the same frequency and orientation as the original SWG, but the contrast is always decreased. The ratio of the image SWG's contrast to the object SWG's contrast is the transfer factor. The transfer factor is always between zero and 1, and different frequencies have different transfer factors. The graph of transfer factor versus frequency is the MTF and is exactly analogous to the frequency response of an audio system.

The MTF of an ideal optical system (no loss of detail) would be a horizontal line. This is impossible to achieve because of diffraction.

The MTF gives a more complete evaluation of optical performance, but it is harder to measure and interpret. Which of two MTFs is better depends on the situation. Still, MTF is an important method of image evaluation.

There are other important methods of image evaluation, such as Strehl ratio, wavefront variance, and root mean square spot size.

21. Apertures

Apertures serve two functions in an optical system. The obvious function is to regulate the amount of light reaching the image, but this is relatively unimportant. The less obvious and much more important function is to control aberrations.

An optical system collects only a small fraction of the light from an object. Some apertures limit the amount of light gathered. This type of aperture may be the edge of a lens, but usually a special aperture of adjustable size is placed in the optical system to control image brightness. The aperture limiting the bundle of rays from an on-axis object point is the *aperture stop*.

The size of the aperture does not change or in any way regulate the size of the image.

The amount of light power per unit area of an image is called the *irradiance*. Irradiance varies linearly with the aperture's area. Thus, a 50% decrease in aperture area does produce a 50% decrease in irradiance. Bear in mind that irradiance varies with aperture area, not aperture diameter. Clinically, pupil size is specified as a diameter. If the pupil size changes from 2 to 3 mm (a 50% change in diameter), the pupil area increases by 125%, more than doubling the retinal irradiance. Although the retinal irradiance more than doubles, the change in brightness is only modest. Consider the point source, lens, and aperture. Some of the rays passing through the lens are blocked by the aperture. It would be convenient to be able to determine which rays traverse the aperture without having to use Snell's law to calculate the exact path of each ray. The *entrance pupil* enables one to determine exactly which object rays reach the image without the need for any calculation or ray tracing. The entrance pupil is the image of the aperture stop formed by all optical elements anterior to the stop. Once the position and size of the entrance pupil are known, it is easy to determine which object rays reach the image. Ignore every optical element between the object and entrance pupil. If an object ray (which does not deviate) passes through the entrance pupil, it will reach the image. If an object ray is blocked by the entrance pupil, it will not reach the image.

Clearly, the iris is the eye's aperture stop. Anatomically, the hole in the iris is the pupil, but optically it is not a pupil but rather a stop. Clinically, one does not measure the actual size of the anatomic pupil. The pupil is viewed through the cornea. That is to say, the clinician measures the size of the image of the pupil formed by the cornea, not the pupil per se. Thus, clinically, pupil size refers to the size of the entrance pupil, which is about 20% larger than the anatomic pupil.

The aperture stop limits rays from an on-axis object point. The stop may or may not be the limiting aperture for off-axis points. For some off-axis points the aperture stop is still the limiting aperture. However, for far off-axis points, some rays traversing the stop are clipped by other lens elements. This is *vignetting.* In old cameras, vignetting was prominent and caused photographs to be dim at the edges. In direct ophthalmoscopy, vignetting limits the field-of-view.

The *exit pupil* is the image of the stop formed by all optical elements posterior to the stop. The major importance of the exit pupil is when using an optical instrument in front of the eye. For example, the best way to use a microscope is to place the eye's entrance pupil at the exit pupil of the scope. The same holds for other visual instruments.

The *chief ray* is the ray from an on-axis or off-axis object point that goes through the center of the entrance pupil. Necessarily, this ray also goes through the center of the stop and through the exit pupil because all three points are conjugate to each other. A *marginal ray* is a ray from any object point that just clears the entrance pupil. The marginal ray will also just scrape by the edge of the stop and exit pupil because these points are conjugate.

If the aperture is at the lens, there is considerable field curvature, and the photograph will be blurry at the edges. By moving the aperture slightly in front of the lens, the field curvature is markedly reduced. The photograph is greatly improved simply by moving the stop a few millimeters.

22. Cylindrical Lenses

Hold a candle about 3 feet in front of a + 4.00 D cylinder with axis horizontal, and note that the "image" is a horizontal line. Change the axis to vertical and observe that the image is now a vertical line.

Consider a point source imaged by a positive cylindrical lens, axis vertical. Rays from the point source fanning out horizontally are converged, but rays fanning out vertically are undeviated. The classic teaching is that a cylinder's power is perpendicular to its axis. However, it is more correct to say that a cylinder's maximum power is perpendicular to its axis. It is also classic teaching to say that a cylinder gives a line image. However, an image is a point-to-point correspondence. A cylindrical lens spreads light from a point source into a line; this is a severe form of aberration called astigmatism. Literally, astigmatism means not stigmatic. However, many aberrations are not stigmatic, so the term is not very descriptive.

Place a + 9.00 D cylinder axis horizontal directly behind a + 4.00 D axis vertical cylinder and image a candle. Not surprisingly, the "image" is a horizontal line close to the lenses and a vertical line farther from the lenses. Both lines cannot be seen on the paper simultaneously; it is necessary to move the paper back and forth between the two lines. The location of each line can be calculated by use of vergence. If the candle is 1 m (-1.00 D) from the lenses, the + 9.00 D cylinder gives a horizontal image + 8.00 D (12.5 cm) behind the lenses. The + 4.00 D cylinder gives a vertical line + 3.00 D (33 cm) behind the lenses.

Move the screen and explore the region between the two line images. Starting at the vertical line and moving toward the lenses, the image becomes an ellipse with the long axis vertical. As the screen moves forward, the ellipse gets rounder, becoming a circle about midway between the lines. Moving farther forward, the image becomes an ellipse with the long axis horizontal. Moving the screen farther forward, the ellipse elongates until the image becomes a horizontal line. The region between the lines is the *conoid of Sturm,* and the circle is the *circle of least confusion.*

Replace the + 9.00 D cylinder with a + 6.00 D cylinder, keeping the axis vertical. The line images become shorter and closer together. Replace the + 6.00 D cylinder with a + 4.00 D cylinder, axis vertical. The candle's image is now clear. The two cylinders act as a + 4.00 D sphere. This is a key point. Two cylinders of the same power with axes perpendicular are equivalent to a sphere of the same power as the cylinders.

Consider the + 4.00 D and + 9.00 D cylinders with axes perpendicular. Four of the nine diopters of the vertical cylinder combine with the horizontal cylinder to give a + 4.00 D sphere. The remaining + 5.00 D give a vertical cylinder. Combine a + 5.00 D cylinder with a + 4.00 D sphere and image a candle. The result is the same as the combination of the + 4.00 D and + 9.00 D cylinders. The combination of a sphere and cylinder is a spherocylinder. Cylindrical power can be combined with spherical power in a single lens by grinding the lens as a toric surface. The *spherical equivalent power* of a spherocylinder is the average of the maximum and minimum powers, which equals the sphere power plus half the cylinder power.

One way of representing a spherocylinder is by graphing the power in each meridian, as in A more convenient representation is the power cross. The *power cross* consists of two lines--one parallel, the other perpendicular to the axis of a spherocylinder. Perhaps the most confusing aspect of spherocylinders is that there are two different ways to designate the same lens; for instance, a + 3.00 D X 030 cylinder combined with a + 7.00 D cylinder X 120 can be considered a + 3.00 D sphere and a + 4.00 D cylinder X 120. Alternatively, this could be a + 7.00 D sphere and a -4.00 D cylinder X 030. These are simply two ways of denoting the same lens. The power cross and the graph of power versus meridian are the same for both designations. It is easy to determine the spherocylinder that results from the combination of two cylinders with axes perpendicular. However, if the axes are not perpendicular, determining the resultant spherocylinder is more complicated.

23. Prisms

A prism is a wedge of glass (or some other material). The sides of the prism are flat and have no optical power. Prisms do not change vergence; they simply change light's direction.

A prism deviates light toward its base. This makes objects appear to be displaced toward the apex.

The prism diopter is a measure of the amount of deviation a prism produces. One prism diopter is a deviation of 1 cm at a distance of 1 m from the prism. The prism diopter is denoted by a superscript triangle.

The problem with prisms is that regardless of the number on the prism, the deviation that is actually produced depends on the way the prism is held in front of the patient. When three different light paths through the same prism, the least amount of deviation occurs when light passes through the prism symmetrically. This is the minimum angle of deviation (MAD) position. In Prentice position, light strikes one prism face at normal incidence. It does not matter if light is normal to the front or back surface because the deviation is the same in both cases. The deviation in Prentice position is greater than the deviation in MAD position. When the prism face is parallel to the frontal plane, the prism is in frontal plane position, and the deviation differs from Prentice and MAD position.

Does the number on the prism represent the MAD, Prentice, or frontal plane deviation? Unfortunately, some prisms are calibrated in MAD position, whereas others are calibrated in Prentice position. Optically, MAD is easy to measure accurately, but clinically it is difficult to use. Prentice position is much more suitable for clinical use. For small deviations there is little difference between the two, but the differences may be important in large deviations. The best clinical practice is to use the same prisms in a consistent fashion.

High-power prisms make spectacle lenses thick and expensive. A useful option is the Fresnel press-on prism. It is also possible to split the prismatic correction between both eyes. Patients may have both horizontal and vertical deviations. If these deviations are small, it may be best to correct them by use of a single prism at oblique axis. The axis may be calculated by adding the horizontal and vertical prism powers vectorially. A Fresnel prism is a collapsed version of a prism. The power of a prism depends on the angle between the faces, not the thickness.

One problem with prescribing large prism powers is prismatic deviation. Gazing through a strong prism at an oblique angle produces a different deviation than when gazing at normal incidence. This can make straight lines appear curved, and some patients find this annoying.

Lenses can induce some prism power. To a first approximation, a lens is a combination of prisms (a pair of prisms). When gazing through an off-center part of a lens, the induced prism is given by Prentice's Rule:

Induced prism = lens power X distance from optical center in centimeters

Induced prism can be used to estimate the power of a spectacle lens. Induced prism is important is prescribing bifocals and in the management of anisometropia.

24. Clinical Examples

This section discusses some clinical applications of the preceding theory. It is impossible to categorize all the clinical applications of optics.

Pathology of the ocular media can be categorized on the basis of its effect on image formation. There are three general classes of pathology: opaque lesions, scattering or contrast-reducing lesions, and aberration-producing lesions.

Examples of opaque lesions include granular stromal dystrophy of the cornea, asteroid hyalosis, and some types of congenital cataract. The important clinical point is that opaque lesions do not affect vision unless the pupil is almost completely obscured or unless the lesion is very close to the retina.

Place a piece of opaque tape in the center of a trial lens and image a candle. The central obscuration has little effect on the image. Light from each object point completely fills the lens. A small opaque lesion blocks some of the light, but most still passes through the lens. The light that does traverse the lens is still redirected to produce a one-to-one correspondence between object and image. At most, an opaque lesion produces a small decrease in image brightness, which, as discussed previously, is barely noticeable.

An opaque lesion blocks some light, but light traversing the unaffected part of the lens still forms an image. The image is slightly dimmer, but otherwise unaffected.

Opaque lesions are usually quite apparent on slit lamp exam but may coexist with other subtler pathology. Problems can arise if visual symptoms are inappropriately attributed to opaque lesions. For example, a patient with a crescent-shaped iris remnant on the lens (from an old posterior synechia that was broken) presents with an arcuate scotoma. The scotoma seemed to correspond to the shape of the iris remnant, which was assumed to be the cause of the scotoma. Two years later, the patient presented with advanced field loss and elevated intraocular pressure (IOP), and the diagnosis of primary open-angle glaucoma was finally made.

When the patient initially presented, it would have been easy to constrict the pupil so that the iris covered the remnant on the lens, and to retest the visual field. If the scotoma had still been present, then it clearly was not caused by the iris remnant. Unfortunately, simple maneuvers for diagnosing optical problems are often overlooked.

Typical scattering lesions include vitreous hemorrhage, posterior capsular cataract, and corneal edema. Light striking the abnormal area of the media is not blocked as in opaque lesions. Light traverses the lesion but is scattered in the process. The scattered light distributes generally over the entire retina. Light that passes through the normal parts of the ocular media still creates an image on the retina, but the image is washed out by the scattered light. The effect is similar to raising the house lights during a movie, only more pronounced. Generally, vision is markedly affected, and these are the easiest lesions to diagnose. Patients complain of rainbows, halos, and glare.

Scattering lesions partially disrupt the one-to-one correspondence between object and image by distributing some light randomly over the image. Light that traverses the unaffected part of the lens still produces an image, but the contrast is somewhat washed out.

Typical aberration-producing lesions include keratoconus, aphakia, subluxed lenses, and postkeratoplasty astigmatism. As discussed, light from a point source is distributed over a small region of the image instead of being confined to a perfect point. Provided the light is spread over only a small area, visual acuity is high. Aberration-increasing lesions cause light from a point source to spread over an abnormally large area and may cause the light distribution to become asymmetric.

Patients with these problems often have near normal acuity but complain of distinct visual phenomena. For example, spectacle-corrected aphakes characteristically complain of pincushion distortion (doorways curve in the middle, appearing too thin to pass through). The visual complaint may be quite variable, depending on the cause of the aberration. Keratoconus patients may complain of a variety of different phenomena because each cone is a different shape and produces different aberrations. The essential feature is not any aspect of the vision per se but rather that the patient is able to describe in vivid detail the visual experience. The visual complaint is specific, not vague. The patient can often draw on paper the appearance of a point source, and this often gives a clue to the problem.

For example, patients post radial keratotomy (RK) may complain of "seeing" the incisions. It was not until RKs were performed with small numbers of incisions that it became clear that the "incisions" the patient was "seeing" and the corneal incisions were not in the same meridians. For instance, if the patient had a four-incision RK with cuts in the 180 and 090 meridians, the patient reported the "incisions he or she saw" in the 045 and 135 meridians. Moreover, some patients "saw" the incisions even when the pupil was much smaller than the optical zone.

The patient cannot be seeing the incisions. If the incisions are opaque, they do not affect the image. If the incisions scatter light, then the contrast is diminished, but this does not cause the patient to see lines in specific meridians. In fact, the patient does not see the incisions at all. The cornea retracts between the incisions, creating four cylinders with axes in the meridians between the incisions. These cylinders create the aberrant image that gives the mistaken impression that the patient is "seeing the incisions."

The importance of apertures is often overlooked. First, it is impossible to selectively "look through" only part of the pupil. Consider a patient with good acuity despite a dislocated intraocular lens (IOL) with a positioning hole in the center of the pupil. The question is often asked, "Which part of the pupil is the patient looking through?" The answer is "all parts." Light from an object point fills the pupil, and some passes through the IOL, some through the positioning hole, and some through the empty pupil. The patient will see well if there is enough light focused on the retina to yield an adequate image despite decreased contrast and possibly glare from the optic's edges. If the patient does see well, it is not because he or she is looking through only the IOL.

Vision is preserved until late in the course of granular dystrophy because the lesions are opaque and do not affect the retinal image until the pupil is nearly totally obscured. However, some explain the preservation of vision by assuming that the patient is somehow "pinholing" by selectively looking through a small part of the cornea between opaque lesions. If the patient were pinholing, then he or she would have an unusually large depth-of-focus, and this could be demonstrated. Patients with granular dystrophy do not exhibit increased depth-of-focus until late in the disease when the pupil becomes nearly a single pinhole.

Of course, it is possible to move the eye so that one looks through only a segment of a bifocal or trifocal spectacle. The eye moving independently of a spectacle, or even a contact lens, can arrange its relatively small pupil so that all the light passing through the pupil passes through only one spectacle segment. The distinction between a bifocal spectacle and a bifocal (or multifocal) IOL is important. At any one time, a patient looks through either the distance or near segment of a spectacle, so all the light on the retina is focused for either near or far. However, with a bifocal IOL, light is always split between two different images simultaneously. There is always some in-focus and some out-of-focus light on the retina.

The importance of the pupil in regulating retinal light levels is often overstated. From dawn to high noon, the amount of ambient illumination varies by thirteen orders of magnitude. The area of the pupil changes by, at most, two orders of magnitude. The pupil may help compensate for small transient fluctuations in illumination, but other mechanisms, such as retinal adaptation, are much more important than the pupil for adjusting to the large variation in light levels that we are exposed to in the course of a day.

Many factors besides light level influence pupil size, indicating that the pupil has other roles than simply regulating retinal illumination. For instance, the pupil constricts during accommodation. Clearly, this is not to regulate retinal illumination, but it does increase depth-of-focus and decrease spherical aberration.

The pupil is also an important consideration in the prescription of visual aids. Two important considerations are magnification and illumination. Galilean telescopes produce upright images and are shorter than Keplerian telescopes, making them attractive as a spectacle-mounted visual aid. However, the exit pupil is inside the telescope. Because of this, some of the light emerging from the exit pupil of the telescope misses the eye's entrance pupil. Thus, some of the light entering the telescope is wasted, and the retinal illumination suffers.

The Keplerian telescope is longer than the Galilean and heavier because it must contain a prism assembly to erect the image that would otherwise be inverted. These aspects make it unsuitable for a spectacle-mounted visual aid. However, the exit pupil is behind the second lens, so the user may place the exit pupil of the telescope in the entrance pupil of his or her eye. Essentially all the light from the telescope enters the eye. When a patient requires both a bright and enlarged image, a hand-held Keplerian telescope may be the best choice.

In a typical astronomical telescope, the aperture stop and entrance pupil are the edges of the objective lens. Thus, the exit pupil is behind the telescope. Most of the light leaving the telescope enters the observer's eye.

It is well known that miosis decreases the visual field. In theory, the small pupil should decrease the general retinal illumination but not alter the field. The decrease in field size is caused by the so-called cosine drop-off law. The beam of light from off-axis points that reaches the retina has a smaller cross-sectional area than the beam from on-axis points. Thus, less light from off-axis points reaches the retina. The visual field is defined by the point where the amount of light reaching the retina falls below threshold. The smaller the pupil, the smaller the field.

Pupils play an important role in ophthalmoscopy. Direct ophthalmoscopy is like looking into a room through an old-fashioned keyhole. The view is limited. The field-of-view can be enhanced by placing a lens in the keyhole to form an image. This is the principle of indirect ophthalmoscopy, and the fundus camera. Indirect ophthalmoscopy may be done binocularly or monocularly. Thus, the essential distinction between direct and indirect ophthalmoscopy is not binocularity. In direct ophthalmoscopy, the observer directly views the retina. In indirect ophthalmoscopy, the observer views an image of the retina.

In both types of ophthalmoscopy, the retina must be illuminated. The illumination and viewing paths should be separate, or light reflected from the cornea obscures the retinal image. Binocular ophthalmoscopy divides the pupil of the eye under examination into three parts. Illumination enters through one part, and each eye of the examiner views the retina through another part (this arrangement is referred to as *dark field illumination*). The headpiece of the indirect ophthalmoscope contains two periscopes that effectively shrink the examiner's interpupillary distance so that both examiner's eyes can peer through separate parts of the patient's pupil.

The size of the retinal image in indirect ophthalmoscopy depends on the power of the condensing lens. The lower the lens power, the larger the image. Examination of the disc is enhanced by the increased axial magnification that accompanies a larger transverse magnification. Because axial magnification increases as roughly the square of the transverse magnification, some examiners use a + 14.00 D instead of the standard + 20.00 D lens to examine the disc for cupping.

Reference

Thall EH. *Geometrical Optics.* In Tasman W and Jaeger EA (eds). Chapter 30. Duane's Ophthalmology on CD-Rom. Lippincott Williams & Wilkins, 2006 edition.

Chapter V

Physical Optics

Abstract

As eye doctors, we measure the optical properties of the eye and study its structures. To enable us to understand our instruments, we are taught that light acts as a stream of tiny particles, moving in straight lines that we call rays, and that these rays follow the laws of geometry. Geometric optics, however, cannot explain why the sclera is white, the iris blue, and the fundus red, or why a cataract is opaque. Study of physical optics is needed to answer these questions. One might think of geometric optics as the workhorse of an ophthalmic practice, whereas physical optics can provide the intellectual excitement. The discoveries of physical optics are rich in the secrets of the universe, and the unraveling of these secrets has allowed us to harness the major forces that surround us (Miller and Schor, 2006).

1. History

The subject of physical optics seemed to gather substantial momentum in 1666, when Isaac Newton directed a shaft of sunlight through a glass prism and collected the transmitted light onto a white surface. The prism had broken the white light into the colors of the rainbow. Although Leonardo da Vinci had actually performed the same experiment in his workshop in Milan 200 years earlier, he feared that the ruling powers might consider the work blasphemous and so he told no one, only recorded the findings in his journal in a mirror writing code. Fortunately, Newton was able not only to report his work, but also to speculate as to its mechanism. Newton had already stated that light rays were a stream of particles, a theory that adequately explained how lenses work. To this he added that white light was simply a combination of many colors, and that the prism refracted each color differently so as to make them all visible.

To some, the presence of many colors in white light suggested that the colored rays had unique qualities. Christian Huygens, a Dutch contemporary of Newton, preferred to liken the process of light to the process of sound waves. Since the pitch of a sound depended on its wavelength, he believed the different colors of light also had different wavelengths. Any new theory of light, however, would also have to explain the facts of geometric optics. Thus, he imagined a light beam as composed of many small, circular wavelets that interacted with each other to form a wavefront. Unless it were to strike an obstacle, this wavefront would travel forward in a straight line. If the wavefront were to strike a piece of glass obliquely, one end of the wave front would strike the glass first. The progress of that end of the front would then be slowed down in comparison to the other end, which would still be in air. In this way, the entire front would be bent, making a smaller angle with the normal. Huygens further suggested that each wavelength, upon entering glass, traveled at a different speed. One could say that he pictured the longer wavelengths as skipping with long strides and the shorter wavelengths, such as violet and blue, as moving more slowly, with short mincing steps, and so were refracted more.

Thus, the nature of light was in doubt until the beginning of the 19th century, when the creative physician-physicist Thomas Young not only demonstrated that the different colors were due to different wavelengths, but also managed to place the magnitude of the wavelength at 1/50,000 inch, which was rather close to the true figure. His simple experiment is repeated in most high school physics courses today. He allowed a point source of light to fall on two closely spaced apertures. Each aperture then served as a source of a cone of light, and the two cones overlapped on a screen. The overlapping region of the screen was made up of alternating light and dark bands. Young explained that light must be a wave because only waves could (1) interfere with each other so as to cancel each other out where dark bands fell; and (2) reinforce each other where the light bands fell. He then used the spacing between the bands to calculate the wavelength. He reasoned that for a bright band to appear, rays coming from both slits must be in phase (*i.e.*, the difference in distance between each slit and the bright band must be a whole number of wavelengths). When he used white light, the band pattern was colored, which allowed him to deduce that the red wavelength was about twice the length of the violet wavelength.

Visible light waves range in size from 400 to 700 nm (1 nm = 1 billionth of a meter). Two waves of the same wavelength constructively interfere if their crests and troughs coincide, producing a resultant wave that is the summation of the two waves' amplitudes. If the crest of one wave coincides with the trough of the other, destructive interference takes place and can lead to complete cancellation. The wave theory also explained why a parallel beam of light seemed to diverge slightly as it passed through a small hole, and why light striking an opaque object cast shadows with indistinct edges.

Recall that Huygens pictured every point on a wavefront as a potential source of a series of waves in all directions, if the wavefront interacted with an obstacle. Thus, as a beam of light goes through an aperture, all the diverging wavelets are cancelled out by their neighbors to the right and left, and only the forward-directed waves are left, with one exception: the edges of the wavefront. At the right end, a right-sided wave has no right-sided neighbor on its extreme side. Thus, the edge of the beam veers sideways. It is almost as though the edge ray meets a friction between its one side and the edge, causing an apparent drag that forces the ray to veer off course. Again, the size of the wavelength is related to this edge effect: the longer the wavelength, the greater the diffraction. This phenomenon is exploited to produce the wide spectrum of colors in modern spectroscopes. A series of closely placed slits (thus yielding many edges) in the form of a diffraction grating produces a vivid spectrum in which red is bent the most and violet is closest to the center. This spectrum is the reverse of that produced by a prism, in which the shortest wavelength (violet) is refracted the most. The edge effect can be a problem in photography, when a large f number (small iris opening) is used to yield a greater depth of field or, as we will see, when the pinhole disc is used to improve visual acuity.

2. Wave Motion

The historical evidence we have recounted so far describes light as a wave motion. This means that when a wave runs over the surface of the water, a piece of cork floating on the surface will bob up and down but will not travel forward. If you jiggle a rope, the hump moves forward but not the rope. These examples describe the essence of a wave as a state of motion that travels forward, forcing vibrations in its path. What, then, vibrates in the direction of a light beam to give the wave? Aristotle suggested that a universal ether filled the universe and that it vibrated. The French physicist Fresnel expanded this idea and pictured ether as a very thin elastic substance that even filled a vacuum. When a portion of the ether was distorted at right angles to a light beam, it snapped back immediately, even though light was traveling at a speed of 186,000 miles/second. It is ironic that by the mid 19th century, almost all the concepts of Aristotelian physics had been discarded, yet the physicists had no choice but to cling to the concept of ether if light was to be considered a wave.

The new idea that would eliminate the mystical ether was supplied by the brilliant Scottish theorist James Clerk Maxwell. Maxwell had been impressed by Michael Faraday's experiments, which had shown that both electrical energy and magnetism could be transmitted without wires or contacts. Faraday had further shown that a varying magnetic field could induce an electric current, and that an electric current could induce a magnetic field.

Maxwell was fascinated by these related forces, which seem to function at a distance. He took Faraday's findings and developed four differential equations to describe the quantitative interrelationship between electricity and magnetism. The equations placed the two forces at right angles to each other in a single electromagnetic field. The equations also suggested that if the changing electrical field induced a changing magnetic field, which, in turn, induced a changing electric field, the resulting electromagnetic radiation had wavelike properties. The equations also predicted the velocity of these radiations to be the same as the speed of light! Although Maxwell embraced the ether theory of the day, we can see that these equations implied that the wavelike properties of light were the same as the oscillating values of an electromagnetic field. Thus, we can imagine the oscillating field of a light beam as oscillating changes in the geometry of space. The concept of an oscillating field could take place in a vacuum, and the unrealistic ether could be abandoned.

Scientific thought has a strange way of going in cycles. Just when the particle theory of light was completely replaced by the wave theory, a type of light particle called a quantum was identified, which appeared to be the true representation of light.

3. Quantum Theory

At the close of the 19th century, interest focused on radiations beyond the visible (*i.e.*, ultraviolet, infrared, radiowaves). This work involved the heating of black elements, since black theoretically absorbed all radiation falling upon its surface. For example, the German physicist Wien studied the manner in which a black-body radiator glowed as it was heated. As the heat rose to 3000 K, the body glowed red; at 5000 K to 6000 K, it glowed yellow; and at more than 8000 K, the radiator glowed blue. Obviously, the heat had been converted to light, but how? At the beginning of the 20th century, the German physicist Max Planck had not only solved this problem, but in so doing had unearthed one of the most important physical principles of the 20th century. Planck had set about carefully measuring the radiant energy and distribution of wavelengths emitted as a black body was heated to higher and higher temperatures. Certainly, as the radiator glowed from red to blue, the frequency of the waves emitted increased. But careful measurement of the radiated energy showed that it climbed at a slower pace compared with the change in frequency. What was happening? In a lecture given in 1900, Planck said, "I find myself driven almost against my will to the assumption, unsuspected till now in physics, that the electromagnetic energy emanating from a source of heat is not continuous, but divided, as it were, into definite portions or quanta." (Dogigi, 1967).

The energy of each quantum was equal to a constant that Planck had uncovered (6.623×10^{-27} erg seconds) times the frequency, which acknowledged a wavelength—yet the final product was a particle of energy. Was Newton right all along? Well, almost. Physicists say that light is a stream of photons and that although light is thus not a moving wave, the probability that a photon will behave in a certain way is best described by a wave equation. This concept is hard to picture, but it does account for all the facts. If Planck had persisted in the theory of the day (*i.e.*, that radiant energy was emitted in a continuous fashion), he could not have explained the fact that the visible energy fell off as the black-body radiator was heated to higher temperatures. Therefore, he made two assumptions: (1) that energy is packed in discrete units, or quanta (*i.e.*, you may have 1 quantum or 2 quanta but never 1½ quanta); and (2) that the energy content of a quantum varies with the frequency of the light. Thus, a violet quantum could have almost twice the energy of a red quantum because violet has double the frequency (*i.e.*, one half wavelength). As the black-body radiator was heated to higher temperatures, energy was accumulating to fill a quantum of violet light. However, one might imagine that during this process, some energy "bled" off to fill the small quantum of red. For the higher frequencies of light, there was a lower probability that enough energy would accumulate to form a complete quantum. Naturally, as the temperature rose, the amount of energy available for radiation became so excessive that quanta for the high-frequency waves had time to form.

Imagine an experiment in which a very dim light source produces one photon at a time. The photon enters one of the two apertures from the Young experiment. The interference pattern will be recorded on film. Over time, millions of photons will reach the film. Each photon will produce a dot of light. The pattern can be thought of as fringes of dots of different densities. Wave theory equations help predict the probability of each photon location in the "interference pattern."

The quantum theory remained half noticed, and not quite believed, until 1905, when Einstein used it to explain the photoelectric effect. For his famous equation, Einstein assumed that electrons on the surface of a metal emitter absorbed light energy, one quantum at a time. If the energy of the quantum was that which was precisely needed to overcome the forces holding an electron to the surface, the electron would be set free and a trickle of current would develop.

The quantum theory applies to the atom as well. It states that the energy of the atom assumes a certain definite spectrum of values characteristic for that species of atom. Usually the atom is in its lowest energy level, or ground state. When the atom is exposed to light of a frequency such that the energy of the photon equals the energy difference between the excited and ground states, the photon is absorbed, producing an excited state. One may also say that the light is in resonance with the atom. In a fraction of a second, the atom will fall back to its previous energy state and emit the energy difference. Einstein realized that every metal is resonant with a critical wavelength for this photoelectric effect.

4. Atomic Structure

If light quanta and electrons interact, they apparently are of a similar magnitude. Is light so fundamental as to be connected to the very structure of the atom? But what is the atom? In 1913, the Danish scientist Niels Bohr presented his model of the structure of the atom. It included a positively charged central nucleus surrounded by shells of swirling negative electrons. He went on to suggest that light had its origin in the atom. He pictured the various shells of electrons as behaving almost like a slot machine, which takes a variety of coins (*i.e.*, the dime slot only takes a dime, the quarter slot only a quarter). The different electron shells will accept only a quantum of energy that corresponds with the innate nature of the shell. When energy is absorbed, an electron of one shell is raised to a new permitted orbit, where it stays for approximately a hundred millionth of a second. As the electron falls back to its original shell, an electromagnetic wave is released. The dimensions of the released wave (*i.e.*, wavelength) are related to the dimensions of the electron shells involved in the interplay.

5. Color

Using this concept, one can explain why certain pigments take on the colors that they do. Molecularly speaking, pigments usually have a ring structure. Electrons move more freely within a ring structure than within a branched molecule. Therefore, the electrons, which are also considered to have wave properties, are allowed to have longer wavelengths, or lower frequencies, in ring molecules. Most molecules resonate with ultraviolet light; however, because of the Planck relationship and the ring structure of the molecule, pigment molecules resonate in a lower energy state and thus absorb visible light. The surface of pigment molecules has been likened to a sieve, and light falling on them to a series of colored balls, each colored ball being a different size. In the case of a red dye, all the colored balls but red would drop through the holes of the sieve and become absorbed, later to radiate in the invisible infrared. The red balls, however, accumulate on the sieve surface. Thus a molecule of pure red dye has its electron shells so arranged that quanta of all the visible wavelengths but red fit snugly into its dimensions and become absorbed. The red, on the other hand, is backscattered to the observer's eyes.

The physical dimensions of light and matter can also explain light scattering. If light strikes a structure larger than 1000 nm, the light is absorbed. If the structure is less than 1 nm, the light passes by unaffected. However, if the object has a size between 1 and 1000 nm, light will be absorbed and re-emitted as a ray of similar wavelength, but in a different direction. This phenomenon of light scattering takes place among the water particles of a cloud and is responsible for the clouds' opaque appearance. (In a subsequent section of this chapter, the principles of light scattering will help unravel the behavior of the edematous cornea and the cataract).

6. Intraocular Light Scattering

Definition

Picture a shaft of light piercing a dusty room. The physicist sees each dust particle as an agglomerate of many atoms and molecules. These, in turn, are composed of negatively charged electrons and positively charged, heavy nuclei. When a stream of photons is absorbed by a dust particle, the electric field in the light beam can be pictured as exerting an oscillating force on both the nuclei and the electrons. The heavy nuclei remain unmoved, but the electrons are displaced from their normal orbits and move rapidly back and forth in synchrony with the driving electric field of the light beam. In so doing, light waves are radiated in all directions. The observer sees the shaft of light because his eye detects the sidewise-scattered light from each particle. If the room were clean of all dust or scattering particles, the beam would be invisible to the observer.

The situation becomes a bit more complicated when the scattering particles are spaced closer together than dust in a room. Certainly, each scattering element radiates light waves in all directions, and the total scattering is the sum of all the waves. But here is where a complication arises. Waves may add constructively or destructively. At any one observation outpost, the net amount of light reaching that point is determined by the sum of the constructive and destructive interference of all waves crossing that point.

Let's stop for a moment for a definition. The quantity that describes what point each wave is in its oscillation cycle is called the *phase of the wave.* The key concept in this definition is that the difference in phase between waves depends, in part, on the spacings of the scattering particles in comparison to the wavelength of light. If, for example, two scattering particles are spaced by distances comparable to one half the wavelength of light, the two scattered waves will be 180° out of phase and the waves will then cancel each other, giving no electric field at the observation point. If, however, two particles are spaced at distances that are small in comparison to the light wavelength, the phases will nearly be the same, and the scattered field will have an amplitude twice as large as each wave individually. Therefore, the final summation of all scattered waves will give a result that depends both on the relative positions of each scattering particle in comparison to the wavelength of light and on the direction of the scattered waves. For example, light is completely transmitted through a transparent medium such as water because the water molecules are tightly packed. This means that all the waves scattered sideways from each of the molecules travel a longer distance and are out of phase with each other and thus interfere destructively with one another in all directions, except the forward direction. In water, side-scatter is eliminated, but forward-directed light waves reinforce each other because their straight-ahead paths have similar lengths.

Another factor important in scattering is the overall regular arrangement of the scatterers. For example, the lens of the normal eye is made up of protein and physiologic fluid. The lens proteins are tightly packed in an orderly fashion, and there is very little change in the density of the scattering particles from point to point in the lens. Thus, the lens is transparent. If a clear lens homogenate is mixed with water, the proteins are dispersed and the density of the proteins fluctuates markedly, producing a random pattern. The result is a great deal of scattering and a milky-appearing solution.

In summary, the relationship between the size of the wavelength of light involved, the spacing of the scatterers, the size of the scatterers, and their arrangement determines the total scattering from a medium. This interaction is analogous to running one's finger over a smoothly polished surface. The surface feels smooth if the irregularities are small in amplitude and are spaced by distances that are small in comparison to the spacing between the pressure-sensitive receptors on the fingertips. The sense of touch has a certain resolving power and cannot respond to small-scale fluctuations. In the case of light and scattering, if the scattering medium has periodic fluctuations in arrangements of scattering components larger than the wavelength of light, then these can be sensed by light waves and scattering can occur. If the spacings of the scattering components of the media are shorter than one half the light wavelength, little scattering can occur.

It is time, now, to apply our theoretic understanding of light scattering. However, in order to explain some natural phenomena we will need to cover one more theoretic point. Lord Rayleigh showed that when light strikes atmospheric particles (particles smaller than the wavelength of light), the amount of light scattering is inversely proportional to the fourth power of the wavelength. Since the blue end of the spectrum is half the wavelength of the red end, the blue end is scattered by a factor of 2^4 or 16 times the amount of the red end. This seems logical, since small particles should interact more completely with smaller wavelengths.

At high noon, the sun's rays pierce the atmosphere in a perpendicular fashion. Thus the shorter wavelengths of the sun's spectrum are more heavily scattered by the atmospheric particles, which splash the color blue all over the sky. This takes some of the blue away from the sun's own appearance, and it looks yellowish. At sunset, the light strikes the atmosphere at an angle and thus must travel a longer distance through the atmosphere. The additional particles scatter not only blue but also a significant amount of the longer wavelengths, and the sun's color goes from yellow to orange to deep red.

When you look at the lens of an elderly patient through the slit lamp, you will notice that the reflection from the anterior capsule is blue-white, whereas the reflection from the posterior capsule is a golden yellow. The double passage of light through the lens has resulted in a loss of blue light due to light scattering, producing the yellow reflection. The more nuclear sclerosis present, the yellower is the reflection. Thus we can think of the crystalline lens as a minus blue filter, because of both its yellow pigment and its preferential scattering of blue light.

This concept of the lens as a minus blue filter was suggested by Dr. Aran Safir (Safir, 1977) and helps to explain why the optic nerve looks more yellow in the phakic eye than in the aphakic eye. In fact, to the medical student, the blue-white appearance of the optic nerve in the aphakic eye may be confused with optic atrophy.

In scleral tissue, we note that the collagen fibers are much larger than those in the cornea. Both the collagen diameters and the spacing between fibers are comparable to a light wavelength. Much scattering occurs in the sclera, resulting in an opaque appearance.

It might be helpful to return to nature for a moment and review what happens when a sunbeam strikes a cloud. Clouds are made up of air and water droplets, both of which are transparent; however, they differ in their optical indices of refraction. Air has a refractive index of 1 and water of 1.333. Thus, these two components, each clear by themselves, produce substantial scattering when the droplets of water are large enough to interact with the light waves and when the droplets are spaced more than one half of a wavelength apart. Light scattering, then, is what makes clouds look cloudy, scleras look white, and cataracts look gray. We will now look at the clinical examples in more detail.

Normal Corneal Scattering

In the normal state (Dogigi, 1967), the cornea is essentially transparent. Experiments show that the corneal stroma scatters approximately 10% of all light incident upon it (Feuk and McQueen, 1971). It is this small amount of scattering that allows us to see the corneal structures under the slit lamp.

But how can the cornea be so clear if it is made of structures as diverse as epithelial cells, collagen fibers (refractive index, 1.47), and a ground substance whose refractive index is close to that of water (1.333)? The epithelial cell layer may be considered as homogeneous units of a protein solution, with each cell so tightly packed against the next that almost no extracellular water accumulates and there is virtually no fluctuation in refractive index throughout the layers. In the stroma, the collagen fibers are approximately 25 nm in diameter, and the spacing between each pair of fibrils is 60 nm. These dimensions are much smaller than a wavelength of yellow light (600 nm) (Miller and Benedek, 1973). Thus, the tiny dimensions and regular arrangement of these fibrils account for the minimal scattering.

Corneal Stromal Edema

In cases of endothelial dystrophy, endothelial trauma, or endothelial incapacitation due to inflammation (*i.e.*, iritis), the pumping action of the endothelium diminishes and the stroma takes on additional fluid and thickens. As interfibrillar fluid increases, the collagen fibers are pushed farther and farther apart. As the lakes of such fluid exceed one half of a wavelength of light in dimension, light scattering increases and the cornea takes on a gray appearance (Miller and Benedek, 1973).

Corneal Epithelial Edema

In cases of advanced endothelial impairment or acute glaucoma, fluid collects between the epithelial cells. Fluctuations in the refractive index develop, and as the spaces between the cells grow, the intensity of the scattering, or haze, grows. Potts and Friedman (Potts and

Friedman, 1959) have shown that in total corneal edema, the epithelial component accounts for the greatest share of light scattering.

Corneal Scars

When discontinuities in Bowman's membrane in ulceration, trauma, or refractive surgery induces scar formation close to the pupillary center, visual acuity decreases. Scars interfere with vision in two basic ways: (1) they cause an irregularity of the corneal surface, producing irregular astigmatism; (2) stromal scars contain either randomly arranged collagen fibers, the diameters of which are five times the diameter of normal corneal fibrils, or unusual material such as hyaluronic acid, which pushes the collagen fibers far apart. This results in backscatter of light, which yields a white appearance to the observer and foggy vision to the patient.

Scattering in the Normal Lens

The normal lens is not as transparent as the normal cornea. This is partially caused by the faint yellow pigment, which absorbs 10% to 40% of all visible blue light. This hint of yellow is augmented by normal Rayleigh scattering, present in the healthy lens. The normal clear lens, composed of tightly packed high-protein-content lens fibers, scatters a small amount of light. With aging, however, large protein aggregates form within the lens fibers, reaching molecular weights of approximately 50×10^6 g/mol.

Cataract

As a cataract develops, a normally uniform background of proteins is disturbed by large lumps of protein aggregates. If these large lumps are uncorrelated in position, and if the aggregates are large enough, significant scattering will produce a turbid appearance. As the protein continues to clump, fluid pools develop between lens fibers, and scattering increases further. At some point in this progression, the clinician decides to describe the patient's lens as cataractous.

Scattering in the Normal Vitreous

The vitreous, a composite of a 1% hyaluronic acid solution, is interspersed with collagen fibers of approximately 10 nm in diameter (Balazs, 1961). These fibers are almost three times smaller than the normal corneal collagen fibers. Since the scattering from each fiber is proportional to the fourth power of the collagen diameter, we can expect the scattering per fiber to be 80 times weaker for vitreous collagen than for corneal collagen. Thus, the effect of the collagen in the vitreous is quite small, and the vitreous will scatter only 0.1% of incident light. With age, vitreous collagen fibrils coalesce, fluid pockets form, and localized scattering develops to the point where the patient notices floating specks and threads.

Retinal Scattering

Because the ubiquitous Müller cells seem to squeeze tightly within the spacings between the retinal cells, the tissue is homogeneous from a refractive index standpoint and scatters about as much light as the cornea.

If, however, the blood supply to a retinal area is interrupted and infarction takes place, the area fed by the occluded vessel becomes milky gray. With infarction, edema fluid accumulates in the nerve fiber layer. Because the refractive index of edema fluid differs from that of the nerve fiber axons, the area loses transparency.

Glare

The term "glare" is often used to describe the contrast-lowering effect of stray light on a visual scene. The outfielder is said to lose a fly ball into the sun because of glare. Extra light thrown onto the retina tends to wash out the contrast of the event we are viewing. For example, every student is aware of the importance of pulling down all the shades and darkening the room if all the details of a slide projected on a screen are to be appreciated. Because of the nature of the light-detecting mechanism at the retina and in the brain, we cannot see intensity differences efficiently in the presence of a high background of light intensity.

This sensitivity to glare is amplified as lens (or corneal) scattering is increased. For example, the older surgeon cannot see the details within a deep surgical wound in the presence of white surgical sponges (Ringrose, 1976). These sponges act as extraneous light sources, which are scattered by the aging crystalline lens onto the macula of the surgeon's retina (Wolf, 1960). Again, the patient with a poorly fitted contact lens who develops epithelial corneal edema reports unusual glare from automobile headlights at night. In cases of cataract or marked corneal edema, the patient has difficulty reading in a bright environment, where all the elements of normal light become sources of glare.

Some time ago, we wondered what percentage of a lens must actually become cataractous or, put another way, how much of the lens must remain clear before scattering and consequent glare reach levels significant enough to impair visual acuity. Although contrast started to drop slightly when almost half the lens was "covered with cataract," contrast dropped suddenly when 80% of the lens became cataractous (Zuckerman et al., 1973).

Thus, light scattering, glare, and visual performance are all tightly bound together.

Clinical Glare Testing

In 1926, the industrial scientist L.L. Holladay (Holladay, 1926) first described the relationship between glare and contrast sensitivity. Holladay developed a mathematical relationship between the glare source (its brightness and angular distance from the target) and contrast sensitivity. In the 1960s, Ernst Wolf (Wolf, 1960; Wolf, 1963; Miller et al., 1967), a Boston visual physiologist, built a laboratory glare tester and showed in a normal population that glare sensitivity increased with age. He also showed that this increase in glare sensitivity was related to the increased light scattering of the normal, aging lens. In the 1970s and early

1980s, Miller, Wolf, Nadler, and others (Miller and Wolf, 1972; Laclaire and Nadler, 1982) built and tested the first clinical glare tester (Miller-Nadler glare tester. With this device, they demonstrated a connection between cataract progress and increased glare sensitivity (Laclaire and Nadler, 1982). The visual acuity is randomly scattered throughout the plot, whereas glare sensitivity increases in an orderly progression. Glare sensitivity also correlated highly with the degree of posterior capsule opacification after extracapsular cataract extraction and intraocular lens implantation (Nadler et al., 1984).

Glare Tester Characteristics

Glare testers offer two types of targets: a standard Snellen visual acuity chart and a variable contrast sensitivity target. The variable contrast targets may be presented as (1) sinusoidal contrast gratings; (2) the Snellen chart printed in different contrasts; or (3) the Landolt ring presented in different contrasts. To determine whether a variable contrast target or a standard visual acuity target would be more valuable in cataract testing, we designed an experiment using scattering filters of progressive severity (simulated cataracts) (Miller and Benedek, 1973; Balazs, 1961). These laboratory experiments suggested that a variable contrast target in the face of a glare source follows cataract progression more smoothly than a conventional visual acuity target.

Quantification of Glare on Contrast Sensitivity

We have asserted that ocular lesions that scatter light degrade contrast sensitivity by splashing extra noninformation containing light onto the retinal image. This can be demonstrated by a simple calculation put forth by Prager and colleagues (Abrahmsson and Sjostrand, 1986).

Suppose we wanted to measure the contrast of the standard projected Snellen chart in both a darkened examining room and a lighted one. Contrast is the difference between the luminance of the target and its background, and can be expressed as a percentage, as follows:

$$\left[\frac{(\text{Background Luminance} - \text{Target Luminance})}{(\text{Background Luminance} + \text{Target Luminance})}\right] \times 100$$

To calculate the contrast of the projected Snellen chart in a darkened room, let us say the background illumination is 97 arbitrary light units, and the target illumination (consisting of letters) is 3 light units. This gives the following:

$$\text{Contrast} = \left[\frac{(97 - 3) \times 100}{(97 + 3)}\right] = 94\%$$

Let us now turn the room lights on, thus placing an additional 50 light units onto both the background and letters of the projected Snellen chart. The new contrast is given by the following:

$$\text{Contrast} = \left[\frac{(147 - 53) \times 100}{(147 + 53)}\right] = 47\%$$

We see that this simple maneuver cuts the contrast in half. Just as the Snellen chart drops its contrast when extra light falls upon it, the retinal image loses contrast when a corneal lesion scatters extraneous light onto the macula There are a number of simple ways to decrease glare and improve contrast:

1) Using side shields on the temples of spectacles prevents glaring sidelong rays from striking the eye.
2) Watching the television set with the room lights off prevents annoying glare from ceiling or lamp light from striking the eye.
3) Wearing polarized sunglasses will cancel out the reflected glare from shiny surfaces (*e.g.*, car hoods, lakes, glossy paper)
4) Wearing a peaked cap or wide-brimmed hat prevents the overhead rays of the sun from striking the eye.
5) Replacing scratched or pitted automobile windshields reduces glare from the sun and oncoming headlights.

Surgical Methods

When these methods fail to help a patient who has glare disability, surgical removal of the scattering lesion should be considered. Significant corneal edema or permanent corneal scars can be treated by a corneal transplant. A significant cataract should be extracted. Finally, an opaque lens capsule after cataract surgery, which produces glare symptoms or reduced contrast sensitivity, requires a capsulotomy. Because the glare disability is proportional to the ratio of the area of capsule opening over the area of capsule opacity, the size of the capsulotomy must be considered. The size of the optimal capsulotomy equals the size of the pupil (Holladay et al., 1985).

7. Diffraction Effects

Laser Interferometry

When a patient develops a cataract and a concomitant decrease in vision, the ophthalmologist must decide whether the visual loss is completely explained by the lens changes. The problem may be compounded by a history of degenerative retinal disease.

If a way could be found to bypass the lens opacity, or any ocular opacity for that matter, and project a resolution target directly upon the macula, the question of the state of retinal function might be answered. It occurred to Green and colleagues (Green, 1970) at the University of Michigan that a proper resolution target could be a set of interference fringes of light and dark bands. The source of the interference fringes could be two tiny light sources, which could be focused directly onto two relatively clear areas in the opaque lens. These tiny sources could then direct their rays, without obstacle, toward the retina, and their light would interfere with each other to produce dark and light bands upon the retina.

Thus, the Michigan group essentially duplicated Thomas Young's original experiment, with a few important changes. The two-point light source came from a safe, low-power HeNe laser. Laser light, being coherent and of one pure color, can come to a very fine point focus and produces vivid interference patterns. The light of the HeNe laser, being red, is also scattered less than other visible wavelengths and thus penetrates the opaque media more cleanly. Finally, Green was able to alter the widths of the dark and light bands by altering the spacing of the two light sources and thus present resolution levels comparable to the scale of the Snellen letters (Green and Cohen, 1971; Gstalder and Green, 1972). The potential acuity meter is another device for testing retinal visual acuity. It projects a small Snellen chart through a small, clear space within an irregular cornea or partially cloudy lens onto the retina. This approach minimizes the influence of the anterior segment problem. It is used to predict postoperative visual function (Tetz et al., 1992).

Haloes

Every medical student is taught that patients with angle-closure glaucoma report seeing colored haloes. Interestingly, similar haloes are more commonly associated with the presence of early cataracts or epithelial corneal edema from poorly fitted contact lenses. In this section, we present the optical derivation of these haloes (Ringrose, 1976).

Lens Haloes

A histologic frontal section of a lens wedge shows cross-sections of lens fibers as stacked like pancakes. This radiating pattern is known as Rabl's lamellae, the fibers being more uniform beneath the epithelium and becoming thicker and irregular as they age and approach the nucleus. At the boundaries between the fibers, the refractive index is different from that in the fibers. Thus, the quasi regular fluctuation in refractive index acts as a radial diffraction grating and produces a circular interference pattern, or halo. The intensity of the halo increases as the separation between fibers widens. This occurs during cataract formation, when fluid accumulates between the fibers. It should also be pointed out that the lens fiber pattern is only regular enough to produce these effects from 2.5 mm from the lens center to the lens periphery. The optics are explained in this manner: thus d in the equation $d \sin\theta = \lambda$ represents the width of the lens fibers. Halo experiments predict the lens fiber diameter to be 10.5 μm, which agrees nicely with histologic measurements. As in all diffraction effects, the longer (red) wavelengths are diffracted more and appear at the edge, whereas the blue wavelengths are closer to the center of the halo.

Finally, it should be noted that the location of the radial scattering elements on the lens periphery also serves as a basis for distinguishing lenticular haloes from those of corneal origin. Ask the patient to view with a stenopeic slit the point source of light producing the halo. As the slit is moved downward, the patient will see only fragments of the halo if it originates in the lens. If the halo is corneal in origin, the whole halo will still be seen, but dimmer with the slit than without.

Corneal Haloes

The ancient sailor knew that a ring around the moon meant foul weather the next day. Rings, or haloes, around the moon are created by ice crystals in the atmosphere, which act as a cosmic diffraction grating. In a similar way, edematous corneal epithelium produces haloes.

When edematous, corneal epithelial edema, the type seen in acute glaucoma, advanced endothelial dystrophy, and contact lens overwear,. the basal epithelial layer acts as a diffraction grating and appears to be the origin of the halo. In physical terms, we have a meshwork of edema fluid of one refractive index surrounding basal cells of another refractive index. If this fluctuation in refractive index has a regular pattern and covers 10 or more cells, it will serve as a diffraction grating. A series of colored rings representing the colors of the spectrum is called one order of interference rings. A second series of colored rings outside of the first is called a second order of rings. The larger the edema pools between epithelial cells are, the brighter is the second order.

The halo itself often consists of two orders of colored rings, the outer order being somewhat fainter.

Pinhole Discs

Diffraction is an edge phenomenon, in which the relative impact of the diffraction is proportional to the ratio of the circumference of the edge to the area of the aperture:

$$\pi D/(\pi D^2/4) = D/4$$

Therefore, as the pupil of the eye or the camera gets smaller, the ratio 4/D gets greater. This effect was brought out clearly in a series of experiments in which we attempted to correct various degrees of refractive error with different-sized pinholes (Miller and Johnson, 1977). The pinhole improves vision by increasing the depth of focus; however, it obscures vision by introducing diffraction effects.

For example, a 0.5-mm pinhole could allow 20/40 (6/12) vision in the presence of an 8 D refractive error, and 20/70 (6/21) vision in the presence of a 12 D error. Yet when our subject, who had no refractive error, looked through a 0.5-mm pinhole, he achieved a visual acuity of only 20/30 (6/9) because of the obscuring effect of the diffraction. The 1-mm pinhole (the one found in the clinician's office) allowed our subject to see 20/40 with a 5 D refractive error and 20/200 (6/60) with a 9 D error. However, it too could produce vision no better than 20/25 (6/7.5) in subjects with no refractive error. This diffraction effect on vision is seen until the pupil size reaches 2 to 2.5 mm.

Metric equivalent given in parentheses after Snellen's notation.

8. Optical Coherence Tomography

Ocular coherence tomography (OCT), a new device, has been used to evaluate intraocular structures based on the low-coherence interference phenomena, similar to the one described by Thomas Young almost two centuries ago.

In OCT, a beam of light is directed onto the tissue or specimen to be imaged, and the internal structure is measured noninvasively by measuring the echo delay time of light as it is reflected from microstructural features at different ranges. Two-dimensional imaging is accomplished by performing successive axial (longitudinal) range measurements at different transverse positions.

The resolution of echo-based devices such as ophthalmic ultrasound and OCT is based on the ratio of the speed of the emitted wave to that of the reflected wave. Traditional ultrasound measurements are achieved with a frequency of approximately 10 Hz and have a 150 μm resolution. New ultrasonic devices increased the resolution by increasing the frequency (up to 100 Hz), but they cannot penetrate more than 4 to 5 mm into the eye. With light-based devices such as the OCT (wavelength, 800 nm), scientists have been able to increase the resolution up to 15 μm. The emitted light beam is split into a reference beam (that goes to a mirror) and a measurement beam (that goes to the patient's eye). The reflected reference and measurement light beam are combined, and their intensity is measured by a photodetector. Positive interference (brighter light) is achieved by moving the mirror (reference light beam) until the distance the light travels to and from the reference mirror precisely matches the distance that light travels when it is reflected from a given structure in a patient's eye.

Dependent on the transparency of the optical media (*i.e.*, cornea-lens-vitreous-retina), the device is limited by opaque media disorders. Its major uses are the observation and analysis of the posterior pole tissue contour (*i.e.*, disc, macula) and the measurement of tissue layers (retina) (Hee et al., 1995)

9. Antireflection Coatings

Approximately 4% of visible light is reflected from either the front or the back surface of a lens. These ghost images can often wash out image contrast. Thus, all fine camera lenses have antireflection coatings.

Surface reflectance depends on the difference in refractive indices for air and glass. For visible light, this is approximately the difference between 1 and 1.5. By selecting a material with a refractive index that falls between these two values (near the geometric mean), and by applying a coating of approximately 0.25 wavelength optical thickness to the surface, it is possible to reduce the reflectance significantly. Magnesium fluoride (MgF_2), a durable substance with an index of 1.38 at 550 nm, is the most commonly used coating material for single-layer antireflection coatings. Instead of one reflection at the air-glass interface, there is now a reflection at the air-MgF_2 interface and a second reflection at the MgF_2-glass interface. These reflections interfere destructively, resulting in a minimum reflectance within the visible spectrum (at normal incidence) of 1.5% or less, as compared with the original 4% for the uncoated glass surface. From the principle of energy conservation, there must be a corresponding increase in overall transmission of a coated surface, including both interfaces.

As a specific example, a ray impinging on the surface of an uncoated aspheric lens (refractive index, 1.523) near its edge at an angle of incidence of 58° would have a reflection loss of 8.3%. Lenses with steep front surfaces tend to produce larger angles of incidence and thus produce stronger reflections. However, by the addition of a single-layer MgF_2 antireflection coating designed for normal incidence, the reflection loss is reduced by more than one half, to 3.6%. Only at angles of incidence larger than 60° does the reflectance of such a coated surface exceed 4%. A practical way to test whether a lens has been coated is to look at the reflected image produced. Coated lenses produce a bluish or greenish, rather than a yellowish, reflection.

High transmission and aesthetics are important reasons why contact lenses are currently so popular. Besides these factors the low reflectance may be beneficial in situations such as reading with a bright light behind and to the side of the head. With normal eyeglasses, the reflected light from the back of the lens would strike an incipient cataract, producing an annoying scattered light on the retina, which decreases the contrast of the retinal image.

In a sense, one might consider the crystalline lens to have a type of antireflection coating. The third Purkinje image (from the front surface of the lens) is quite dim. Because the intensity of the reflected image is proportional to the difference in refractive indices between the lens and the surrounding media, a dim reflected image is the result of a small difference between lens and surrounding media. The refractive index of the outer layers of the mammalian lens is close to that of the aqueous. The refractive index gradually increases toward the nucleus. A reflection from a synthetic intraocular lens is quite noticeable, however, because of the large jump in refractive index from aqueous (1.33) to implant (1.48).

10. Polarization Phenomena

Since the time of Thomas Young, light has been considered a wave phenomenon. The waves vibrate in a plane perpendicular to the line of motion of the light. Thus, if a light ray emerged perpendicular to the plane of this paper, the light waves would be considered to be moving up and down, right and left, and in every conceivable diagonal direction, and all within the plane of this paper. For simplicity, physicists vectorially divide all the directions of vibration into up-and-down components and equal side-to-side components. Such light is considered *unpolarized.*

To remove one component, it should be possible to locate a transparent material whose molecular anatomy resembles a picket fence. In such a case, the up-and-down component of the wave might squeeze through, but the side-to-side vibrations would collide with the pickets and be redirected, producing two separate light rays. Such a material (crystals of calcium carbonate known as Iceland spar) was discovered in 1669 by the Dutch physician Erasmus Bartholinus (Miller and Benedek, 1973). We now know that as light penetrates the crystal, vibrations parallel to the planar carbonate groups are slowed down, as if bumping into these molecular "pickets," to a greater degree than the vibrations perpendicular to these groups. The result is an ambivalent crystal that refracts light waves vibrating in one direction differently than it refracts those vibrating in a perpendicular direction. In 1828, the British physicist William Nicol glued two pieces of Iceland spar together in such a way that light waves vibrating in one direction passed through the crystal; the other waves were refracted differently and so struck the crystal-glue interface and were reflected out of the way. Thus, light emerging from a Nicol prism would be considered *plane polarized,* representing about half the original light intensity. If this light then passed through a second Nicol prism, aligned in a similar fashion, the light would pass through unchanged. However, if the second Nicol prism, called an *analyzer,* were rotated by a small angle, the molecular pickets would eliminate some of the plane-polarized light. Finally, if the second Nicol prism were rotated in an orientation 90° from the first, no light would get through.

In 1932, Edwin Land made available an inexpensive substitute for the Nicol prism, which he called *polaroid.* Polaroid is made of an extremely thin layer of many fine crystals of iodine and quinine sulfate. This compound, known as herapathite, after its discoverer W.B. Herapath, is unique in that it strongly absorbs one of its double-refracted beams so that light vibrating in only one direction gets through. Land succeeded in lining up all the crystals in one direction and imbedding them in plastic sheets, which could be manufactured on a commercial basis.

As a sunglasses material, polaroid not only attenuates the light, but also eliminates reflected glare. When light is reflected from the surface of water, it is partially polarized (*i.e.*, part of the reflected rays are plane polarized). If the axis of the polaroid sunglasses is oriented perpendicular to this direction, much of the reflected light will be absorbed.

The polarization principles have been around for more than 100 years, with some ophthalmic applications. The three-dimensional (or stereoscopic) vision seems to be related to the capacity of our brain to interpret slightly different images from both eyes. Nature uses the interocular distance itself as a source for the disparity by providing two different observation angles for real objects. An artificial way to recreate this angular disparity is through the use of polaroid glasses and polarized printed images. The light from each picture vibrates in a different direction, and each polarizing lens allows only one direction of vibration to be transmitted to each eye. Therefore two slightly different images are received by the brain and interpreted as a stereoscopic object. This is the principle of the Titmus test to access stereopsis, mainly in children with strabismus.

The polarization phenomenon can also be used to create a disappearing reticule to be placed in the surgical microscope eyepiece. Let us assume that a surgeon would like to measure an ocular structure during an operation (*i.e.*, pupil diameter), or the size of a corneal reflection (which can be converted into a measure of corneal power). A measuring reticule, in one of the eyepieces of the microscope, would be needed; however, the presence of the ruled reticule during the surgery might annoy the surgeon. How can the reticule be made to disappear and then reappear? Let the marks of the measuring reticule be made of a polarizing material. Let the reticule also be rotatable. Now place a polarizing filter over the microscope light. If the light reflected from the eye is polarized with the same orientation as the markings of the reticule, then the markings will be invisible. If the reticule is rotated 90° then it will be easily seen.

Haidinger Brushes

We humans also possess a polarization sensor in our eyes, although it is very primitive. The first description of this polarization effect was made by the German mineralogist Wilhelm Karl von Haidinger, in 1844. Haidinger brushes are entoptic phenomena seen best when a uniformly blue background (*e.g.*, the sky) is visualized through a polarizing element. The brushes look like two yellow sheaths of wheat extending out 2° to 3° from the point of fixation and separated by bright blue quadrants. Understanding the source of the brushes has challenged some of the greatest minds in science and ophthalmology over the years (*e.g.*, Helmholtz, Brewster, Stokes, Gullstrand).

The best explanation, so far, was presented by Ulf Hallden (Hallden, 1957) of Uppsala, Sweden, who was able to model the phenomenon with pieces of polaroid and cellophane. He believed that the initially polarized light travels through the nerve fiber layer of Henle in the macula, which functions as a yellow filter. The yellow filter effect is accomplished by the nerve fibers, which are double refracting (birefringent) and of a thickness that allows constructive interference for the two sets of waves of yellow and blue. Finally, the radial polarizer (analyzer) located in the photoreceptors absorbs the light wherever the radial elements are perpendicular to the vibration of the polarized light. Yellow light comes through, and light in adjacent quadrants is diminished.

The Haidinger brush phenomenon has been made into a clinical test for macular function. The test consists of a blue light with a rotating polaroid element covering the light. The yellow brushes are usually seen to be revolving if the macula is functioning at 20/100 (6/30) level or better. The brushes are even said to be seen in patients with dense amblyopia if the anatomy of the macula is intact (Sloan and Naquin, 1955).

Photoelasticity

One of the most important practical applications of polarized light is in the field of photoelasticity. This is the study of the stresses and strains in transparent plastics. These stresses and strains produce unusual colored patterns when they are examined between crossed polaroid elements.

If a material with only one refractive index is placed between crossed polaroids, the field remains dark. If a doubly refracting material is placed between crossed polaroids, the initially polarized light is rotated by the material and gets through the analyzing polaroid. For example, glass annealed improperly, or glass case hardened for added strength, develops a crystalline structure and becomes doubly refracting. When such glass is placed between crossed polaroids, it exhibits the typical interference pattern of glass under strain. Before the advent of plastic eyeglass lenses or glass lenses that were chemically hardened, this test was the only way to determine whether a lens labeled “safety glass” was truly casehardened.

Corneal Birefringence

Finally, it should be noted that both the cornea and the lens are birefringent. For example, illuminating the cornea with polarized light and analyzing the reflected light with a crossed polaroid produces a striking pattern composed of two black parabolas, which closely resemble a Maltese cross, surrounded by one or two orders of colored rings near the limbus. The pattern is apparently the result of the arrangement of the double-refracting collagen lamellae in the cornea and is typical of biaxial, birefringent crystals. The pattern is also dependent on local corneal thickness and is altered in keratoconus (Miller and Weinstein,

1955) and collagen shrinkage produced by the Holmium laser. Elevation of intraocular pressure does not significantly alter the position of the collagen fibrils and thus does not alter the interference pattern (Maurice, 1962). As yet, no evolutionary advantage has been ascribed to the birefringence of the cornea, nor has a clinical test been devised that exploits this unique characteristic.

11. Eye Colors

Iris

The color of the iris is a result of three variable factors in each patient: (1) the density of the posterior pigmented epithelial layer; (2) the density of the stromal pigment cells; and (3) the fiber size and arrangement of the stromal collagen. In the blue eye, light incident on the iris is mostly backscattered by the stromal fibers. The larger radial fibers, which are wrapped in heavy bundles like shreds of white paper, backscatter white light, acting as small reflectors with no preference for any wavelength. The fine gossamer stromal collagen fibers, seen as cottony wisps between the radial bundles, backscatter light in the typical Rayleigh fashion (*i.e.*, inversely proportional to the fourth power of the wavelength). Thus, they give a blue appearance. Incident light that manages to squeeze between the stromal fibers is absorbed by the melanin of the pigment epithelium and contributes a darker background to the stromal light scattering. Thus, the blue iris always looks bluer in the periphery, where the heavy whiter appearing fibers fan out and the fine fibers predominate, and appears lighter near the pupil, where the heavy radial fibers are concentrated.

Those irises that represent the spectrum from green to dark brown are characterized by heavier and heavier sprinklings of melanin pigment within the iris stroma. For example, a light dusting of melanin in the stroma will give a yellowish appearance. Thus, yellow plus the blue from the stromal light scattering yields a green appearance. As the melanin concentration gets heavier, more light becomes absorbed by the pigment, producing the dark brown color characteristic of melanin.

Scleral Whiteness

The heavy, irregularly spaced, transparent collagenous bands that make up the sclera are surrounded by ground substance of a different refractive index. Such a combination produces marked light scattering. Because the collagen fibers are large in relation to the wavelength of light, they do not scatter in a Rayleigh fashion; they scatter all wavelengths alike, yielding a white appearance. In a patient with scleral thinning, the sclera will look blue. In such an instance, the remaining scleral fibers are finer and thus preferentially backscatter blue light. This effect is even more pronounced because the underlying heavily pigmented choroid provides a dark background.

Fundus

The fundus varies from a pinkish red in the lightly pigmented patient to a dusky red in the heavily pigmented patient. Light incident on the eye penetrates the transparent retina and is partially absorbed by the pigment granules in the retinal pigment epithelium. A combination of (1) some white light slipping between the pigment granules and (2) the yellow-to-red wavelengths, which can penetrate the melanin pigment, arrives in the choroid. Light striking the multiple layers of melanin pigment in the choroid tends to be absorbed, yielding a dark backdrop, similar to the pigment epithelium of the iris. The blue and green components of the light striking the blood of the choroidal vessels are absorbed, and the light that returns to the observer is primarily yellow-red, which is the distinctive characteristic of the pigment oxyhemoglobin. In lightly pigmented areas, some incident light may penetrate the choroidal structures and arrive at the sclera, which will backscatter the light much as a sheet of white paper would. Lightly pigmented fundi predominantly represent a combination of scleral backscatter and hemoglobin absorption and reflection, modulated by the pigmentation present. In the darker fundi, there is little scleral effect, and the color primarily depends on melanin and hemoglobin absorption and reflection.

The preferential absorption of specific wavelengths by various fundus layers has been exploited to improve, by contrast enhancement, the visualization of certain fundal components and pathologic lesions (Behrendt and Duane, 1966; Potts, 1965).

For example, nerve fiber bundles are best visualized with light from 475 to 520 nm, depending on the fiber density and fundus pigmentation. These wavelengths are heavily absorbed by the retinal pigment epithelium and thus yield a dark background, whereas the nerve fibers themselves efficiently reflect the blue end of the spectrum. Therefore, the red-free filter of the ophthalmoscope, by eliminating the red end of the spectrum, brings out the nerve fibers around the disc more clearly against a dark background. Hoyt and co-workers (Hoyt et al., 1973) photographed the fundus with red-free light and demonstrated areas of nerve bundle atrophy adjacent to healthy nerve bundles.

Retinal blood vessels are seen with the greatest contrast within the 550- to 580-nm spectral band. These wavelengths are maximally absorbed by the hemoglobin pigment and appear very dark against a light background when these filters are used in an ophthalmoscope or retinal camera. Such filters also improve the contrast of the pale physiologic cup against the pink optic nerve head.

Choroidal nevi are best seen in red light (about 650 nm), which can effectively penetrate the retinal pigment epithelium and choroid. Thus, monochromatic photography that uses black-and-white film and red light sometimes can provide higher contrast and better resolution than color photography (Delori and Gragoudes, 1976).

The existence of the yellow macular pigment has been known since the eighteenth century (Polyak, 1941). It acts as a broad band blue filter, influencing color appearance, color matching, and color vision tests (Ruddock, 1970). This probably is achieved through compensation for the eye's chromatic aberration and a reduction of atmospherically scattered blue light. It also may serve as an ultraviolet filter. The composition of the yellow pigment seems to be a combination of carotinoids (Bone et al., 1985) and is primarily located in the outer plexiform layer with some in the inner cone segment.

12. Fluorescence

You may have noticed how a freshly laundered white shirt, if illuminated by ultraviolet or blue light, will glow in the dark. This glow, known as fluorescence, may last a short time after the exciting light is turned off. On a molecular or quantum level, the following probably happens. A quantum of blue or ultraviolet light (short wavelength, high energy level) is absorbed by the "fluorescing material." The photon interacts with the outer electrons, raising the energy from a ground state to some excited level. As the energy level drops back to the ground state, a small amount is lost as vibrational-rotational energy. The major loss, however, results from the emission of a photon. This photon has a 10% to 20% longer wavelength. Thus, the fluorescent process can be seen as capturing nonvisible ultraviolet photons and turning them into less energetic visible light, or capturing blue light and converting it into the less energetic green or yellow light.

How is fluorescence related to the eye? The fluorescence of fluorescein dye is a good example. Another interesting example is the natural fluorescence of the crystalline lens. If the lens is excited with a nonvisible ultraviolet wavelength (say, 300 or 350 nm), a faint blue fluorescence will be observed. This is thought to be primarily related to the accumulation of tyrosine and tryptophane residues, and is responsible for the filtering effect of ultraviolet light as one ages. The increased tryptophane and tyrosine levels are thought to be related to oxidation of lens biomolecules. This oxidation may be driven, in part, by cumulative light exposure.

The lens also shows a second type of fluorescence, obvious to any examiner who has observed the human lens with blue slit-lamp illumination. The blue exciting light creates a yellow-green fluorescence. These fluorescing proteins are thought to be the result of lens metabolism (Yu et al., 1988).

The blue light-induced fluorescence increases with age (Carlyl et al., 1988). Thus, as a person ages, less blue light reaches his or her retina. This induced fluorescence appears in all parts of the lens. After age 50, the 442-nm induced fluorescence seems to decrease. In a sense, this is an artifact. The lens scatters more light. The shorter (blue) wavelengths, are scattered more than the longer ones. Thus, less blue light reaches the nucleus and posterior cortex, and less fluorescence is induced. This same study showed that diabetic lenses fluorescence more than age-controlled normal lenses. Finally, the study showed that the fluorescence increased with cataract severity.

Recent studies have been able to correlate corneal and lens fluorescence with degree of diabetic retinopathy; this may be a powerful tool for the clinician in the early diagnosis of the condition. The basis for a clinical device is termed *redox fluorometry*. This term is derived from the fact that nicotinamide adenosine dinucleotide (NAD) and flavin adenosine dinucleotide (FAD) participate in the energy production chain in the cell receiving electrons and becoming reduced. The reduced substances exhibit a strong fluorescence at 450 and 500 nm, respectively. The cellular concentration of these substances is determined by the difference between the rate at which they are produced and the rate at which they are used in the stages of cellular respiration. There is less cellular activity when less glucose enters the cell due to lack of insulin (diabetes), and this results in a higher degree of fluorescence.

In a study of 94 insulin-dependent diabetes mellitus patients and 46 healthy controls, a positive correlation between corneal autofluorescence and minimal background retinopathy, background retinopathy, and (pre-) proliferative retinopathy was shown. Another study analyzed the populations of a geographically based survivor group of 161 mixed early- and late-onset diabetics (and 133 nondiabetic controls) and a second group of 104 early-onset insulin dependent diabetics (and 138 nondiabetic controls). Powerful associations ($p < 10^{-6}$) were found between the presence of diabetes and increased lenticular autofluorescence in both populations (Sparrow et al., 1992).

13. Densitometry of Scheimplug Photographs of the Lens

As a cataract progresses, it scatters more light. As we have seen, the mechanism for this increased light scattering is the development of large protein aggregates in the lens. The size and concentration of these aggregates can be measured with the quasi elastic light scattering analysis (Benedek, 1969). Another objective method of following the progression of the cataract is to measure the total backscattered light. With the slit-lamp beam, the observer can easily see the increase in backscattered light as the cataract progresses. However, because of the limited depth of focus of the normal slit-lamp microscope, it is impossible to take a sharp and undistorted picture of the entire lens. If the Scheimpflug principle is used, sharp slit-lamp photographs of the entire lens is possible (Drews, 1964; Brown, 1969). Once such pictures are taken, a densitometric trace of the photo will accurately document the level of light scattering of the lens.

The *Scheimpflug principle* states that the plane of an obliquely positioned object intersects the plane of the image (Scheimpflug, 1906). In the case of the crystalline lens, the slit-lamp beam slices through the lens in an oblique direction. The observer sees only the front or back of the lens in focus because the oblique section through the lens is wider than the depth of focus of the slit lamp. There is a plane in image space, however, that will be conjugate with the oblique object plane. This plane intersects the object plane. The principle is used by tilting the slit-lamp objective and/or the film plane. Thus, a special Scheimpflug slit lamp camera will have the film plane not where the observer is, but off to the side, so that the extension of its plane will intersect the oblique plane through the lens, somewhere in space.

14. The Doppler Shift

The Doppler shift has been called a kind of cosmic speedometer. By measuring the Doppler shift of a telescopic image of a star, one can tell just how fast it is moving away from you. This is possible because the star is sending us light, as a wave phenomenon. The wave can be described in terms of wavelength or frequency. Frequency can be thought of in terms of the number of waveforms appearing in a set interval. Take the situation of a train receding with the whistle blowing. The whistle is sending out its characteristic sound (*i.e.*, a waveform that has a certain frequency). Let us say the frequency is 10 cycles/second. When the train is very close to us, the sound wave does not have far to travel, and so all 10 cycles do appear in 1 second. As the train speeds away, its distance from us gets longer. Thus, although the whistle blows at 10 cycles/second, by the time we hear the sound, it has taken more than 1 second for the first to the last cycle to reach us. In 1 second, we may register only 9 cycles. Therefore, the frequency is lower and consequently its wavelength (read this as pitch for sound) is longer (c = 1/f). This implies that we can calculate the speed of an object moving away from us by measuring the change in frequency or wavelength.

In 1929, the American astronomer Edwin Hubble noted that the galaxies were rushing apart and that the universe was expanding. Hubble had actually looked at the galactic spectra and noted that the light was shifting to the red. Using the Doppler effect, he calculated the speed of recession of the galaxies. This same principle can be used to measure the velocity of blood in the retinal circulation in a noninvasive way. The laser Doppler velocimeter directs monochromatic light to a retinal blood vessel. The moving blood cells within the vessel backscatter the light. This light shows a shift in frequency that is proportional to the blood velocity. In the laser Doppler velocimeter, the backscattered light is made to interfere with the original light to best bring out the frequency shift.

The resulting interference produces an oscillating intensity of light, as registered by the photomultiplier. The original work was done on polystyrene spheres flowing through plastic tubes (Riva et al.,1972). The results showed that the fluid did not flow with just one velocity, but that a frequency shift profile occurred across the flowing fluid. Nevertheless, for a specific part of the flow profile, the frequency shift was proportional to the velocity of blood flow and the angle made by the analyzer with the direction of the tube.

After many years of debugging the apparatus, results in 1989 in living human patients showed that blood flow velocity in the retinal vessels could be obtained (Feke et al., 1989). The values for blood flow in retinal arterioles must be obtained during diastole, and the reading should be obtained in the center of the vessel. Usually, two readings along the vessels are recorded. Because the vessels are narrow, multiple scattering is not a problem, but the blood flow does vary with the diameter of the vessels. The method showed that the average retinal blood flow was 26 ± 4 g blood/min/100 g tissue, which agrees well with invasive measurements.

The Doppler effect has also been used to better understand field loss in normal-tension glaucoma. A study showed that compared with normal subjects, patients with chronic open-angle glaucoma had a statistically significant ($p < 0.05$) decrease in mean end-diastolic velocity and an increase in mean resistive index in all retinal vessels studied (Rankin et al., 1995). The patients with normal-tension glaucoma showed similar changes. Thus, open-angle glaucoma is associated with a decreased mean flow velocity and an increased mean resistive index in the retinal vasculature.

References

Abrahmsson M, Sjostrand J. Impairment of contrast function as a measure of disability glare. *Invest Ophthalmol Vis Sci* 1986;27:1131-1136.

Balazs EA. Molecular morphology of the vitreous body. In Smelser GK (ed): The Structure of the Eye, p 306. New York, *Academic Press,* 1961

Behrendt T, Duane TD. Investigation of fundus oculi with spectral reflectance photography: depth and integrity of fundal structures. *Arch Ophthalmol* 1966; 75:375-379.

Benedek GB. Optical mixing spectroscopy with applications to problems in physics, chemistry, biology and engineering. In Jubilee Volume in Honor of A Kastler: Polarization, Matter and Radiation. Paris, *Press Universitaire de France,* 1969

Bone RA, Landru JT, Tarsis SL. Preliminary identification of the human macular pigment. *Vis Res 1985*; 25:1531-1535.

Brown N. Slit-image photography. *Trans Ophthalmol Soc UK* 1969; 89:397

Carlyl LR, Rand LI, Bursell SE. In vivo lens autofluorescence at different excitation wavelengths. *Invest Ophthalmol Vis Sci* 1988;29(suppl):150

Delori FS, Gragoudes ES. Examination of the ocular fundus with monochromatic light. *Ann Ophthalmol* 1976;8:703-709.

Dogigi J: The Magic of Rays. New York, *Knopt*, 1967.

Drews C. Depth of field in slit lamp photography: an optical solution using the Scheimpflug principle. *Ophthalmologica* 1964; 148:143-150.

Feke GI, Tagawa H, Deupree DM et al. Blood flow in the normal human retina. *Invest Ophthalmol Vis Sci* 1989; 3:58-65.

Feuk T, McQueen D. The angular dependence of light scattering by rabbit cornea. *Invest Ophthalmol 1*971;10:294-299.

Green DG, Cohen MM. Laser interferometry in the evaluation of potential macular function in the presence of opacities in the ocular media. *Trans Am Acad Ophthalmol Otolaryngol 1971;75:629-637.*

Green DG. Testing the vision of cataract patients by means of laser generated interference fringes. *Science* 1970; 168:1240-1242.

Gstalder RJ, Green DG. Laser interferometry in corneal opacification. Preoperative visual potential estimation. *Arch Ophthalmol* 1972; 87:269-274.

Hallden U. An explanation of Haidinger brushes. *Arch Ophthalmol* 1957;57:393-399.

Hee MR, Izatt JA, Swanson EA et al. Optical coherence tomography of the human retina. *Arch Ophthalmol* 1995;113: 325-332.

Holladay J, Bishop J, Lewis J. The optimal size of a posterior capsulotomy. *Am Intraocular Implant Soc J 1985*; 11:18-20.

Holladay LL. The fundamentals of glare and visibility. *J Optical Soc Am* 1926;12:492

Hoyt W, Frisen L, Newman NM. Funduscopy of nerve fiber layer defects in glaucoma. *Invest Ophthalmol* 1973;12:814-829.

Laclaire J, Nadler MP, Weiss S et al. A new glare tester for clinical testing. *Arch Ophthalmol* 1982;100:153-158.

Maurice D: The cornea and sclera. In Davson H (ed). The Eye, Vol 1. New York, Academic Press, 1962

Miller D, Benedek G. Intraocular Light Scattering. *Springfield, Charles C Thomas*, 1973

Miller D, Johnson R. Quantification of the pinhole effect. *Surv Ophthalmol* 1977; 21:347

Miller D, Schor P. Physical optics. Chapter 31. In Tasman W, Jaeger EA (eds). Duane's Ophthalmology on CD-Rom. *Lippincott Williams é Wilkins,* 2006 edition.

Miller D, Weinstein D. An investigation of corneal phenomena under crossed polaroids. Masters Thesis, Columbia University, New York, 1955

Miller D, Wolf E, Geer S et al. Glare sensitivity related to the use of contact lenses. *Arch Ophthalmol* 1967;78:448-450.

Miller D, Wolf E, Jernigan ME et al. Laboratory evaluation of a clinical glare tester. *Arch Ophthalmol* 1972;87:324

Nadler D, Jaffe N, Clayman H et al. Glare disability in eyes with intraocular lenses. *Am J Ophthalmol* 1984; 97:43-47.

Polyak SL. The Retina. Chicago, University of Chicago Press, 1941

Potts AM, Friedman BC. Studies on corneal transparency. *Am J Ophthalmol* 1959;48:480-487.

Potts AM. Monochromatic ophthalmoscopy. *Trans Am Ophthalmol Soc* 1965; 63:276-293.

Prager TC, Holladay JT, Ruiz RS. The other side of visual acuity testing: Contrast sensitivity. *CLAO J* 1986; 12:230-233.

Rankin SJ, Walman BE, Buckley AR et al. Color Doppler imaging and spectral analysis of the optic nerve vasculature in glaucoma. *Am J Ophthalmol* 1995;119:685-693.

Ringrose NH. White sponges and surgical wound illumination. *Med J Aust* 1976; 2:893-896.

Riva C, Ross B, Benedek GD. Laser Doppler measurements of blood flow in capillary tubes and retinal arteries. *Invest Ophthalmol Vis Sci* 1972; 13:936-944.

Ruddock KH. Light transmission through the ocular media and its significance for psychophysical investigation. In Jameson D, Hurvich LM (eds): Handbook of Sensory Physiology. Berlin, *Springer-Verlag*, 1970

Safir A. Personal communication, 1977

Scheimpflug T. Des photoperspaktFograph undspine *Anwendung. Photogr* 1906;43:516

Sloan L, Naquin H. A quantitative test for determining the visibility of Haidinger brushes: Clinical application. *Am J Ophthalmol* 1955; 40:393-406.

Sparrow JM, Bron AJ, Brown NA et al. Autofluorescence of the crystalline lens in early and late onset diabetes. *Br J Ophthalmol* 1992; 76:25-31.

Tetz MR, Klein U, Volcker HE. Measurement of potential visual acuity in 343 patients with cataracts: a prospective clinical study. *Ger J Ophthalmol* 1992;1:403-408.

Wolf E, Gardiner JS. Studies on the scatter of light in the dioptric median of the eye as a basis for visual glare. *Arch Ophthalmol* 1963;37:450

Wolf E. Glare and age. *Arch Ophthalmol* 1960; 64:502-514.

Yu N-T, Cai M-Z, Ho DJ-Y et al. Automated laser-scanning microbeam fluorescence/Raman image analysis of human lens with multichannel detection: evidence for metabolic production of green fluorophor. *Proc Natl Acad Sci USA* 1988; 85:103-106.

Zuckerman JL, Miller D, Dyes W et al. Degradation of vision through a simulated cataract. *Invest Ophthalmol* 1973; 12:213-224.

Chapter VI

Biology of the Eye

Abstract

Theoretically, ametropia might result from an anomalous dioptric apparatus or from an abnormal axial length of the globe. A dioptric apparatus that brings parallel rays of light to focus either in front of or behind the retina produces myopia or hyperopia, respectively. Obviously, the concept of too strong or too weak a refracting system is relative to a fixed axial length, but ametropia could equally well arise from a fixed dioptric power of an eye and a variable axial length. It is also obvious that refractive errors might arise from a mismatch between these two factors, and there is evidence to support each of these three views. In fact, ametropia is sometimes classified as being refractive, axial, or combination in type.

1. Axial Length as the Determinant of Refraction

These theoretic possibilities have considerable practical implications. For almost the past 100 years, it has been widely accepted that refractive error is generally the result of anomalies in axial length (Stenstrom, 1948; Sorsby et al., 1957; Sorsby et al., 1961; Sorsby and Leary, 1970). For all practical purposes, the hyperopic eye is a short eye, and the myopic eye is a long eye, although a mismatch between an eye's axial length and its dioptric power also results in ametropia (Sorsby, 1957). These assumptions have led to an enormous amount of work aimed at disclosing the mechanism whereby the axial length of the eye remains short in some cases and grows abnormally long in others, with most attention having been given to the latter question (Mutti et al., 1996).

Steiger (Steiger, 1913) broke with the older views on the nature of emmetropia and refractive error. No longer regarding average values as constants, he postulated instead a wide range of refractive errors on the basis of distribution actually observed in the corneas of 5000 eyes, that is, a distribution conforming to a normal (or binomial) curve. His measurements, which showed corneal values extending from 39 to 48 diopters (D) and a lack of any fixed corneal value for emmetropia, enabled Steiger to calculate the axial length in emmetropia as theoretically extending from 21.5 to 25.5 mm.

The rather simple scheme postulated by Steiger is no longer tenable, as it led to a theoretically normal distribution of refractive error, but his seminal work is the starting point of current ideas about the ocular components and refractive error. Current views are based on knowledge of the distribution of the refractive error in the general population and on the measurement of the various individual components of refraction (corneal power, anterior chamber, crystalline lens anterior and posterior surface curvature and thickness, vitreous chamber depth, and axial length).

2. Refractive Error Distribution

A number of curves giving the distribution of the different refractions in various sample populations are available. Some of these curves are derived from clinic-based patients and are, therefore, potentially biased. Others deal with specialized populations, such as children or specific ethnic groups. Curves substantially free from selection bias are few. The distribution of refractive error in British national service recruits was reported in (1033 men) in 1957 (Sorsby et al., 1960) and showed significant deviations from a normal distribution. No comparable curves are available for women.

There are significant deviations from a normal distribution. The peak of the distribution is at approximately +1.00 D of hyperopia and represents a disproportionate number of people with low hyperopia (leptokurtosis). Moderate myopia and hyperopia are underrepresented in the actual data relative to the theoretic normal distribution, and high myopia and hyperopia are overrepresented. In this general population, a high proportion has no refractive error by any practical definition. Seventy-five percent of the sample of national service recruits had refractive error between 0.00 and +1.90 D.

The considerable excess of emmetropic and nearly emmetropic refractions and in other samples excludes the possibility that such refractions are the result of a random combination of components of refraction, whereas the probable excess of high myopes and high hyperopes suggests that these fall outside the mechanism that produces coordinated emmetropic and nearly emmetropic eyes.

3. Optical Components of Refraction

Normal Distribution and Age/Gender Effects in Childhood

Sorsby's original work (Sorsby et al., 1957) shows that although refractive error was not normally distributed but followed the pattern showing the peak of the distribution at approximative +1.00 D, all the individual components were normally distributed. The Orinda Longitudinal Study of Myopia (Zadnik et al., 1993), now continuing as the Collaborative Longitudinal Evaluation of Ethnicity and Refractive Error (CLEERE) Study (Zadnik et al., 2003), is the first study to measure all the ocular components in school-aged children.

Table 1. Ocular Components in Children as a function of age and gender (adapted from Zadnik K, Manny RE, Yu JA, et al. for the CLEERE Study Group: Ocular component data in schoolchildren as a function of age and gender. Optom Vis Sci 2003;80:226-)

Components	Girls					Boys				
	Age (years)									
	6	8	10	12	14	6	8	10	12	14
RE (D)	+0.88	+0.64	0.00	-0.16	-0.46	+0.81	+0.53	+0.34	+0.32	-0.11
VCP (D)	44.57	44.49	44.46	44.39	44.14	43.55	43.75	43.65	43.68	43.47
HCP (D)	43.71	43.67	43.65	43.61	43.14	42.82	43.01	43.05	42.99	42.75
ACD(mm)	3.51	3.57	3.61	3.69	3.64	3.57	3.65	3.70	3.73	3.69
LT (mm)	3.54	3.47	3.41	3.41	3.43	3.53	3.46	3.43	3.39	3.52
CLP (D)	24.67	23.50	22.56	22.02	22.61	23.79	22.71	21.66	21.13	22.16
AL (mm)	22.33	22.65	23.07	23.27	23.48	22.82	23.14	23.43	23.55	23.69

Legend: RE=refractive error in diopters, spherical equivalent; VCP=vertical corneal power in diopters; HCP=horizontal corneal power in diopters; ACD=anterior chamber deep in mm; LT= lens thickness in mm; CLP=calculated lens power; AL= axial length in mm.

As would be expected with the continued ocular growth of children, there was a significant effect of age on refractive error (spherical equivalent ($p < .0001$)). Children 6 or 7 years old were more hyperopic than children 9, 10, 11, 12, 13, or 14 years old. Similarly, children 8 years old were more hyperopic than those aged 10 to 14 years, and the mean spherical equivalent for 9-year-olds was greater than for 14-year-olds. Using *a priori* criterion for significance ($p < .005$), there was no difference in the spherical equivalent values obtained from girls and boys ($p = .0118$).

For corneal power in both the vertical and horizontal meridians, there was a significant effect of gender. Girls, on average, had corneas 0.74 D steeper in the vertical meridian ($p < .0001$) and corneas 0.63 D steeper in the horizontal meridian ($p < .0001$) compared with boys. There was no effect of age on corneal power in either meridian ($p = .16$).

Both age and gender were significantly associated with anterior chamber depth ($p < .0001$ for both). Children 6 and 7 years old had significantly shallower anterior chambers than did children 9 to 14 years of age. In addition, children aged 8 years had significantly shallower anterior chambers compared with children aged 12 or 13 years. Girls had anterior chambers that were, on average, 0.08 mm shallower than the anterior chambers of boys.

Although the crystalline lens showed a significant thinning effect with age ($p < .0001$), there was no difference in lens thickness between girls and boys ($p = .66$). The mean lens thickness was significantly greater for children aged 6 and 7 years compared with children aged 8 through 13 years. There was also a significant difference between the mean at age 8 years and the mean at age 12 years.

Both Gullstrand lens power and calculated lens power showed significant effects of age and gender. Girls, on average, had Gullstrand lens powers that were 0.28 D stronger and calculated lens powers that were 0.80 D stronger than those of boys ($p < .0001$ for both). As with the other components discussed above, mean differences in both lens power variables were observed as a function of age. The mean Gullstrand lens power was significantly stronger in children aged 6 and 7 years compared with children aged 8 to 14 years, in children aged 8 years compared with children aged 10 to 13 years, and in children aged 9 years compared with those aged 12 years. Calculated lens power differences were observed for children aged 6 compared with those aged 7 to 14 years, children aged 7 years compared with those aged 9 to 14 years, children aged 8 years compared with those aged 9 to 13 years, and children aged 9 years compared with those aged 12 years.

Similar results were also obtained when comparing the average vitreous chamber depth between the genders ($p < .0001$) and among the age groups ($p < .0001$). The mean vitreous chamber depth for children aged 6 years was significantly shorter than for children aged 8 to 14 years. Children aged 7 and 8 years had significantly shorter vitreous chambers than those aged 9 to 14 years, and the mean for 9-year-olds was significantly different from the mean for 13-year-olds. As with anterior chamber depth, girls had vitreous chambers that were shorter (by an average of 0.32 mm).

Axial length also showed significant effects of age and gender ($p < .0001$ for both). Girls had eyes which were, on average, 0.40 mm shorter when compared with the boys. Eyes of children aged 6 years were significantly shorter than eyes of children aged 8 to 14 years. Children aged 7 and 8 years had significantly shorter eyes compared with children aged 9 to 14 years. There was also a significant difference between the mean axial length when children aged 9 years were compared with those aged 13 or 14 years and when the 10-year-olds were compared with the 13-year-olds.

4. Refraction and Its Components during the Growth of the Eye

Ocular growth presents a fascinating picture in the context of the development of refractive error. The eye is approximately 17 mm long at birth. From birth to age 6 years, the eye grows by approximately 5 mm, loses 4 D of corneal power, and loses 20 D of lens power. Through the process of emmetropization, this growth occurs so that the distribution of refractive error becomes narrow, there is a preponderance of emmetropes, and the prevalence of myopia is only 2% by age 6 years. The interesting future of ocular development is that during the next 8 years, when the average eye will grow only an additional 1 mm, the prevalence of myopia will increase more than sevenfold, to 15% by age 15 years (Mutti et al., 1996).

Rapid Infantile Phase of Ocular Growth

The optical and structural components of the eye undergo their most rapid development in infancy. The average newborn eye on ultrasonography is about 17 mm in length (Fledelius, 1992; Gernet, 1964; Larsen, 1971; Larsen, 1971; Larsen, 1971; Luyckx, 1966; Blomdahl, 1979) with a corneal power of about 49 D (Inagaki, 1986; Insler et al., 1987; Mandell, 1967; York and Mandell, 1969).These dimensions change rapidly over the next 9 to 18 months of age. The general pattern of change is that the anterior and vitreous chambers and overall axial length of the eye increase, the radius of curvature of the anterior and posterior lens surfaces flatten, the cornea and lens decrease in equivalent power, and the crystalline lens thins. Rates of change then slow as the eye approaches its juvenile ocular dimensions.

Slow Juvenile Phase of Ocular Growth

Ocular component data collected from children enrolled in the Orinda Longitudinal Study of Myopia between 1989 and 1993 as a function of age showed declining on average of refractive error in the vertical meridian from low hyperopia toward emmetropia with increasing age. Refractive error in the vertical meridian declines, on average, from low hyperopia toward emmetropia with increasing age, with the typical distribution, leptokurtic for near emmetropia and more myopes than hyperopes, evident. The summary curve for central corneal curvature in the vertical meridian did not show no effect with age. Previously Zadnik et al. reported thinning of the crystalline lens between the ages of 6 and 9 years (Zadnik et al., 1995). The typical decrease in crystalline lens power occurring during school ages was showed, presumably to compensate for the axial length increases that occur concurrently. It is when the thinning and flattening of the crystalline lens are outpaced by excessive or anomalous axial elongation during this slow phase of ocular growth that myopia occurs.

5. Heredity

Although much of the experimental side of myopia research has examined the responsiveness of the growth of the eye to the visual environment, a considerable body of clinical evidence suggests that the majority of the variance in refractive error can be explained by genetic factors. Many studies have shown that myopia can be induced by depriving the eyes of form vision in neonates of several species: the tree shrew (Norton, 1990), marmoset (Troilo et al., 2000), monkey (Smith and hung, 1999), and chick (Wallman and Adams, 1987). Analogous situations to form deprivation may occur in humans that explain the induction of myopia in various clinical situations, for example, cataract, vitreous hemorrhage, corneal scarring, and ptosis (Rabin et al., 1981). Form-deprivation myopia probably explains very little about human refractive error because it is unidirectional (only producing myopia) and only occurs with pathology present. The more important experimental procedure supporting a role for environment in refractive error is nearly constant exposure of an infant animal eye to lenses that simulate refractive error (Schaeffel et al., 1988). Applying lenses with more plus power than the animal's refractive error simulates myopia, whereas using minus lenses simulates hyperopia. The eyes of young animals compensate for these simulated refractive errors by changing their rate of axial growth, speeding up to produce a compensatory myopia in response to minus lenses or slowing down to become hyperopic in response to plus lenses. Yet despite this consistent experimental finding across species, the relevance to human refractive error is still unclear. Because the relevance of animal lens experiments can only be as large as the role for environment, this question can be answered partly by examining the evidence for the relative influence of heredity and environment in the etiology of human refractive error.

Hereditary influences are suggested by family studies of refractive error. A parental history of myopia appears to be a risk factor for myopia in children. The prevalence of myopia in children with two myopic parents is 30% to 40%, whereas it is only 20% to 25% in children with one myopic parent and less than 10% in children without a myopic parent (Gwiazda et al., 1993). Quantification of this association would be useful.

The primary measure of hereditary influence is *heritability*, or h^2, defined as the proportion of total phenotypic variance in a trait that can be explained by genetic factors. Heritability can be estimated from family studies. Heritabilities are calculated by doubling either the slope or correlation between refractive errors as a function of family relationship (Plomin et al., 1990). This doubling factor is used because siblings, parents, and children each share half of the other's genetic variance. The heritability presented is the average across studies weighted by the number of subjects in a study. Heritability ranges from 0.36 to 0.86, depending on family relationship. It is 0.36 between parents and children, increasing to 0.59 between siblings.

The higher heritability between siblings compared with that between parents and children may be explained by two effects. One is that the environment between siblings is more similar than that between parents and their children. If environment helps to shape refractive error, a more similar environment would increase the correlation and inflate estimates of heritability. A second possibility is that the effect is due to age. Because the prevalence of myopia increases with age, siblings are more similar in refractive error because they are more similar in age than parents and children.

Heritability may also be estimated from studies of twins. Twin studies have the dual advantage of using subjects matched in age who are also very similar in their environments. Although environmental similarity may inflate estimates of heritability for monozygotic and dizygotic twins, the analytic technique of doubling the difference in the correlation between monozygotic and dizygotic twins is reported to essentially cancel the effects of their shared, assumed equal environment. Twin studies were examined in a similar manner to family studies and are reported. Heritability for monozygotic twins is calculated directly from the slope or correlation for refractive error of each twin. Doubling is not needed because monozygotic twins share all genes. There are two features worth noting. One is the high values for heritability from twin data: 0.74 for dizygotic twins and 0.80 for monozygotic twins. The second feature is how little these estimates differ from 0.86 when estimated by doubling the difference between monozygotic and dizygotic twins. The small impact on heritability of removing the effects of environment by this technique suggests a limited role for environmental contributions to the association between the refractive error of twins and siblings.

Eye size and shape are evaluated if they are different in premyopic elementary schoolchildren based on their parental history of myopia and the extent to which familial patterns of eye size and shape are associated with environmental factors by adjusting for parent-reported near work. With prevalent cases of myopia excluded and grade in school and near work controlled for, children with two myopic parents had longer eyes and less hyperopic refractive error (analysis of covariance, $p \leq 01$) than children with only one or no myopic parent.

The impact of environment may also be estimated in clinical studies through assessments of near work. It is particularly useful to assess the impact of parental history of refractive error and near work in the same subjects in order to gauge the relative impact of a parental history of myopia and near work. This approach has been used in studies in both the United States and Asia. In our sample of 366 eighth-grade children enrolled in the Orinda Longitudinal Study of Myopia (Mutti et al., 2002), the odds of being a myope increased by

6.40 times when a child had two myopic parents compared with children without a myopic parent. In contrast, the odds of being a myope only increased by about 2% per diopter-hour (D-hr) (Zadnik et al., 1994) per week of near work. One D-hr = (3 × (hours spent studying + hours spent reading for pleasure)) + (2 × hours spent playing video games or working on the computer at home) + (1 × hours spent watching television). This study also estimated the relative impact of both parental history of myopia and near work. The total range of near work performed by children can be approximated by four standard deviations for D-hrs, or roughly 100 D-hrs. A child would have had to increase the time spent in near work by over half the total range of time in near work (61.3 D-hrs) to equal the effect of one myopic parent on the risk of myopia. Nearly the entire range of near work (94.7 D-hrs) equaled the effect of two myopic parents on the risk of myopia.

Results from Asia appear to be similar. In a sample of Singaporean conscripts with a highly myopic average refractive error of –6.10 D, Saw and colleagues (Saw et al., 2001) found that parental myopia was significantly related to myopia but not to past or current near work. Parental myopia became nonsignificant when adjusted not for near work but for educational level and placement in a gifted track in school. In a sample of Chinese schoolchildren in Singapore, odds ratios for parental myopia were higher (3.44 for two compared with no myopic parents) than for near work (1.43 for reading more than two books compared with fewer than two books per week) (Saw et al., 2002).

Despite a long history of association with myopia, near work describes very little of the variance in refractive error compared with heredity. Models of refractive error that include a near work variable generally have R^2 values between 2% and 12% (Angle and Wissmann, 1978; Angle and Wissmann, 1980; Richler and Bear, 1980; Zadnik et al., 1994).This compares poorly with the heritability of 0.86 from the twin studies. These three types of clinical measures—heritabilities from family and twin studies, odds ratios for parental refractive error and near work, and R^2 values for near work alone—all suggest that refractive error is predominantly genetic in etiology, with smaller contributions from the environment.

Are heritability estimates for refractive error inflated? At least theoretically, environment may masquerade as heredity by either the inheritance of near work habits or by the inheritance of a susceptibility to the effects of environment. In the former case, the tendency for myopia to run in families might be due to a shared, intense near work environment within a family rather than because of shared genes. In the latter situation, a child could perform intense near work but would not develop myopia if he or she did not possess the susceptibility genes, whereas another child with the genetic susceptibility to near work who performed the same level of near work would have a higher risk of myopia. Both of these possibilities were evaluated in our Orinda Longitudinal Study of Myopia database, with little evidence for either. Adjustment for near work had almost no effect on the univariate odds ratio for parental myopia because near work was not associated with the number of myopic parents, arguing against an inherited environment. Likewise, there was no significant change in the odds ratio for near work as a function of the number of myopic parents, arguing against inherited susceptibility. Both findings suggest that there should be genes for refractive error underlying its high heritability.

The search for such genes has borne fruit for pathologic forms of myopia, myopia in excess of –6.00 D. Bornholm disease, an X-linked form of myopia characterized by myopia of more than –6.00 D, deuteranopia, and moderate optic nerve hypoplasia, has been linked to the distal part of the X chromosome at Xq28 (Schwartz et al., 1990). Knobloch syndrome, which includes severe myopia and encephalocele has been mapped to 21q22 (Sertie et al., 1996) and shown to be caused by defects in the collagen XVIII gene (Sertie et al., 2000). Other recent molecular genetic studies of families with two or more individuals with –6.00 D or more of myopia have found significant linkage with regions on chromosome 18p11.31 (Young et al., 1998), 12q21-23 (Young et al., 1998), and 7q36 (Naiglin et al., 2002). Perhaps not surprisingly, a complex-trait myopia may be characterized by heterogeneity. Loci identified by Young and coworkers in highly myopic families were not associated with high myopia in another study (Naiglin et al., 2002).To date, no loci have been associated with juvenile, less myopic refractive errors. Again, loci identified by Young and coworkers were not associated with juvenile myopia (Mutti et al., 2002). Identification of such loci is clearly one test that a genetic hypothesis for refractive error must meet.

References

Angle J, Wissmann DA. Age, reading, and myopia. *Am J Optom Physiol Opt* 1978; 55:302-308.

Angle J, Wissmann DA. The epidemiology of myopia. *Am J Epidemiol* 1980;111:220-228.

Blomdahl S. Ultrasonic measurements of the eye of the newborn infant. *Arch Ophthalmol* 1979;57:1048-1056.

Fledelius HC. Pre-term delivery and the growth of the eye. An oculometric study of eye size around term-time. *Acta Ophthalmol* 1992;204(Suppl):10-15.

Gernet H. Achsenlänge und refraktion lebender augen von neugeborenen [Axis length and refraction of the living eye in newborn infants]. *Albrecht von Graefes Arch Ophthalmol* 1964; 166:530-536.

Gwiazda J, Thorn F, Bauer J, Held R. Emmetropization and the progression of manifest refraction in children followed from infancy to puberty. *Clin Vis Sci* 1993; 8:337–344.

Inagaki Y. The rapid change of corneal curvature in the neonatal period and infancy. *Arch Ophthalmol* 1986; 104:1026-1027.

Insler MS, Cooper HD, May SE, Donzis PB. Analysis of corneal thickness and corneal curvature in infants. *CLAO J* 1987; 13:182-184.

Larsen JS: The sagittal growth of the eye. I. Ultrasonic measurement of the depth of the anterior chamber from birth to puberty. *Acta Ophthalmol* 1971; 49:239-262.

Larsen JS. The sagittal growth of the eye. II. Ultrasonic measurement of the axial diameter of the lens and the anterior segment from birth to puberty. *Acta Ophthalmol* 1971;49:427-440.

Larsen JS. The sagittal growth of the eye. IV. Ultrasonic measurement of the axial length of the eye from birth to puberty. *Acta Ophthalmol* 1971 ; 49:873-886.

Luyçkx J. Mesure des composantes optiques de l'oeil du nouveau-né par échographie ultrasonique. *Arch Ophthalmol* (Paris) 1966;26:159

Mandell RB. Corneal contour of the human infant. *Arch Ophthalmol* 1967; 77:345-348.

Mutti DO, Mitchell GL, Moeschberger ML, et al. Parental myopia, near work, school achievement, and children's refractive error. *Invest Ophthalmol Vis Sci* 2002; 43:3633-3640.

Mutti DO, Semina E, Marazita M, et al. Genetic loci for pathological myopia are not associated with juvenile myopia. *Am J Hum Genet* 2002; 112:355-360.

Mutti DO, Zadnik K, Adams AJ. Myopia. The nature versus nurture debate goes on. *Invest Ophthalmol Vis Sci* 1996;37:952-957.

Naiglin L, Gazagne C, Dallongeville F, et al. A genome wide scan for familial high myopia suggests a novel locus on chromosome 7q36. *J Med Genet* 2002; 39:118-124.

Norton TT. Experimental Myopia in Tree Shrews, pp 178–199. Chichester, UK, *John Wiley and Sons,* 1990

Plomin R, DeFries JC, McClearn GE. Behavioral Genetics, pp 256–259, 315–325. New York, WH Freeman and Company, 1990

Rabin J, Van Sluyters RC, Malach R. Emmetropization: a vision-dependent phenomenon? *Invest Ophthalmol Vis Sci* 1981; 20:561-564.

Richler A, Bear JC. Refraction, nearwork and education. A population study in Newfoundland. *Acta Ophthalmol* 1980;58:468-478.

Saw SM, Wu HM, Seet B, et al. Academic achievement, close up work parameters, and myopia in Singapore military conscripts. *Br J Ophthalmol* 2001; 85:855-860.

Saw SM, Zhang M, Hong R, et al. Near-work activity, night-lights, and myopia in the Singapore-China study. *Arch Ophthalmol* 2002;120:620-627.

Schaeffel F, Glasser A, Howland HC. Accommodation, refractive error, and eye growth in chickens. *Vision Res* 1988;28:639-657.

Schwartz M, Haim M, Skarsholm D. X-linked myopia. Bornholm eye disease. Linkage to DNA markers on the distal part of Xq. *Clin Genet* 1990;38:281-286.

Sertié AL, Quimby M, Moreira ES, et al. A gene which causes severe ocular alternations and occipital encephalocele (Knobloch syndrome) is mapped to 21q22.3. *Hum Mol Genet* 1996;5:843-847.

Sertié AL, Soss V, Camargo AA, et al. Collagen XVIII, containing an endogenous inhibitor of angiogenesis and tumor growth, plays a critical role in the maintenance of retinal structure and in neural tube closure (Knobloch syndrome). *Hum Mol Genet* 2000; 9:2051-2058.

Smith EL, Hung L-F. The role of optical defocus in regulating refractive development in infant monkeys. *Vision Res* 1999; 39:1415-1435.

Sorsby A, Benjamin B, Davey JB, et al. Emmetropia and Its Aberrations. London, Her Majesty's Stationery Office, 1957

Sorsby A, Benjamin B, Sheridan M. Refraction and Its Components During the Growth of the Eye From the Age of Three. London, Her Majesty's Stationery Office, 1961

Sorsby A, Leary GA. A Longitudinal Study of Refraction and Its Components During Growth. London, Her Majesty's Stationery Office, 1970

Sorsby A, Sheridan M, Leary GA, Benjamin B. Vision, visual acuity and ocular refraction of young men. *Br Med J* 1960;1:1394-1398.

Steiger A. Die Entstehung der spharischen Refraktionen des menschlichen Auges. Berlin, Karger, 1913

Stenstrom S. Investigation of the variation and the correlation of the optical elements of human eyes. *Am J Optom Arch Am Acad Optom* 1948; 25:218

Thall EH. Geometrical Optics. In Tasman W and Jaeger EA (eds). Chapter 30. Duane's Ophthalmology on CD-Rom. *Lippincott Williams & Wilkins,* 2006 edition.

Troilo D, Nickla DL, Wildsoet CF. Form deprivation myopia in mature common marmosets *(Callithrix jacchus). Invest Ophthalmol Vis Sci* 2000;41:2043-2049.

Wallman J, Adams JI. Developmental aspects of experimental myopia in chicks: susceptibility, recovery and relation to emmetropization. *Vision Res* 1987; 27:1139-1163.

York MA, Mandell RB. A new calibration system for photokeratoscopy. Part II—corneal curvature measurements. *Am J Optom Arch Am Acad Optom* 1969;46:818-825.

Young TL, Ronan SM, Alvear AB, et al. A second locus for familial high myopia maps to chromosome 12q. *Am J Hum Genet* 1998; 63:1419-1424.

Young TL, Ronan SM, Drahozal LA, et al. Evidence that a locus for familial high myopia maps to chromosome 18p. *Am J Hum Genet* 1998; 63:109-119.

Zadnik K, Manny RE, Yu JA, et al. for the CLEERE Study Group. Ocular component data in schoolchildren as a function of age and gender. *Optom Vis Sci* 2003; 80:226-236.

Zadnik K, Mutti DO, Adams AJ, et al. Parental history and myopia: taking the long view [letter to the editor—in reply]. *JAMA* 1994; 272:1256

Zadnik K, Mutti DO, Friedman NE, Adams AJ. Initial cross-sectional results from the Orinda Longitudinal Study of Myopia. *Optom Vis Sci* 1993; 70:750-758.

Zadnik K, Mutti DO, Fusaro RE, Adams AJ. Longitudinal evidence of crystalline lens thinning in children. *Invest Ophthalmol Vis Sci* 1995; 36:1581-1587.

Zadnik K, Satariano WA, Mutti DO, et al. The effect of parental history of myopia on children's eye size. *JAMA*1994; 271:1323-1327.

Chapter VII

The Optics of Myopia

Abstract

The prevalence of myopia is about 20% in the United States population, but varies with age, sex, race, ethnicity, occupation, environment, and other factors in various sampled populations (Curtin; 1985; Mutti and Zadnik, 2000). In the average ophthalmic practice, myopes represent an even larger proportion of patients because of their lifelong dependence on visual aids. The refractive power of the cornea and crystalline lens, modified slightly by anterior chamber depth, determines the refractive power of the eye. In combination with the axial length, these elements determine the refractive state of the eye. The distribution for axial length shows an excess above the normal random distribution at approximately 23.5 mm and a skew toward increased axial lengths (Stenstrom, 1947). By what appears to be an active process of "emmetropization," these components tend to develop and correlate so that most eyes become emmetropic. Animal experiments in primates and other vertebrates have shown that normal postnatal eye growth is dependent on form vision (to the retina) and that with normal development and normal visual input, eyes "seek to become emmetropic." (Raviola and Weisel, 1985; Whitmore, 1991; Whitman and Curtin, 2006).

1. The Angle Kappa

The angle between the visual and pupillary axes of the eye is defined as the *angle kappa*. The visual axis in emmetropic eyes is normally slightly medial to the pupillary axis. This is defined as a *positive angle kappa*. In higher grades of myopia, a temporal shift in the visual axis with respect to the pupillary axis is seen, resulting in a negative angle kappa. Patients with a negative angle kappa may have the illusory appearance of esotropia on cursory examination (pseudoesotropia). This temporal shift of the visual axis in high myopia probably relates to an asymmetric expansion of the posterior segment of the globe. These illusory shifts in the visual axis can be distinguished easily from true tropias by cover testing.

2. The Correction of Myopia

The optical correction of myopia with spectacles, particularly the higher degrees, presents several considerations that must be addressed by the practitioner. Minus lenses cause image minification and "barrel" distortion in addition to prismatic image displacement. These problems are more pronounced in larger diameter lenses. Although these do not present an adjustment problem to myopes accustomed to wearing spectacles, changes in prescription may bring on their unpleasant optical effects. The thick-edged lenses necessary for higher myopic corrections can present cosmetic problems for some patients. These considerations should be discussed with patients to ease the transition to, and permit a more realistic expectation of their vision with, stronger spectacles.

The minus spectacle lens operates at an optical disadvantage when compared with the plus lens, and this is increasingly so with higher degrees of refractive error. A minus lens requires substantially greater power to correct a given refractive error than would a plus lens at the same vertex distance. Image minification also becomes more marked with greater lens powers of myopic correction and with increases in lens vertex distance. Light rays originating from a point more than 6 meters in front of the eye are considered for practical purposes to be parallel on entering the pupil. At any point closer to the light source, the rays are said to have vergence, which is measured in diopters. The vergence of a light ray is equal to the reciprocal of its distance, in meters, from its point of origin. Thus, the vergence of light rays at a given point measured in diopters is inversely proportional to the distance from the focal point of those rays. This focal point may be in front of or behind a given reference point, resulting in divergent (i.e., minus vergence) or convergent (i.e., plus vergence) light rays, respectively. The divergence of light rays 20 cm from an object of regard with a vergence of-5.0 D is 10 times greater than the divergence of light from the same object at 200 cm with a vergence of -0.5 D. A minus lens diverges parallel rays of light. Parallel rays of light entering a -2.0-D lens have a vergence of -2.0 D on leaving the lens, as though the source of the light rays were 50 cm in front of the lens. The optical correction of myopia is accomplished by interposing a minus lens between the cornea and the far (or focal) point of the eye so that the focal point of the lens coincides with the far point (or focal point) of the eye. The closer the minus lens is placed toward the far point, the stronger it must be. Conversely, the closer the minus lens is placed toward the eye, the weaker the lens required to correct the myopia. To minimize optical disadvantages, the minus lens spectacles should be fitted as close to the eyes as possible. The higher the degree of myopia, the greater the optical benefits of a reduced vertex distance (i.e., the distance between the corneal surface and the lens). It is important to reduce vertex distance when refracting patients with moderate to high myopia (greater than 5 D) and to note this measurement on the spectacle prescription.

Minus lens design affects the position of its principal planes. The biconcave lens of equal curvatures has its principal planes between its two surfaces. The meniscus lens, which has one surface convex and the other concave, has its principal planes toward the side of the lens on which the minus power is present. By placing its concave surface toward the eye, the effective vertex distance with the latter type of lens is decreased, which can have definite optical advantages. In the past, meniscus lenses of increasingly stronger base curves had thicker edges, were heavier, produced bothersome image changes, and were cosmetically less acceptable.

Newer lenses of higher refractive index, manufactured in both glass and plastic, can now be made in aspheric single vision and aspheric progressive (multifocal) spectacles. Aspheric lenses for myopic corrections have a thinner edge for improved cosmesis and provide superior optics. When viewing through aspheric spectacles off the optical axis, there is less distortion, improved visual acuity, less chromatic aberration, and, in the case with the aspheric surface on the back of the lenses, an enlarged visual field.

Image Minification

The effect of minus lenses on image size. The angle subtended by the light rays at the nodal point of the eye determines the size of the retinal image. It can be seen that the stronger the correcting concave lens, the smaller the size of the image projected onto the retina. This produces minification of the object. Theoretically, this image minification effect would be more marked in refractive myopia than in axial myopia. Because proportionately stronger minus lenses are needed at greater vertex distances, poorly fitted spectacles with excessive vertex distances increase image minification in the patient with myopia.

There is a strong reciprocal relationship between increased vertex distance of spectacle correction and the degree of image minification in myopia. The ultimate reduction of vertex distance afforded by contact lens correction in the higher grades of myopia results in an increased image size of approximately 20% over that produced by spectacles. Axial errors are seen to yield small increases in image size with spectacle correction when compared to refractive myopia (Ringrose, 1976).

Lens Tilting

To avoid coma, reflections, and image distortion and to accommodate the human facial anatomy, spectacles are best fitted so that the plane of the corrective lenses is perpendicular to the line of sight. Spectacles used for both distance and near are fitted with a downward "pantoscopic tilt" of approximately 7.5 degrees to the visual axis. This represents a compromise of sorts between the visual tasks that involve viewing straight ahead for distance and downward for near. The effect of tilting a minus spherical lens is the production of a minus cylinder at the axis of rotation (180 degrees). The cylindric power increases with both the degree of the tilt and the power of the lens. In addition, there is an increase in the myopic spherical refraction equal to approximately one third of the induced cylindric increase (Wolf, 1960). An undercorrected myope is therefore able to obtain better distance acuity by tilting his or her glasses.

As an example, the effect of tilting a -10 D lens 10 degrees along the horizontalaxis results in an optical correction of -10.10 -0.31 × 180 degrees with a spherical equivalent of -10.25 D. If this same lens is tilted 30 degrees, the resultant effective optical correction is -10.95 - 3.65 × 180 degrees with a spherical equivalent of -12.78 D. It is not uncommon to see undercorrected myopes tilt their spectacles to attain better distance vision.

Convergence and Accommodation

If an object of regard is brought toward a fully corrected myope with normal binocular fixation, the increase in divergence of the light rays from the object results in their being focused behind the retina. This stimulates ocular accommodation and convergence so that the image is brought into focus at both foveae. Both accommodation and convergence are altered with the use of minus spectacle lenses.

Minus spectacle lenses have the effect of base-in prisms when the visual axes of the eyes are convergent. From Prentice's rule, the amount of prism in diopters is equal to the displacement, in centimeters, from the optical center of the lens times the dioptric power of the lens.

$$P = d \times p$$

where P = prismatic power in prism diopters, d = displacement in centimeters from the optical center of the lens, and p = lens strength in diopters. In the case of a bilateral -15 D myope who is looking 3 mm nasal to the optical center of the lens, $p = 0.3 \times 15$, or $p = 4.5$ prism diopters of inducedbase-in prism in each eye for a total of 9 prism diopters base-in for both eyes. Thus, the convergence required for binocular fixation at near is reduced with minus spectacles. This is a consideration when fitting a high myope with contact lenses who shows a mild degree of convergence insufficiency. Correcting this patient's vision with contact lenses might produce symptoms by increasing the convergence necessary to maintain near vision.

The range of accommodation in the uncorrected myope is reduced in nonlinear proportion to the myopic error. This range is defined as the distance from the far point to the near point (i.e., point of focus using maximal accommodation) of the eye and represents the distance over which a clear focus can be achieved. The amplitude of accommodation, conversely, is defined as the difference in the refraction of the eye between these two values expressed in diopters. Without correction, a myope has the advantage of a closer near point. Thus, for special vocational or avocational needs that demand extended periods of work at a close near point, the removal of glasses often may be advantageous. Medium and high myopes learn of this advantage early in life and instinctively resort to uncorrected near vision for fine, detailed near work. Another maneuver used by many presbyopic myopes is that of sliding their spectacles down on their nose to increase vertex distance. This reduces the effective power of the minus lens and affords better near vision.

Spectacle correction with minus lenses also requires less accommodative effort to maintain clear near vision (Balazs, 1961). The greater the minus power and the greater the vertex distance of the lens from the eye, the less the accommodation necessary to see a near object clearly. For the hyperope, conversely, the greater the plus power lens and the greater its vertex distance, the greater the accommodative effort required to see an object at the same distance. With correcting spectacles at a vertex of 15 mm, a corrected + 10 D hyperope requires 3.9 D of accommodation to focus on an object 33 cm from his or her eyes, whereas this amount is only 3 D for the emmetrope. A corrected -10 D myope, however, requires only 2.1 D of accommodation to focus on the same object.

Clinically, the increased accommodative effort required at near for a spectacle-corrected myope who first starts to use contact lenses frequently induces acute asthenopic symptoms.

The possibility of near-vision problems should always be explained carefully to prospective myopic contact lens users, especially those who are approaching presbyopia.

Bifocal Spectacles for Myopia

The base-in prismatic effects of single-vision myopic spectacle lenses at near require modest adjustments in the patient's accommodative-convergence to accommodation ratio (AC/A). Image jump and object displacement due to the presence of two optical centers in bifocals, however, can present formidable adjustment difficulties. As the visual axes are shifted inferiorly and nasally to the optical center of the lenses when reading, both base-down and base-in prisms are induced.

The best choice of bifocal lens segments is one that reduces the vertical prismatic displacement. One-piece bifocals, such as the Ultex design, achieve increased positive refraction of their lower segments by a reduction of minus power on the posterior surface of the lens. The optical centers of the lower segment in these lenses are located well below the bifocal line. The base-down prismatic effect in the reading position increases directly with the size and power of the segment.

This, combined with the base-down prism of the minus lens carrier, produces an additive effect. Thus, when gaze passes from distant to near objects across the bifocal line, there is a pronounced base-down prism effect with resultant image jump upward and associated object displacement. Both these effects of the Ultex design are usually unacceptable to the wearer.

The flat top bifocal, the most widely used bifocal, greatly reduces or almost eliminates these effects. In these bifocals, the optical center of the bifocal segment is located as near as possible to the bifocal line. The truncated circular segments of these bifocals come in sizes of 28 mm, 35 mm, and 45 mm in diameter, with the smaller being the most used. The larger segments have a deeper shelf across the top of the bifocal segment that can make them less attractive.

In binocular myopes with roughly equal amounts of refractive error in each eye and who are in the habit of performing some or all of their near work without lenses, the best approach for optical correction often can take the form of avoiding bifocals altogether. A reverse half-spectacle, in which the patient reads below the distance-correcting spectacle, can be an ideal solution. This should always be considered in patients with -2 to -4 D of myopia.

Progressive Addition Lenses

Progressive lenses offer a single continuous field of view without the annoying image jump or the disruption of vision by a line across the lens. The disadvantage of these lenses is the astigmatic blurring of images when gaze is directed medially or laterally from the central vertical line of symmetry. The popularity of these lenses is steadily increasing as new presbyopes are being introduced to this type of multifocal.

3. Anisometropic Myopia

The optical correction of anisometropic myopia presents the same prismatic difficulties described above, with additional problems due to the unequal prismatic effects between the eyes. When gaze is not directed through the optical centers of unequal myopic spectacle lenses, horizontal and, more important, vertical phorias or tropias can be induced. Fusional vergence amplitudes can overcome the effects of these lenses so that the patient is asymptomatic. At times, however, it may be necessary for these patients to turn their heads rather than their eyes to keep the visual axis near the optical centers of the lenses. This is done instinctively if these situations are presented early in life. Whereas the anisometropic and presbyopic adult usually has little problem adjusting to new, carefully centered single-vision reading glasses, the transition to a bifocal can be a considerable problem. This can be handled in one of two ways. Different-type bifocal segments with different locations of their optical centers can be dispensed so that at the usual reading position, the induced prism between lenses is neutralized. Another easier method is to reduce the vertical prism induced in the lower half of a minus lens by eliminating some of the base-down prism of the stronger lens. This is done by "slabbing off" to produce a biprism lens. It has the effect of removing a portion of the base-down prism of the minus carrier lens.

Another problem encountered in high anisometropic myopia is that of unequal image minification by the correcting lenses. This can result in sizable amounts of aniseikonia, which can adversely affect binocular vision. Changes in base curve, thickness, and vertex distance of the spectacle lenses can be made to compensate for some of the difference in image size between the two eyes. Contact lenses are the best solution if they can be worn, as they result in the greatest reduction of image size disparity between the two eyes. Because most patients have this problem from birth, neurophysiologic adaptive processes usually facilitate wearing spectacles asymptomatically if they are provided at an early age. Patients who suddenly have a substantial change develop in their spectacle correction, such as from retinal detachment surgery or asymmetric progression of myopia, usually become symptomatic because of aniseikonia. These cases require special consideration when dispensing new spectacles.

The ability of many patients, notably children, to fuse in the presence of high degrees of myopic anisometropia may be attributed to "Knapp's rule," which holds that in axial myopia, correcting lenses placed at the anterior focal plane of the eye produce no change in retinal image size (Bennett, 1984). Regardless of the reason offered, many patients with anisometropic myopia exhibit some grade of fusion while wearing spectacles.

Knapp's rule. With placement of the spectacle correction at the anterior focal distance of the eye, image size remains unchanged in eyes with axial refractive errors.

It should be clear from all of the forgoing that myopes, especially those with higher errors, need special attention to detail in the selection and fitting of their correcting spectacles. In addition to recording the vertex distance of refraction and the notation of the need for slab-off bifocals, the ophthalmologist should take a moment to advise the patient regarding the choices now available regarding spectacle frame styles and lens types. For example, the patient should know that large frames require large-diameter lenses, which are thicker and heavier, more subject to warpage, and more apt to be dispensed with incorrect lens centration. The thick edges of high minus lenses can be camouflaged to some degree by tinting the lens edges the same color as the frame. Placing the lens further back in the frame by advancing its bevel also is effective in this regard. The use of newer high refractive index lens materials as well as aspheric lens designs allows for more than a 40% reduction in edge thickness and overall weight. Cost may be the only restraint keeping these lenses from being the only ones available on the market today.

Finally, the clinician should always advise the optician to avoid, or at least minimize, any changes in the base curves and thickness of spectacle lenses. If a notable increase in correction is prescribed, necessitating different base curve and lens thickness, it is always best to warn the patient that there may be some difficulty in adjustment to the new spectacles. Some of the effects produced by base curve changes are peripheral distortion, tilting, and increased minification of objects. Head movements accentuate these disturbing visual phenomena, especially peripheral distortion. The patient may experience an effect of "floating" and, not infrequently, experience nausea. A moment of explanation can minimize patient concern after new spectacles are obtained.

4. Visual Field Alterations

While contracting image size, minus spectacle lenses theoretically increase the visual field. In actuality, this may not be the case because the thick edges of the minus lenses and the spectacle frame may each produce peripheral field restriction. The location of the blind spot in myopic eyes may vary with spectacle correction. The minification of the visual field should move the blind spot closer to the fixation point. In clinical practice, however, this effect often is neutralized by an increase in the distance between the optic nerve and the fovea that often develops in many myopic eyes.

High grades of myopia, in particular, can produce a number of unusual field defects. Concentric contraction occurs occasionally and is thought to be caused by a generalized depression of retinal sensitivity. This field change has been found to occur most often with elevated intraocular pressures. Comet and ring-shaped scotomata somewhat like those seen in glaucoma also are encountered in pathologic myopia. These defects may arise from the sharp, sloping walls of a posterior staphyloma. The sentient retinal elements in this situation are not aligned properly with the pupillary center. A resultant Stiles-Crawford effect with reduced retinal sensitivity results.

Hemianopic and quadrantic defects also occur in myopic eyes with posterior staphyloma. These defects are of importance as they may be mistaken as evidence of neurologic disease in those patients who have not had a careful fundus examination. The most common of these defects is bitemporal hemianopsia. This defect is produced by bilateral nasal staphylomas that arise at the optic nerves and involve the fundus areas nasal to it. Most frequently, these staphylomas are inferonasal. The resultant defect is initially relative and is because of ectasia of the affected fundus area. With the subsequent development of chorioretinal degeneration, the visual field will show corresponding absolute defects. Relative field defects can be eliminated by retesting the affected field with increased minus power to correct for staphyloma depth.

Contact Lenses

The optical benefits of contact lenses over spectacle correction in high myopia include image magnification, the elimination of prismatic object displacement with its attendant “barrel” distortion, and the elimination of image degradation caused by the spherical aberration of spectacle lenses with off-axis viewing (coma) (Michaels, 1985). As we have observed earlier, when the optical correction in myopia is brought closer to the corneal surface, image minification decreases. With a contact lens at the corneal surface, image minification is reduced to a minimum. The prismatic effects and spherical aberration of spectacle correction are eliminated because the optical axis of the contact lens moves with the visual axis of the eye. As noted earlier, the increase in accommodation and convergence effort with the use of contact lenses must be taken into consideration when dispensing lenses.

Contact lens technology has advanced significantly in the past decade. Rigid polymethylmeth-acrylate contact lenses have been virtually replaced with daily and extended-wear rigid gas-permeable lenses. Better quality daily and extended-wear toric soft contact lenses are in turn replacing rigid gas-permeable lenses. Many patients who were pre-vious polymethylmethacrylate or rigid gas-permeable contact lens failures can now wear soft contact lenses comfortably. Custom toric soft lenses can correct very high degrees of myopia (up to 20 D at the corneal surface) and astigmatism (up to 10 D at the corneal surface), making comfortable contact lens correction a possibility for most patients. Sufficient patient motivation and normal external ocular anatomy, however, are still essential for successful contact lens wear. Fitting myopes and other patients with high degrees of refractive error, including astigmatism, can be very challenging but also quite rewarding. Refer to a detailed exposition of this subject elsewhere in this text.

Refractive Surgery

The correction of myopia by photorefractive keratoplasty, laser *in situ* keratomileusis, intrastromal corneal ring implants (Schanzlin et al., 1997), phakic intraocular lens implants (Alio et al., 1999), and even clear lens extraction for very high myopia (Colin et al., 1999) have been gaining acceptance among surgeons and patients as the risks for these procedures decrease. With a good surgical outcome and the improvements in medical technology allowing for high-quality optical devices, these methods of optical correction of myopia are superior to spectacle correction by their reduction or elimination of lens aberrations and by their increase in image size relative to spectacle correction. Obviously, the benefits of these methods of optical correction must be weighed against the risks, the downside of which can be considerable.

References

Alio JL, de la Hoz F, Perez-Santonja JJ et al. Phakic anterior chamber lenses for the correction of myopia: A 7-year cumulative analysis of complication in 263 cases. *Ophthalmology* 1999:106:458–466.

Bennett AG, Rabbetts RB. Clinical Visual Optics. London: *Butterworths,* 1984:275–276.

Colin J, Robinet A, Cochener B. Retinal detachment after clear lens extraction for high myopia: Seven year follow-up. *Ophthalmol* 1999:106:2281–2284.

Curtin BJ. The Myopias: Basic Science and Clinical Management. Philadelphia: *Harper & Row,* 1985;39-59.

Michaels DD. Visual Optics and Refraction. St Louis: *CV Mosby,* 1985:65–66.

Mutti DO, Zadnik K. Age related decreases in the prevalence of myopia: longitudinal change or cohort effect? *Invest Ophthalmol Vis Sci* 2000:41:2103–2107.

Raviola E, Weisel TN. An animal model of myopia. N Engl J Med 1985;312:1609–1615.

Schanzlin DJ, Asbell PA, Burris TE et al. The intrastromal corneal ring segments: Phase II results for the correction of myopia. *Ophthalmology* 1997:104:1067–1078.

Stenstrom S. Variations and correlations of the optical components of the eye. In Sorsby A (ed): Modern Trends in Ophthalmology. 2nd ed. New York: *Hoeber*, 1947:87.

Whitman WG, Curtin BJ. The optics of myopia. Chapter 42. In Tasman W, Jaeger EA (eds), Duane's ophthalmology on CD-Rom. *Lippincott Williams & Wilkins,* 2006 edition.

Whitmore WG. The etiology of myopia. *Curr Opin Ophthalmol* 1991:2:72–77.

Chapter VIII

Diagnosing Myopia

Abstract

The purpose of diagnosing a patient with myopia refractive error is to improve visual acuity, visual function, and visual comfort by correcting the refractive error when appropriate (AAO, 2010-2011).

Goals (AAO,2007; AAO, 2010-2011):

- Determine the patient's visual needs
- Identify and quantify any refractive errors
- Discuss with the patient the nature of the refractive error, appropriate alternatives for correction, and the risks and benefits of each approach
- Inform patients, especially those with high refractive errors, about the potentially increased incidence of associated pathologic conditions
- Correct symptomatic refractive errors with eyeglasses, contact lenses, or surgery as desired by the informed patient and as deemed appropriate by the physician
- Provide the patient with follow-up care and management of any side effects or complications resulting from the correction provided

A comprehensive medical eye evaluation includes history, examination, diagnosis, and initiation of management. Included within each part of the evaluation is a series of items particularly effective for the detection, diagnosis, and choice of appropriate therapy for ocular, visual, and systemic disease. The items listed are basic areas of evaluation or investigation and are not meant to exclude additional elements when appropriate. For example, because history taking is an interactive process, additional questions and evaluation may be suggested by the patient's responses.

The history should incorporate the elements of the comprehensive medical eye evaluation in order to consider the patient's visual needs and any ocular pathology. In general, a thorough history may include the following items, although the exact composition varies with the patient's particular problems and needs:

- Demographic data (e.g., name, date of birth, gender, and where appropriate, ethnicity or race)
- The identity of the patient's other pertinent health care providers
- Chief complaint and history of present illness

- Present status of visual function (e.g., patient's self-assessment of visual status, visual needs, any recent or current ocular symptoms, and use of eyeglasses or contact lenses)
- Ocular history (e.g., prior eye diseases, injuries, surgery, including refractive surgery, or other treatments and medications)
- Systemic history: pertinent medical conditions and previous surgery
- Medications: ophthalmic and systemic medications currently used, including nutritional supplements
- Allergies or adverse reactions to medications
- Family history: pertinent familial ocular and systemic disease
- Social history (e.g., occupation, smoking history, alcohol use, family and living situation as appropriate)
- Directed review of systems

The comprehensive eye examination consists of an evaluation of the physiologic function and the anatomic status of the eye, visual system, and its related structures. This usually includes the following elements:

- Visual acuity with current correction (the power of the present correction recorded) at distance and when appropriate at near
- Measurement of best corrected visual acuity (with refraction when indicated)
- External examination (e.g., lids, lashes, and lacrimal apparatus; orbit; and pertinent facial features)
- Ocular alignment and motility
- Pupillary function
- Visual fields by confrontation
- Slit-lamp biomicroscopic examination: eyelid margins and lashes, tear film, conjunctiva, sclera, cornea, anterior chamber, and assessment of peripheral anterior chamber depth, iris, lens, and anterior vitreous
- Intraocular pressure measurement preferably with a contact applanation method (typically a Goldmann tonometer)
- Examination of the fundus: vitreous, retina (including posterior pole and periphery), vasculature, and optic nerve
- Assessment of relevant aspects of patient's mental and physical status

Examination of anterior segment structures routinely involves gross and biomicroscopic evaluation before and after dilation. Evaluation of structures situated posterior to the iris requires a dilated pupil. Optimal examination of the peripheral retina requires the use of the indirect ophthalmoscope or slit-lamp fundus biomicroscopy. Optimal examination of the macula and optic nerve requires the use of the slit-lamp biomicroscope and accessory diagnostic lenses.

The evaluation of myopia requires an assessment of both the refractive status of the eye, the patient's current mode of correction, symptoms, and visual needs. Refraction is often performed in conjunction with a comprehensive medical eye (American Academy of Ophthalmology Preferred. Practice Patterns Committee. Preferred Practice Patterns Guidelines. Comprehensive Adult Medical Eye Evaluation, 2005) Evaluations of myopia include visual acuity, refraction, and refinement. The depth of the corneal lesion can be measured using an optical pachymeter (Campos et al., 1993). The combination of manifest refraction, slit-lamp examination, and keratometry is generally sufficient for detecting most anterior abnormalities.

1. Measuring Visual Acuity

Distance Visual Acuity

Distance visual acuity is usually measured in a dimly lit room as the patient looks at a chart of high-contrast characters. Distance acuity should be measured separately for each eye with current correction. Distance refraction should be performed with accommodation relaxed. Near acuity is usually measured while the patient looks at a well-lit reading card of high-contrast characters held at a specified near working distance, typically 14 inches or 30 cm.

Types of visual acuity testing:

a) *Minimum Visible Acuity :* measures brightness discrimination; the person's ability to detect small differences in the brightness of two light sources. Minimum visible acuity is determined by the brightness of the object relative to its background illumination as opposed to the visual angle subtend by the object.
b) *Minimum Perceptible Acuity*: measures detection discrimination. Minimum perceptible acuity is concerned with simple detection of objects, not their identification or naming. An example of this type of acuity testing is determining if a child can see and grasp a small candy bead held in the examiner's hand.
c) *Minimum Separable Acuity*: measures the resolution threshold, or smallest visual angle at which two separate objects can be discriminated. Landolt C, and grating acuity are examples of minimum separable tasks.
d) *Vernier Acuity (hyper acuity)*: a precise form of visual discrimination still under study. Hyper acuity has been coined to classify the high precision (within a few seconds of arc) with which vernier alignment task can be performed. This level of precision is well above resolution or recognition acuity thresholds.
e) *Minimum Legible Acuity:* measures the individual's ability to recognize progressively smaller objects (letters, numbers or objects) called optotypes. The angle that the smallest recognized letter or symbol subtends on the retina is a measure of visual acuity. This type of acuity testing is used most often clinically.
f) *Snellen Acuity* uses a notation in which the numerator is the testing distance (in feet or meters) and the denominator is the distance at which a letter subtends the standard visual angle of 5 minutes. A 20/20 letter (6/6 in meters) subtends an angle of 5 minutes when viewed at 20 feet (6 meters). A 20/20 "E" from a chart meant to be viewed at 20 feet is about 9 mm tall. Each leg and space between the legs is about 1.7 mm tall. The 20/20 "E" subtends 5 minutes of visual angle; each leg and space is 1 minute (1/60 degrees) – 0.017 degrees of visual angle. For the Landolt "C", the opening in the "C" is about 1.75 mm (1 minute of arc). Snellen eye chart measures the minimum legible acuity.

Table 2. Visual Acuity Conversion Chart (Equivalent Visual Acuity Measurements)

Distance			LogMAR Acuity Chart				Near				
Snellen 20 feet	Equivalent 6 Meters	Decimal Fraction	Line Number	LogMAR	Spatial Frequency (Cycl/deg)	% central Visual Efficiency	Jaeger Standard	Inches (14/)	Centimeters (35/)	Revised American Point Type	M Notation
200	60.0	0.10	10	1.00	3.00	20	14	140.0	350.0	23	4.0
160	48.0	0.13	9	0.90	3.75	30	13	112.0	280.0	21	3.2
150	45.0	0.13	-	0.88	4.00	32	-	105.0	262.5	-	3.0
125	3.,5	0.16	8	0.80	4.80	40	12	87.5	218.8	14	2.5
114	34.2	0.18	-	0.76	5.26	44	11	79.8	199.5	13	2.3
100	30.0	0.20	7	0.70	6.00	50	10	70.0	175.0	12	2.0
80	24.0	0.25	6	0.60	7.50	60	9	56.0	140.0	11	1.6
70	21.0	0.29	-	0.54	8.57	63	-	49.0	122.5	-	1.4
63	18.9	0.32	5	0.50	9.52	65	8	44.1	110.3	10	1.3
60	18.0	0.33	-	0.48	10.00	67	7	42.0	105.0	9	1.2
50	15.0	0.40	4	0.40	12.00	75	6	35.0	87.5	8	1.0
40	12.0	0.50	3	0.30	15.00	85	5	28.0	70.0	7	0.80
32	9.6	0.63	2	0.20	18.75	90	4	22.4	56.0	6	0.64
30	9.0	0.67	-	0.18	20.00	91	3	21.0	52.5	5	0.60
25	7.5	0.80	1	0.10	24.00	95	2	17.5	43.8	4	0.50
20	6.0	1.00	0	0.00	30.00	100	1	14.0	35.0	3	0.40
16	4.8	1.25	-1	-10	37.50	100	-	11.2	28.0	-	0.32
12,5	3.8	1.60	-2	-20	48.00	100	-	8.8	21.9	-	0.25
10	3.0	2.00	-3	-30	60.00	100	-	7.0	17.5	-	0.20

Adapted from: Holladay, 1997 and Ferris et al., 1982.

Snellen fraction visual acuity measurement is indicated to determine level of vision quantitatively. Standard eye lane with Snellen acuity chart typically placed 20 feet, (6 meters in the metric system) in front of the patient either directly or with mirrors. An alternative system is the EDTRS chart which is placed 4 meters in front of the patient. Patient uses occluder to test each eye individually and is instructed to read the smallest possible line. Attention is directed to maximizing the patient effort in order to minimize subjectivity related to effort. The vision is recorded as a fraction; the numerator of the fraction represents the distance (either feet or meters) from the patient to the chart; the denominator is the distance at which the letter subtends the standard visual angle of five minutes; the smallest line for which the patient is able to read at least half the letters is recorded as the denominator. For higher accuracy, +/- notation is used to identify the number of letters made on the next smallest line or missed on the recorded line respectively. The fraction is sometimes reported in decimal notation or metric terms and sometimes converted to a logMAR (logarithm of the minimal angle of resolution) equivalent. In interpretation of this diagnostic procedure: it must be remembered that there is some level of subjectivity to this test and that there are alternative methods for assessing vision (AAO, 2010-2011). If the largest number could not be identified at 4 meters, the chart was brought closer to the subject, then counting fingers, hand motion, or light perception vision was assessed. Table 2 shows visual acuity conversion chart, an equivalent visual acuity measurements.

Although most normal eyes should have a corrected acuity of 20/20 to 20/25 or better, it may not be possible to achieve this level of acuity in patients with high myopia, even with optimal refraction. A pathologic etiology for high myopia may exist, whether the refractive error is transient or permanent. A suddenly acquired refractive change may signal a systemic or local disease, or a drug or medication effect (Wilkins and Fraunfelder, 1990). Excellent acuity does not exclude serious eye disease; all patients should have a comprehensive medical eye evaluation at the recommended intervals (American Academy of Ophthalmology Preferred. Practice Patterns Committee. Preferred Practice Patterns Guidelines. Comprehensive Adult Medical Eye Evaluation, 2005; American Academy of Ophthalmology Preferred. Practice Patterns Committee. Preferred Practice Patterns Guidelines. Pediatric Eye Evaluations, 2007).

2. Near Distance

Near vision should be measured in each eye before cycloplegia for patients with high hyperopia, presbyopia, or complaints about near vision. If the patient is presbyopic, the needed reading add is determined at the near distance preferred by the patient.

Near Vision Testing

Indications: patients presenting for refractive surgery evaluation, or routine examination including refraction, particularly in those aged 40 and above; patients with near distance symptoms of blurred vision or discomfort.

Pre-procedure evaluation: ophthalmic and social history with particular regard to vocation, hobbies and lifestyle.

Instrumentation and Technique

A handheld reading card is typically used at approximately 14 to 16 inches or the patient's preferred reading distance. The handheld card has Jaeger (J) numbers or points (P) which are used by printers to denote letter sizes commonly used in printed material. These are helpful notations to avoid confusing a near acuity measurement with a distance measurement. The M unit has also been developed and is particularly useful in low vision patients to calculate comparable distance acuity. Ideally, the patient is tested for both the uncorrected and best-corrected state at an appropriate distance as determined by the patient's needs. One technique recommends testing at 40 cm allowing for easy comparison between near and distance vision measured at 4 m

Another important component of near vision is the accommodative amplitude.

Near point of accommodation: The eye is corrected for distance and the near blur point is determined. Far point (infinity) allows near point to be calculated in diopters of amplitude.

Prince rule: A reading card and ruler calibrated for diopters and centimeters are used along with a +3.0 diopter lens; The far point becomes 33 cm in an emmetropic eye and the near point is 3D closer; near point minus far point equals amplitude

Plus and minus spheres: Reading target is placed at 40 cm; progressively stronger minus spheres are placed until near blur; this is followed by successively stronger plus lenses until blur; the difference between the lenses at the two endpoints is the amplitude.

Range of accommodation: this measures the useful range of near vision when a certain lens is employed and helps determine the functional capabilities of a near lens

Considerations in interpretation: subjective nature of measurement and range of near point needs will vary from patient to patient (AAO, Basic and Clinical Science Course. Section 3: Optics, Refraction, and Contact Lenses, 2010-2011).

Tests of accommodation are performed monocularly. When measuring the accommodative amplitude, it is assumed that you are testing an emmetropia, or someone who is corrected with spectacles, so that their far point is at infinity.

Target size, target illumination, and speed of target approach will affect the measurement of the amplitude of accommodation. The push up method works well for emmetropes, or fully corrected ametropes:

a) **Near point of accommodation "Push Up Test":** For this test, use relatively small letters (0.4M or 0.5M) to help better control accommodation. Slowly move these letters closer to the eye until they become blurry. Measure the distance the letters became blurry. This is the near point of accommodation.
b) **Prince Rule:** A scaled accommodative ruler is used. Normally it is done with +3.00D sphere over the distance correction. A standard reading card is used and moved slowly towards and away from the individual to locate both the near and far points as in the push up method.
c) **Spherical Lens Test:** Spherical lenses are used in this test. The individual focuses on a stationery target while plus or minus lenses are used to measure the accommodative

amplitude. A reading card is put at a convenient distance, say 40 cm, and the individual fixates on threshold size type (0.5M). Plus lenses are added until the print is blurred and then minus spheres are gradually added until the print blurs again. The difference is the accommodative amplitude.

Always test for accommodate relaxation with plus lenses before performing accommodative stimulation with minus lenses. This is because some individuals cannot adequately relax accommodation after exerting a maximum accommodative effort.

During the act of accommodation, there is a thickening of the lens and a decrease in its diameter (vertically and horizontally), with at the same time, a protrusion forward of the center and a relative flattening of the periphery, the whole process being accomplished by an axial movement of the lens substance which is evident, particularly in the central regions (Duke-Elder, 1938).

When wearing contact lenses, the convergence requirement is the same as that of an emmetrope, because the lenses rotate with the eye and the line of sight remains relatively well directed through the center of the lenses. When an ametrope wearing spectacle lenses centered for his distance pupillary distance fixates a near object, the amount of convergence required is not only a function of his intrapupillary distance and the distance of the object, but will also be a function of the refracting power of the spectacle lenses. As a myope converges to bi-fixate a near object, his line of sight departs from the center of his spectacle lenses and encounters increasing amounts of base in prismatic effect. The spectacle wearing hyperope encounters base out prismatic effect, as he converges to bi-fixate a near object. Thus, to bi-fixate a given object at a distance less than infinity, the bespectacled myope converges less than the emmetrope or the contact lens wearer, while the hyperope wearing spectacles converges more than the emmetrope or the contact lens wearer. Therefore, the myope who discards his spectacle lenses in favor of contact lenses, must converge more to bi-fixate a given near object, while the hyperope will converge less under the same conditions.

3. Refraction

The physicist defines refraction as the bending of light rays as they pass through substances of different densities. In eye care, the term refraction is used to describe the process of measuring a patient's refractive error and determining the optical correction needed to focus light rays from distant objects onto the retina and provide the patient with clear vision.

The process of refraction included refractometry, a multifaceted measurement of refractive errors with a variety of specific instruments and techniques, in addition to the clinical judgment required to prescribe appropriate optical correction. Ophthalmic medical assistants are often responsible for many of the measurements involved in refractometry, the ophthalmologist alone provides the clinical judgment needed to verify the refractometric results, assess related patient needs, and prescribe appropriate correction. Because considerable skill and experience are required to perform the complex steps of refractometry well, this section provides only general descriptions and principles of these processes.

(The processes of) Refractometry may be divided into following separate steps:

1) Retinoscopy
2) Keratmotry
3) Autorefraction
4) Wavefront
5) Lensometry
6) Refinement
7) Binocular balancing

These steps may be performed manually with a variety of instruments and materials or partly with automated refractors. The automated units can be moderately accurate and very efficient, but their utility will depend on their ability to produce the specific kinds of information the ophthalmologist needs to determine the appropriate correction. Performance of manual refractometry is an important skill for ophthalmic medical assistants. Even in practices where automated refractors are used, knowledge of the principles and methods of manual refractometry is required to use the equipment properly.

Whether manual or automatic, refractometry may be performed either with or without the use of cycloplegic drops, solutions of drugs that temporarily paralyze the ciliary muscle and thus block accommodation. Each eye should be evaluated independently. The refraction may be done objectively by retinoscopy, with an autorefractor, or with a wavefront analyzer; or it may be done subjectively. In cooperative patients, subjective refinement of refraction using a phorometer or trial lens set is preferred. Determination of vertex distance and precise astigmatic axis is especially important in patients with high myopia.

The reproducibility of subjective refraction has been found to be within 0.50 D for spherical equivalent, sphere power, and cylinder power (Zadnik et al., 1992; Goss and Grosvenor, 2007). This may be accomplished by using manifest (noncycloplegic) refraction with fogging or other techniques to minimize accommodation with care not to provide excess minus power correction to the patient. In some cases, a cycloplegic refraction can be useful especially in younger patients (American Academy of Ophthalmology Preferred. Practice Patterns Committee. Preferred Practice Patterns Guidelines. Pediatric Eye Evaluations, 2007).

Cycloplegic refraction is indicated for patients in whom accommodation cannot be relaxed and for patients whose symptoms are not consistent with the manifest (noncycloplegic) myopia. It is advised for patients when the accuracy of the refraction is in question for any reason. In adults, the most frequently used cycloplegic agents are tropicamide and cyclopentolate. Tropicamide provides a more rapid onset of action and a shorter duration of effect while cyclopentolate provides greater cycloplegia that can allow a more accurate refraction but a longer duration of effect (Hofmeister et al., 2005). A significant difference between manifest and cycloplegic refraction is frequent in children; in adults, a substantial difference between manifest and cycloplegic refraction may require a post-cycloplegic refraction on a subsequent day where the cycloplegic refraction is used to guide the final manifest prescription. The post-cycloplegic refraction is performed when full accommodation has returned.

3.1. Retinoscopy

The refractive state of the whole optical pathway is estimated by retinoscopy. Retinoscopy is the initial step in refractometry. It is used to determine the approximate nature and extent of a refractive error and to estimate the type and power of the lens needed to correct the error. Retinoscopy is sometimes referred to as objective refractometry because it requires no participation or response from the patient. Retinoscpy allows the clinician to objectively determine the spherocylindrical refractive error, irregular astigmatism, and also evaluate opacities and irregularities of the cornea and lens. For some patients, such as children, retarded individuals, and others unable to communicate well, retinoscopy is one of ways to determine the refractive error.

In performing retinoscopy, the examiner uses a retinoscope, an instrument consisting of a light source and a viewing component. A mirror in the retinoscope directs an adjustable beam of light at the patient's eye, while the examiner observes the eye through the viewer. Two basic types of retinoscopes are available: one produces a spot light; the other, a streak. Most retinoscopes today use a streak projection system. This streak of light is reflected from a mirror. Additionally, the streak can be moved in relation to a convex lens in the device by way of the sleeve. This allows the light to leave the device as if it were coming from a point behind the retinoscope (plano mirror setting) or as if it were coming from a point between the examiner and the patient (concave mirror setting). For Copeland retinoscopes, the plano position is with the sleeve up, while the Welch Allyn retinoscope is in the plano position with the sleeve down. Normally, the examiner will use their right eye to perform retinoscopy on the patient's right eye and their left eye for the patient's left eye. The examiner should align themselves just off-center to minimize lens reflections and to allow the patient to visualize the distance target to relax their accommodation. The patient should be instructed to look at a distance target such as a large Snellen letter (20/200-20/400). When doing retinoscopy, the examiner is attempting to put the far point of the patient's eye at the plane of the examiner's pupil. When the reflex shows "against" motion, the far point plane lies between the patient's eye and the examiner's eye, indicating myopia. When the reflex shows "with" motion, the far point lies outside the interval between the patient's eye and the observer's eye, indicating hyperopia, emmetropia or mild myopia.

One eye is examined at a time in retinoscopy. If the patient's accommodation has not been blocked by cycloplegic drops, the patient is instructed or otherwise guided to fixate (gaze steadily at) a distant object. The examiner projects the streak of light from the retinoscope directly into the patient's eye. The light beam passes through the optical system of the eye and is reflected back by the patient's retina, appearing as a "retinoscopic reflex" in the patient's pupil. The examiner, who sees the reflex as a red-orange glowing line, watches its movement while sweeping the light across the pupil. As the light sweeps across the pupil, the different types of refractive errors of the eye produce characteristic movements of the reflex. Reflexes produced by the streak retinoscope can be: (A) Normal. (B) "With" motion: the reflex moves in the same direction as the streak of light, indicating a hyperopic eye. (C) "Against" motion: the reflex moves in the direction opposite to that of the streak, indicating a myopic eye. (D) Neutralization point: there is no apparent movements of the reflex, and the pupil is filled with a red glow. The direction in which these reflexes move is affected by the retinoscopic lighting effect chosen by the examiner. Retinoscopes allow the user to select either one of two lighting effects by raising or lowering a sleeve on the instrument handle to change the instrument's optical system. The plano (flat) mirror effect produces slightly divergent rays. The concave mirror effect produces convergent rays. The most commonly used retinoscopes require the sleeve to be raised to achieve the concave mirror effect. These positions are referred to as "sleeve up" and "sleeve down" respectively. When the plano mirror effect of the retinoscope (usually "sleeve up") is being used, the hyperopic eye usually causes the retinoscopic reflex to move in the same direction as the streak of light. This movement is termed with motion. The myopic eye usually causes the reflex to move in the opposite direction from the streak, termed against motion. An astigmatic eye causes different types or degrees of movement in the two principal meridians; astigmatic retinoscopic reflexes vary greatly and can be difficult to interpret, and further discussion of them is beyond the scope of this text.As might be imagined, with and against motions are reversed if the examiner uses the concave mirror effect. However, for the purposes of this text, the succeeding discussions will assume that the plano mirror effect is in use. The examiner can affect movement of the retinal reflex by placing corrective lenses between the patient's eye and the retinoscope. The objective is to find the lens power that will "neutralize" the reflex and fill the pupil with light. The lens that achieves this neutralization point is the approximate correction for the patient's refractive error. Such a lens will neutralize the reflex regardless of the retinoscope's movement or the mirror effect used. If the eye has an astigmatic error, neutralization will have to be done for both the maximum and the minimum meridians and the axis identified.

During retinoscopy and neutralization, the examiner selects various lenses to introduce before the patient's eye by means of a trial set and trial frame or with a refractor, also called a phoropter, which stores a range of trail lenses that can be dialed into position. When "with" motion is observed (hyperopia), plus lenses are added sequentially until sufficient power is present to achieve the neutralization point. When "against" motion occurs (myopia), minus lenses are added until the neutralization point is reached.

Because the examiner must be much closer to the patient than 20 feet (optical infinity) to perform retinoscopy and neutralization, an additional adjustment to the dioptric power of the neutralization lens must be made to correct for the distance between the examiner and the patient (the "working distance"). The amount of adjustment needed can be easily calculated using a variation of the formula D = 1/F previously discussed: D = 1/working distance in meters. As an example, if the working distance is 50 cm, then D = 1/0.5m= 2 D.

3.2. Keratometry

Performed with a device called keratometer or ophthalmometer, keratometry is the measurement of a patient's corneal curvature. As such, it provides an objective, quantitative measurement of corneal astigmatism, measuring the curvature in each meridian as well as the axis. Keratometry is also helpful in determining the appropriate fit of contact lenses. The appearance of irregular mires on attempted keratometry is characteristic, sometimes precluding measurement to an aligned endpoint. This is a measure exclusively of the anterior corneal surface irregularity, but it may be affected by the tear film (Kaimbo Wa Kaimbo, 2012). The major limitation to keratometry is the assumption that the cornea is a spherocylindrical surface with a single radius of curvature in each meridian, and with a major and minor axis separated by 90 degrees. Additionally, keratometry measures only four points approximately 3 mm apart and provides no information about the cornea central or peripheral to the points measured. Finally, mild corneal surface irregularities can cause mire distortion that precludes meaningful measurement (Wilson & Klyce, 1991). In most cases, the curvature over the visual axis is fairly uniform, and this simple measurement is sufficiently descriptive. However, keratometry is not useful for measuring corneas that are likely to depart from spherocylindrical optics, as commonly occurs in refractive surgery (Arffa, Klyce & Busin, 1986), keratoconus, and many other corneal abnormalities.

3.3. Autorefraction (Automated Refractors)

In the 21st century, we are faced with an ever-more automated world, and the ophthalmic practice has paralleled this move toward automation. The retinoscope, really little more than a light filament, lens, and mirror, is now joined by many more sophisticated (and certainly more expensive) devices developed to help us obtain information regarding the refractive state of our patients. One family of such instruments consists of the automated refractors—tabletop or hand-held devices that perform an objective refraction in a matter of seconds at the touch of a button. The largest advantage of the automated refractor is that clinic personnel who have almost no knowledge in the art of refraction can use it. For the average patient, automated refractors are reasonably accurate when compared with the retinoscope and generally agree within ½ D (Salvesen and Kohler, 1991; Grosvenor et al., 1985). If automated refractors err, they tend to overestimate minus sphere by a fraction of a diopter. This discrepancy probably stems from the fact that patients accommodate in response to their sense that the automated refractor is at a closer distance to the patient than is the 6 meter far point used in retinoscopy. This is true even though the devices are designed to relax accommodation while fixing on an artificial distant target (Wirstschafter and Schwartz, 2006). Automated refractors analyze the focal power of emitted light from the eye and convert it into a dioptric correction. They are very fast, require minimum skill levels to operate, and are fairly accurate (Rosenberg, 1991). They are also very expensive. Certain high-end models have subjective refraction capability so that the correction can be refined in the instrument. Portable and hand-held automated refractors are now available.

3.4. Wavefront Analysis

Wavefront Analysis and Retinal Raytracing

This emerging method measures the refractive status of the whole internal ocular light path at selected corneal intercepts of incident light pencils (Harris, 1996). By comparing the wavefront of a pattern of several small beams of coherent light projected through to the retina with the emerginging reflected light wave front, it is possible to measure the refractive path taken by each beam and to infer the specific spatial correction required on each path. Wavefront analysis and retinal raytracing are used to measure the lower and the higher-order optical aberrations of the entire eye. Wavefront analysis is the study of the shape of light waves as they leave an object point and how they are affected by optical media. An ideal optical system with no aberrations would produce a flat wavefront. Any aberration would distort the shape of the wavefront. There are different methods to measure the wavefront. In

Hartmann-Shack aberrometry a single spot of light is lit on the retina, and the wavefront of the existing light is calculated. This method is considered outgoing aberrometry. In the Tscherning aberrometry the ingoing light passes through a mask of holes before entering the eye. The resultant array of spots on the retina is captured with a high-magnification camera, and the wavefront of the entering light is calculated. This method is considered ingoing aberrometry. Retinal raytracing is another example of ingoing aberrometry. Here a laser beam is used to scan across the pupil. At each laser beam position, the amount of deviation is measured, and the degree of aberration can thereby be calculated (Varssano, 2012; Kaimbo Wa Kaimbo, 2012).

3.5. Lensometry

Lensometry is a procedure used to measure the prescription of a patient's existing eyeglass lenses or the power of contact lenses. This technique is often called neutralization, but should not be confused with neutralization as the word applies to retinoscopy. Lensometry is performed with a specialized instrument known as a lensmeter.

Lensometry measures four principal properties of lenses:

1) Spherical and cylindrical power of lenses in diopters;
2) Axes if the lenses have a cylinder component;
3) Presence and direction of a prism incorporated into the lenses;
4) Optical centers of the lenses.

Lensometry performed on a patient's eyeglasses before refraction can provide a starting point for current refraction. This information is also useful in revealing changes in refractive error. Lensometry also serves to confirm that a patient's new glasses have been made in accordance with the doctor's prescription.

Autorefraction and keratometry could be obtained using the Autorefractor Keratometer. Spherical equivalent (SE) is calculated as the sum of the spherical power and half of the cylindrical power.

3.6. Refinement, Subjective Refractometry

The second step in refractometry is refinement. Also performed on one eye at a time, refinement consists of a group of procedures that provides a very precise measurement of refractive error and appropriate lens correction. It serves to refine (confirm) the information produced by retinoscopy. Refinement is sometimes referred to as subjective refractometry because it requires patient participation and reaction ("I can see better with this lens than with that one"). Because of the subjective nature, refinement is not possible with infants, some toddlers, and other patients who are unable to communicate adequately.

In this first step of the process, the patient views letters of various sizes on a special visual acuity chart placed at a distance of 20 feet from the patient. (This is usually the standard eye chart of letters or numbers that is familiar to many people though school or driver's-license screening procedures.) The examiner leads the patient by presenting a choice of lenses in the refractor or trial frame while asking a series of questions about the relative clarity of the images seen on the chart. The patient's responses guide the examiner to selecting the most appropriate lens to correct the refractive error in each of the patient's eyes.

Binocular Balancing

Performed on both eyes, balancing (sometimes called binocular balancing) helps ensure that the optical correction determined by refractometry for distance vision does not include an uneven overcorrection or undercorrection for the two eyes. Such an anomaly can result from errors introduced by the patient's natural accommodation. Obviously, then, this procedure is unnecessary in patients who have undergone cycloplegic refraction or in patients whose accommodation is minimal or absent (patients over 60 years of age or those who have had cataracts removed). It also is not possible inpatients with unequal visual acuity.

One technique used for balancing involves "fogging" the end-point refractive correction in both eyes with plus spheres. A -0.25 sphere is then placed before one eye and then the other, alternating rapidly between the two. If the patient reports a clearer image with the -0.25 sphere before one eye, the initial correction for the two eyes is not in balance and the refractometrist must consider making particular adjustments accordingly.

Subjective Refraction

One of the most common reasons that patients seek eye care is to obtain correction of their refractive error. However, refraction is also a diagnostic tool used to differentiate decreased acuity caused by uncorrected or incompletely corrected refractive error from blurred vision related to eye disease.

In most cases, the final determination of the refractive correction is based upon the patient's appreciation of the lens power that provides the clearest vision at the desired viewing distance. This procedure, subjective refraction, is a time-honored combination of the technical skill required to select a lens that produces a sharply focused image on the retina tempered with the fine art of determining the best overall correction, incorporating other factors such as the balance between the two eyes, the patient's visual needs, the patient's age, and the rate of change of the refractive error. The concepts and procedures described here refer to neutralization of the refractive error with spectacles, but most of these principles and techniques also apply to correction using contact lenses.

Subjective refraction is usually performed after an in-depth history has been obtained,(Amos, 1991) which includes ascertaining that clear vision has been achieved previously, describing visual symptoms and any relief provided with the current correction, and specific visual requirements related to work and avocations. It should be performed before any other test that might alter the patient's responses because of physical changes to the eye, such as Goldmann tonometry and gonioscopy. Any examination procedure that uses bright lights, such as ophthalmoscopy or slit-lamp evaluation, can produce a photostress response. Refraction should be done either before performing these tests or after an appropriate recovery period.

Cycloplegic Refraction

Cycloplegic eye drops can be used to eliminate accommodation during the examination. In most cases, the results of a cycloplegic refraction are not prescribed as a correction. Rather, this type of examination is used in selected circumstances to determine the baseline refractive status of the eye. There are two common situations in which this is valuable.

- In young individuals who are suspected of accommodative spasm, especially when it is accompanied by esophoria or esotropia, it is important to prescribe the strongest plus power correction in order to relax accommodation. A follow-up examination, not under cycloplegia, is usually required to determine the maximum amount of lens power that can be tolerated in the natural state.
- Protocols for refractive surgery usually dictate that the cycloplegic refractive power of the eyes be determined prior to undergoing the procedure (Azar, 1997).

Procedure

Although a totally subjective test is possible, most examiners use a baseline starting point, such as an evaluation of the patient's previous eyeglasses, retinoscopy, or the results of an automated refraction, which they then refine to meet the patient's requirements. In general, the goal is to determine the maximum plus power correction that provides clear vision at far and a near correction that provides clear vision at the desired distances. Many methods have been developed to determine the "best" correction.

Instrumentation

Most practitioners rely upon the manually operated refractor or phoroptor that contains a battery of lenses arranged in wheels that can be positioned in front of the patient's eyes; the lenses can be changed quickly to provide a wide array of plus and minus spherical lenses as well as a range of cylindrical lenses, available in both minus cylinder and plus cylinder configurations, that can be rotated to the appropriate axis. Earlier in this century, when most ophthalmic lenses were manufactured in plus cylinder form, it made sense to use plus cylinder examination lenses that mimicked the final lens design as closely as possible. Contemporary ophthalmic lenses are made in minus cylinder form, so it now makes sense to refract using minus cylinders.

A trial frame can be used to mount loose trial lenses in front of the patient's eyes. Trial frame refraction is a time-consuming procedure, and because of the thickness of individual lenses, especially at stronger powers, a power shift is induced when several lenses are stacked together. This error can be minimized by placing the strongest spherical lens in the rear well closest to the patient's eye. A variation of this technique is to use a clip-on trial lens holder, which can be mounted on the patient's current glasses or on a "loaner" pair of glasses made up in a spherical power close to the patient's required correction. This works exceptionally well when the existing eyeglasses contain a strong spherical or cylindrical component. The most practical use of a trial frame or clip-ons is to allow the patient to experience the change in correction before investing in a new pair of glasses.

Monocular Subjective Refraction

There are three basic components in the operation of a spectacle lens: the spherical power, the astigmatic cylinder power, and the axis. An accurate determination of the spherical component is predicated on having fully corrected the astigmatic error to ensure that a point focus is obtained with the final correcting lens. Therefore, subjective examinations proceed in that order. In eyes with astigmatism, each of the principal meridians produces a linear image at its focal distance. In the space between foci, the interval of Sturm, the image has a progressive change in its elliptic profile. At the focal distance of the dioptric average of the two principal powers, the image is round and is called the circle of least confusion. In an eye uncorrected for astigmatism, the best acuity occurs when the circle of least confusion falls upon the retina. At all other points within the astigmatic pencil, the image is distorted along the principal meridians whereby each point source produces an oval image (Borish, 1975).The oval images of two or more adjacent point objects overlap along onc of the principal meridians and appear darker along their long axes. Some refractive techniques use this effect to neutralize subjectively the astigmatic focus.

The Jackson Cross-Cylinder test

The Jackson cross cylinder is a common refinement instrument used to confirm first the axis and then the power of a correcting cylindrical lens for astigmatism. The cross cylinder is a special lens consisting of two cylindres of equal power, one minus and one plus, with their axes set at right angles to each other. The technique requires choices and responses by the patient, and is extremely accurate.The Jackson Cross-Cylinder (JCC) test is perhaps the most commonly used method for subjectively determining the presence of astigmatism and for refining the power and axis of a refractive cylinder (Polasky, 1991). It relies on the principle of placing the circle of least confusion on the retina. A crossed cylinder is a lens whose principal powers are equal and opposite in sign. The standard power JCC has powers along its principal meridians of +0.37D and −0.37D to produce an astigmatic range of 0.75 D. Each end of the minus axis is marked with a red dot, whereas the plus axis has white dots. The rotating handle in the manual lens and the pivot axis in the refractor-mounted JCC is 45° away from the principal meridians to allow the lens to be flipped quickly into two primary positions. When the circle of least confusion lies on the retina, meridians are equally out of focus.

Duochrome Test

Another technique commonly used to refine the final sphere is the duochrome test, which makes use of the chromatic aberration of the eye (Borish, 1970). White light entering the eye is refracted according to its component wavelengths. In an emmetropic eye, blue light focuses about 1 D myopic, whereas red light focuses about 0.5 D hyperopic but equidistant from thc retina. The duochrome test uses a pair of colored filters built into the projector chart, the peak transmission of one at 530 μm (green) and of the other at 670 μm (red). In corrected emmetropia, a matched presentation of letters is equally blurred on each side of the chart. With the best spherocylindrical correction, the patient is asked to look at the letters on the green side. They remain in focus only whcn accommodation is relaxed. Because the letters on the red side can be made clearer by accommodating for them, the patient is asked to look quickly at the letters on the red side and then back at the green and compare their clarity. If the letters on the green side are clearer, the correcting sphere is changed by 0.25 D in the plus direction. If the letters on the red side are clearer, 0.25 D is added in the minus direction. This test is sensitive enough for 0.25 D to cause a reversal in clarity. When letters on the green side of the chart are clearer, more spherical plus power needs to be added.

Binocular Balance

The entire procedure is repeated for each eye to produce two monocular subjective prescriptions. Assuming that the patient has clear, single binocular vision, the effects of compensating for an existing heterophoria or the effects of summation of vision from both eyes may alter the lens powers chosen for the binocular subjective prescription (West and Somers, 1984). The process is usually accomplished in two steps.

The first is to ensure that equal accommodative effort is present between the two eyes. If the best-corrected vision is approximately the same in each eye, vision is fogged with +0.75 D lenses. Sufficient vertical prism is placed in front of each eye to produce two separate images of the isolated 20/40 (6/12) line. The patient is asked to compare the clarities of the upper line and the lower line. If they appear equally blurred, +0.25 D is added to one eye and they are compared again. The other eye should now see slightly more clearly. The lens is removed and the process repeated for the other eye. Adjustments are made until the images are as equally blurred as possible. If there is no pair of lenses that produces an equality of blur between the two eyes, the pair that gives the slightly better image in front of the dominant eye is often preferred.

The best acuity line is then isolated on the chart. The fogging lenses are reduced from both eyes by 0.25 D at a time, allowing sufficient time between stages for the patient to adjust to the lens change. In the same way as with the monocular subjective test, the lens power that gives best acuity without inducing accommodation is usually the final choice. The duochrome test offers an alternative method of determining the lens powers that produce a sharp unaccommodated retinal image.

The same technique can be employed with eyes that have a moderate discrepancy in best-corrected vision, either from amblyopia or from some other abnormality. The lens powers can be balanced using a larger line of letters, for example, the 20/80 (6/24) line, and then reduced to the best binocular acuity, which is that of the better eye. This solves the dilemma of trying to determine the best monocular subjective correction in an eye with poor visual discrimination.

Binocular refraction is an infrequently used technique in which both eyes are fixating while the monocular refraction is measured. Most contemporary devices use some form of vectographic separation in which a polarized target is presented to each eye through interposing polarized analyzers with a different axis in front of each eye (Grolman, 1966). This has the advantage of mimicking the normal form of seeing, incorporating all of the patient's binocular efforts including horizontal and vertical phorias (Eskridge, 1971). In addition, this method offers the only way to identify a cyclophoria in which the astigmatic axes of the eyes are different under binocular conditions than when observed monocularly (Rustein and Eskriage, 1990).

Trial frame confirmation of the final prescription is often overlooked but is an extremely valuable verification of the comfort and acuity of the new lens power. Although an examination room of length 20 ft (6 m) is considered to be the equivalent of optical infinity, 0.17 D of accommodation is still required at that distance. It is psychologically reassuring for the patient to step out of the examination room and view the end of the hallway or, better still, the other side of the street through the new lenses. This small investment of time may save lengthy follow-up visits that could result from miscommunication in the examination room.

If the cylinder correction is similar to that of the patient's old glasses, it is relatively straightforward to have the patient hand-hold spherical trial lenses in front of the glasses and compare vision with and without the change in prescription. This is a simple way to determine which is the more satisfactory lens correction when there is a discrepancy between the monocular subjective and the binocular subjective tests. As the monocular subjective test's endpoint is best acuity and the binocular subjective test's endpoint is equality of accommodation, some patients may have a slight difference in right and left eye acuities through the binocular prescription. This refinement offers them the opportunity to observe the difference between the two corrections and to make a practical choice between them.

If there is some doubt about the visual comfort of the change, the lenses can be held in position with a clip-on lens holder while the patient takes the opportunity to walk around and adjust to the difference. In some cases, it may be beneficial to allow patients to borrow the lenses and holders overnight in order to evaluate the lens changes in their own environment. It is important to mark the right and left lenses and, if cylinders are required, to provide a sketch to help align the axis marks.

A similar procedure can be used when the change in correction is a spherocylinder. It is unwieldy to place and remove more than one lens in front of the patient's glasses. If the new cylinder axis is different from that of the old eyeglasses, a calculation of resultant cylinder axis and power is required to determine the appropriate lens to hold in front of the glasses. In such a situation, it is more practical to place the new correction in a trial frame and to let the patient alternately view at a distance through the trial frame and the old glasses. The trial frame interpupillary distance, the vertical lens position, and the pantoscopic angle should be adjusted correctly, especially with strong lens powers.

Subjective Refraction: Fogging (Kaufman, 2006)

Optical Principles of the Method

There are two components to this subjective technique: fogging to eliminate accommodation. Optically, fogging means artificial blurring of vision, identical to the naturally occurring state of myopia. It is accomplished by placing convex lenses in front of the eye. Fogging induces relaxation of accommodation because conditions are so arranged that accommodation would blur visual acuity further. A myope, of course, is naturally fogged. If the fogging is too extreme because of the amount of myopia present, concave lenses may be required to reduce the blurring to a level that permits the use of this method.

Technique

Regan and Regan (Regan, 1955) and later Regan and Boeder (Regan, 1958) outlined the steps in this method of refraction:

1) Measure the visual acuity with and without the present correction.
2) Apply adequate fogging lenses to both eyes.
3) Occlude one eye when the blurred vision is static.
4) Reduce the fog until the astigmatic axis can be seen.
5) Determine the axis on the number 1 astigmatic dial.
6) Set a number 2 dial at the determined axis and neutralize with minus cylinders.
7) Reduce the sphere to maximal visual acuity.
8) (Optional) Remove the cylinder and redetermine the axis on the number 1 dial.

9) Refract the fellow eye in the same manner.
10) Balance the refraction.

Steps 1 to 4

After visual acuity for distance has been measured, the fogging process is begun. Remember that the patient with normal vision unaided by lenses probably has little astigmatic error but, if young, may be significantly hyperopic. In a myope, as previously mentioned, the fog may be adequate to begin with and may even have to be reduced with minus lenses to bring the patient's vision to a level suitable for testing with the dials. In less myopic patients or in hyperopes, sufficient myopia is simulated and accommodation is relaxed by adding plus spheres in front of the eye.

The end point of the fog is difficult to determine. An old pair of the patient's spectacles is useful in determining the approximate working range. Visual acuity is often not a reliable index of the adequacy of the fog, because acuity varies considerably depending on the degree of astigmatism. One way of approaching fogging is to continue to add plus lenses, having the patient close the eyes between changes, until the denominator of the Snellen notation of visual acuity is doubled (*e.g.*, 20/20 to 20/40 (6/6 to 6/12)).

Metric equivalent given in parentheses after Snellen notation.

Retinoscopy also provides a useful estimate of the proper fog. Neutralize the most hyperopic or least myopic meridian and place this spherical correction in front of the eye, being careful *not* to deduct for the working distance. If retinoscopy is done at 2/3 meter, a fog of 1.5 diopters (D) will result.

Unless large astigmatic errors make it necessary, it is better not to produce a blur worse than 20/100 to 20/200 (6/30 to 6/90). For the average patient, a wait of 1 or 2 minutes after fogging induces relaxation of accommodation. However, in a hyperope who has never worn glasses, 10 or 15 minutes may elapse before satisfactory relaxation of accommodation occurs.

Once the desired degree of fogging has been induced, the process is reversed by gradually removing the fogging lenses. As the fog is reduced, watch carefully for an increase in visual acuity with each decrease in fogging. If acuity does not increase as expected, attention should be directed to the astigmatic dial; the astigmatism is probably decreasing the vision. In a person with 3 or 4 D astigmatism, reducing the fog by as much as 1 D may not help acuity, although the patient will still be able to select the axis of astigmatism accurately.

Step 5

If fogging has been correctly performed, enough myopia will have been induced to suppress accommodation but not enough to impair the intensity of the black lines on the astigmatic dial. Because it is easier for a patient to recognize the differing sharpness of radiating lines than to appreciate differences in visual acuity using letters as test objects, this is a highly sensitive test for astigmatism. In regular astigmatism, lines that run in the same direction as the meridian of the greatest refractive error appear sharply defined. A line therefore appears sharply outlined when it is accurately refracted in the meridian at right angles to it. (Another way of stating this is that the clearest lines are in the axis of least refractive error, the axis closest to the retina.) Thus, a patient with uncorrected myopic astigmatism at the 180-degree axis sees the vertical line at the 12- and 6-o'clock positions most clearly.

Make sure the patient's head is not tilted. Superimpose a pointer over the number 1 chart and ask the patient to select the *darkest* and *clearest* lines on the dial and to indicate his or her choice. Hold the pointer parallel to and alongside the axis you are pointing out, and ask the patient how many lines on either side of the pointer appear equally dark. Adjust the pointer to the center of any such group of lines. With larger degrees of astigmatism (*e.g.*, 2 D), one to three lines are clearer. When astigmatism is small (*e.g.*, less than 1 D), the patient often selects a larger number of lines as darker or clearer.

Sometimes a patient may not discern any difference among the lines on the dial. If no darker or clearer lines are noted, check the accuracy of the patient's observations by placing a -0.50 D cylinder at the 90-degree axis before the fogging lens. The patient should report that the vertical lines are darker. Likewise, when the cylinder is at the 180-degree axis, the horizontal lines should come into focus. Often such a maneuver clarifies what the examiner is testing for and makes astigmatism apparent for the first time. Now when the cylinder is removed, the patient can recognize slightly darker or clearer lines on the number 1 dial.

Step 6

Set the number 2 dial so that one line is parallel to the axis determined previously. This line, of course, appears sharper than the line at right angles to it. Now introduce minus cylinder in 0.25 D steps with the cylinder axis parallel to the less dark or less clear line. (A good way to choose the proper minus cylinder axis is to multiply the lowest clock hour of the sharp line by 30 degrees. For instance, with a line running from the 2-o'clock to the 8-o'clock position, $2 \times 30 = 60$-degree axis.) Minus cylinder is added until both lines on the number 2 dial are equally sharp and clear. At this point the patient's astigmatism has been corrected.

The axis of astigmatism may be double-checked by using a Jackson cross cylinder. The amplitude of astigmatism may be checked by adding -0.25 D of cylinder first at one axis and then at the perpendicular axis for comparison. This ensures that the patient sees equally clear lines and does not require more or less cylinder to equalize the lines.

Remember to protect the fog as minus cylinder is added by adding + 0.25 D of sphere for every 0.50 D of minus cylinder that is given. Protecting the fog means keeping the astigmatic focal lines in the vitreous by maintaining the myopic state. If this is not done, the focal lines may be moved too close to the retina so that the adequate fog is lost and accommodation is stimulated.

Step 7

When astigmatism has been corrected, reduce the fog in gradual steps. The goal is to improve visual acuity to 20/15 (6/5) by the least reduction in sphere that can accomplish this. Remove 0.25 D of fog, and check the resultant visual acuity. Repeat this procedure until no further improvement occurs.

Step 8

If desired, the final prescription may be checked by reusing the dials. Removal of the correcting minus cylinder (the power of which has already been checked) produces the so-called perfect fog. The posterior focal line is now on the retina, and refinement of the axis to within 2.5 degrees is now possible by repeating the use of the dials.

Step 9

Examination of the second eye is done in the identical manner and is facilitated by the patient's familiarity with the test and the fact that the examiner has a good idea of what to expect, because most patients have similar refractive errors in both eyes.

Step 10

Balance the Refraction

Possible Problems

Several circumstances may render this subjective method of refraction inaccurate. If the patient's vision is so poor that 0.50 D of cylinder is not recognizable, or if the fog is too strong to allow discrimination of the proper axis, then the method will fail. If the fog is insufficient, accommodation will interfere with measurement of astigmatism. A patient with miotic pupils creates a pinhole effect, and one who squints induces a stenopeic slit; therefore, both miosis and squinting influence the final refraction. Finally, some patients cannot or will not cooperate with the technique. Children who cannot respond accurately to the examiner's questions cannot be refracted well with this method. Senile or mentally deficient patients are also poor candidates. Some patients are simply no good at making decisions, and their responses to subjective testing are therefore unreliable. In all these patients, techniques that rely more on the examiner's objective measurements (*e.g.*, retinoscopy) are more reliable.

Cycloplegic Refraction

Indications

Cycloplegic refraction is useful in measuring refractive errors in patients under 20 years old, whose powerful accommodative ability may contribute to false measurements and lead to inadequate correction of their refractive problem. When performed without cycloplegic drugs, as is the case with most other patients, the measurement is referred to as a manifest refraction. The ophthalmologist usually determines whether manifest or cycloplegic refractometry is more appropriate for a given patient (Apt and Gaffney, 2006).

The refracting power of the eye results from the *static power* of the eye (the combined ability of the cornea and the lens to bend incoming rays of light) and the *accommodative power* of the eye (the variable force of accommodation that alters the path of light rays by causing the ciliary body to change the curvature of the lens). The total increase in plus power that accommodation produces is known as the amplitude of accommodation. Cycloplegia inhibits the accommodative power of the eye by blocking the action of the ciliary muscle, allowing the static or objective refractive error of the eye to be measured. The best way to obtain paralysis of accommodation is to use cycloplegic drugs. Cycloplegic drugs are called anticholinergic because they block the muscarinic action of acetylcholine. This action inhibits cholinergic stimulation of the iris sphincter and ciliary muscle, which results in mydriasis and cycloplegia.

The younger the patient, the greater the patient's amplitude of accommodation and the more difficult it is to inhibit it. Because of the powerful accommodation and the inability of young pediatric patients to respond with accurate subjective responses, cycloplegic refraction rather than manifest or subjective refraction usually is necessary. In older children and adults, noncycloplegic methods of inhibiting accommodation, such as fogging, become more practical clinically, but cycloplegics can be used selectively to help determine the refractive state of the eye.

Indications

Cycloplegia is necessary for controlling accommodation and obtaining an accurate refraction in young children. No other technique, such as fogging, can replace cycloplegia for preciseness in determining refractive errors in early childhood because it does not depend on patient cooperation or fixation distance.

Cycloplegic examinations not only allow refractive error to be determined, they also dilate the pupil, preparing the patient for an ophthalmoscopic examination. All children require a thorough ophthalmoscopic examination, which enables the physician to look for opacities in the ocular media and abnormalities in the inner eye.

In older children and young adults, cycloplegic refraction can confirm the diagnosis of accommodative spasm, which is a constant or intermittent, involuntary increase in ciliary contraction. Ciliary spasm may be caused by spasm of the near reflex or high ciliary tonus, or secondary to factors such as hyperopia or convergence insufficiency (Michaels, 1987). Patients with low hyperopia may present as myopic during examination; this so-called pseudomyopia can be identified by cycloplegic evaluation.

Although indicated for all patients with ocular motility disorders, cycloplegic refraction is indispensable to the clinician in diagnosing and managing accommodative vergence anomalies. The role of accommodation in esotropia is well recognized. A fully accommodative deviation exists when no tropia is present after accommodation is fully relaxed. Most esotropic vergence disorders are partly accommodative and are characterized by an abnormal accommodative-convergence ratio. Treatment includes blocking accommodation by the use of plus lenses and miotics.

The entire hypermetropic refractive error is usually prescribed in the spectacle correction of children with esotropia who are less than 5 years of age. Complete blockade of the ciliary hypertonus is necessary to eliminate all accommodation-induced convergence. If adjustment to the full hypermetropic correction is not prompt, a short course of a cycloplegic drug such as atropine is useful. The key to determining the full hypermetropic correction is a proper cycloplegic refraction, repeated one or two times several months apart. In most cases of esotropia with hypermetropia in children less than 5 years of age, atropine or scopolamine preferably is used to ensure that no residual accommodation goes unrecognized. Several investigators have shown atropine to be more effective than cyclopentolate in blocking accommodation in young esotropic children (Rosembaum et al., 1981; Ingram and Barr, 1979).

The indications for cycloplegic refraction are limited in adults. As amplitude of accommodation gradually decreases with age, a closer agreement between cycloplegic and manifest refraction findings takes place.

The 17 diopters of accommodation of a 3-year-old child decreases to 14 diopters at 10 years of age, 10 diopters at 25 years of age, 6 diopters at 40 years of age, and 2 diopters or less at age 50.

Cycloplegia may be necessary in handicapped or mentally disabled individuals because of their unresponsiveness to subjective refraction; it also may be used to objectively evaluate the suspected malingerer or hysteric. Young adults with asthenopic symptoms who use their accommodation to compensate for their hyperopic refractive error may require a cycloplegic examination when the manifest refraction reveals too little hyperopia to account for their symptoms. Blurred vision or headaches after sustained reading or changing focus from near to far may be caused by latent hyperopia. With the advent of modern laser refractive surgery, cycloplegic refraction has become a valuable preoperative test for accurately determining refractive error.

Cycloplegia can be used in pharmacologic occlusion therapy when the nonamblyopic eye is sufficiently hypermetropic that effective blurring of vision can be obtained by instilling a cycloplegic drug in that eye alone.

The success of this penalization therapy can be determined in the office by blurring the sound eye with a short-acting cycloplegic agent, removing the spectacle correction, and evaluating the fixation preference. If under test conditions the patient switches from using the good eye to using the amblyopic eye, chances are excellent that he or she will also do so during treatment and that penalization will force the amblyopic eye to be us

Indications for Cycloplegic Refraction are as follows:

- Accurate refraction in young children
- Distinguish true myopia from pseudomyopia
- Diagnose accommodative spasm
- All forms of strabismus, particularly esotropia
- Pharmacologic occlusion therapy in amblyopia
- Latent hyperopia
- Mentally disabled or uncooperative patient
- Visual acuity not consistent with manifest refraction
- Suspected malingering or hysteria
- Opacities in the ocular media
- Preoperative refractive laser patients

Undesirable Effect

Because it is so difficult to fully suppress ciliary body function, cycloplegic findings are not always consistent or complete. Retinoscopy findings are more uncertain because of the ocular aberrations caused by the wide mydriasis that accompanies cycloplegia. Repeated refractions often are necessary to achieve accurate results.

Cycloplegic refraction after childhood may require a post-cycloplegic manifest refraction in those children found to have significant hypermetropia. Eyeglasses cannot be prescribed based on cycloplegic findings alone because visual acuity may be reduced when the eye returns to its normal state of accommodative tonus. In those patients without a motility problem, the amount of reduction in plus lens correction is determined by the difference in manifest and cycloplegic refractions and the age and visual demands of the child.

A cycloplegic refraction is inconvenient because the loss of accommodation and mydriasis may last several hours to several days after the examination. Pilocarpine does not effectively reverse the cycloplegia or mydriasis produced by anticholinergic cycloplegic drugs such as atropine and cyclopentolate (Havener, 1983; Nelso and Orton, 1987). For these reasons, and because the resultant miosis and ciliary spasm can cause significant discomfort, the use of miotics to counteract anticholinergic drops is no longer advised.

All cycloplegic drugs have potentially serious systemic side effects, especially in infants and children. Both allergic and toxic reactions may occur with their use. Specific adverse effects are included in the comments section for each individual cycloplegic drug described later in this chapter. Several references in the literature detail these side effects (Havener, 1983; Apt and Gaffney, 1990; Apt, 1995; Bartlett and Jaanus, 1995; Bartlett and al, 1998; Ellis, 1985; Gilman et al., 1990; Jose et al., 1984; Spencer, 1990). Proper techniques of drug instillation can greatly reduce the hazards of cycloplegics.

One drop of each drug is sufficient, if instilled directly into the eye, because the eye normally holds only about one fifth of 1 drop. Overflow onto the skin should be blotted away quickly; gentle eyelid closure for several minutes after drug instillation should be attempted. Digital pressure should be applied at the periphery of the nasolacrimal system at the medial canthus for several minutes, if possible. A second set of drops may be indicated 5 minutes or so later in darkly pigmented irides. The lowest dose necessary to produce adequate cycloplegia should always be used.

Cycloplegic drugs can precipitate an attack of acute angle closure glaucoma in predisposed patients. A slight transient rise in intraocular pressure of little clinical significance may occur in glaucoma patients with open angles. Patients with open-angle glaucoma receiving miotics, however, may experience a distinct rise in intraocular pressure after the instillation of a cycloplegic drug when the miotic effect is counteracted.

Here are some undesirable effects of cycloplegic refraction:

- Findings can be inconsistent and incomplete.
- A second post-cycloplegic examination may be necessary.
- Inconvenient because mydriasis and cycloplegia cannot be reversed quickly.
- AC/A ratio is increased; muscle balance and near-point testing cannot be performed.
- Local and systemic toxic and allergic side effects are potentially significant.
- Acute glaucoma can be precipitated.

Cycloplegic Protocol

Tropicamide 0.5% can be used in infants up to 3 months of age, and 1% may be used thereafter to enhance the cycloplegic effect when cyclopentolate is used (Miranda, 1972). A topical anesthetic (0.5% proparacaine) may be instilled initially to improve the absorption and effectiveness of the cycloplegic drop and to avoid the stinging sensation caused by subsequent drops (Mordi et al., 1986; Keller and Chang, 1976). Phenylephrine drops can be added to enhance mydriasis for ophthalmoscopy.

Choice of Cycloplegic Agent for Infants and Children

- Preterm to 3 mo: Cyclopentolate 0.2% and phenylephrine 1%
- 3 mo to 1 yr: Cyclopentolate 0.5%; atropine 0.5%; scopolamine 0.25%
- 1 to 9 yr: Cyclopentolate 1%; atropine 0.5%; scopolamine 0.25%
- 10 yr and adults: Cyclopentolate 1%; atropine 1%

Current Cycloplegic Agents

Atropine Sulfate

PREPARATIONS. Solution, 0.5%, 1%, and 2%; ointment, 1%; atropine in oil, 0.25% (not commercially available).

DOSAGE FOR CYCLOPLEGIA. One drop of 0.25%, 0.5%, or 1% solution 2 or 3 times daily for 1 to 3 days before examination and in the morning of the examination. The ointment form (preferred in infants; 1/8-inch strip of ointment) should be used twice a day for 1 to 3 days before examination.

ONSET AND DURATION OF ACTION. Full mydriasis occurs in about 30 minutes; cycloplegia occurs in 60 to 180 minutes. Maximal cycloplegia is reached within 36 hours (usually after the fourth dose) and lasts up to 1 to 2 weeks. The cycloplegic effect is more profound when more than one drop is instilled. Atropine is less effective in eyes with darkly pigmented irides.

CONTRAINDICATIONS. Atropine is best avoided in lightly pigmented children, children with Down syndrome, or brain-damaged infants because of a possible increased sensitivity to the drug (Apt and Gaffney, 1990). The drug should not be used in patients with angle closure glaucoma or patients with a tendency toward increased intraocular pressure because of a narrowed iris angle.

COMMENT. Systemic toxicity, which can lead to death, may occur from an idiosyncratic response after the instillation of only 1 or 2 drops in each eye or from overdosage after multiple instillations of the drug. Parents must be advised of the early signs of toxicity (fever, skin rash, rapid and irregular pulse, dry mouth and nose, and delirium) so that administration of atropine is not continued. Instructions that can be given to parents for use at home. In the event of systemic atropine toxicity, prompt treatment with physostigmine salicylate (Antilirium) reverses both central and peripheral anticholinergic effects. The dosage of physostigmine salicylate is 0.02 to 0.03 mg/kg up to 2 mg IV, IM, or SC; the dose is repeated in 30 minutes and then every 1 to 2 hours as needed. Generally, atropine should be reserved for esotropic children less than 5 years of age. Its potential for toxicity in infants and children make its use undesirable unless esotropia is present or cycloplegia is inadequate with other drugs.

*The traditional dosage regimen of atropine solution instilled three times daily for 3 days before examination is usually not necessary to obtain maximum cycloplegia. Furthermore, the 3-day dosage routine may lead to toxicity in young pediatric patients. Maximum cycloplegia usually is reached within 36 hours after four divided doses of atropine have been given. Therefore, a more practical dosage regimen is 1 drop of atropine solution three times on the day before and once on the morning of the examination.

Traditional Instructions for Cycloplegic Refraction

1) These are atropine eyedrops. They permit accurate refraction (determination of the need for eyeglasses) and examination of the inside of the eye.
2) Some children react to these drops by becoming flushed, and develop a fever, skin rash, and rapid pulse. If the child's temperature rises above 100°F (oral), stop using the drops. If the child shows any reaction other than a slight flushing of the face, discontinue use of the drops and call the office immediately.
3) These drops will cause the pupil to enlarge and may temporarily blur near vision. On bright days sunglasses may be helpful in reducing the glare caused by the large pupils; nothing need be done for the near blur.
4) Instill drops as follows (*Important:* Use only *one* drop):
   - 3 days prior to appointment: 1 drop in both eyes morning and afternoon
   - 2 days prior to appointment: 1 drop in both eyes morning and afternoon
   - 1 day prior to appointment: 1 drop in both eyes morning and afternoon
   - Day of appointment: 1 drop in both eyes in morning on awakening
5) These drops should be used only in the eyes of the person for whom they were prescribed. Nobody else should use them and they should be discarded after this routine has been completed.
6) Like many common medicines such as aspirin, these drops can be extremely dangerous, and possibly even fatal, to a small child if swallowed. Be sure to keep these drops out of reach of all children. They are safe if used as directed.

Homatropine Hydrobromide

PREPARATIONS. Solution, 2% and 5%.

DOSAGE FOR CYCLOPLEGIA. One drop of 2% solution in each eye, repeated once in 5 to 10 minutes.

ONSET AND DURATION OF ACTION. Onset of cycloplegia occurs in 10 to 30 minutes, with peak cycloplegia occurring in 30 to 60 minutes. Cycloplegia lasts 1 to 3 days.

CONTRAINDICATIONS. Similar to those for atropine.

COMMENT. Homatropine is a weaker cycloplegic agent than either atropine or scopolamine. The drug is infrequently used because its cycloplegic action is less complete than that of atropine and lasts longer than that of cyclopentolate, which is at least as effective. Systemic toxic reactions are similar to those from atropine. Physostigmine salicylate reverses the systemic toxicity of homatropine (see the dosage recommended in the comment on atropine).

Scopolamine Hydrobromide

PREPARATION. Solution, 0.25%.

DOSAGE FOR CYCLOPLEGIA. Although one drop in each eye twice daily for 2 days before refraction is often prescribed, we prefer one drop in each eye the night before and 1 hour before examination.

ONSET AND DURATION OF ACTION. Maximal cycloplegia occurs within 1 hour and lasts 3 to 7 days.

CONTRAINDICATIONS. Similar to those for atropine.

COMMENT. The cycloplegic strength of 0.25% scopolamine hydrobromide and 1% atropine sulfate solutions are similar, and therefore, scopolamine can be substituted when atropine allergy occurs or when contraindications to atropine are present. Central nervous system (CNS) toxicity perhaps is more common from scopolamine. The systemic signs and symptoms of scopolamine toxicity are the same as those for atropine. Systemic toxicity is treated with physostigmine salicylate (see the dosage recommended in the comment on atropine).

Cyclopentolate Hydrochloride (Cyclogyl)

PREPARATIONS. Solution, 0.5%, 1%, and 2%.

DOSAGE. One drop of 0.5% solution in small infants. In other children or darkly pigmented infants, 1 drop of 0.5% or 1% solution, followed in 5 to 10 minutes by a second drop. The drug causes a marked transient stinging sensation after instillation, which can be minimized if preceded with a drop of proparacaine.

ONSET AND DURATION OF ACTION. Onset of cycloplegia occurs in 15 minutes, with maximum cycloplegia reached in 30 to 75 minutes. Because the period of maximum cycloplegia is brief, refraction must be performed within 1 hour after instillation of the drug. However, to be certain that refraction is performed at the time of maximum cycloplegia, one must test for residual accommodation (at least 2 diopters or less).

CONTRAINDICATIONS. The 2% concentration should be avoided, especially in newborns and young infants, to prevent toxicity. If a darkly pigmented patient exhibits resistance to cyclopentolate, it is better to use another cycloplegic such as atropine or scopolamine than it is to instill the 2% concentration several times. Premature and small infants are particularly susceptible to CNS, cardiopulmonary, and gastrointestinal toxicity from all concentrations of cyclopentolate (Jones and Hodes, 1991). As with atropine, systemic toxicity is seen more often in patients with brain damage, a history of seizures, Down syndrome, or light pigmentation.

COMMENT. Cyclomydril is a commercially available combination of 0.2% cyclopentolate and 1% phenylephrine. Although the concentration of cyclopentolate in Cyclomydril is low, the drug has been used by some workers as an adequate cycloplegic agent in preterm infants and newborns because although some accommodation function is present, it is not consistently or fully used. After the age of 3 months, 0.5% or 1% cyclopentolate is used. Systemic toxicity induced by cyclopentolate eyedrops is similar to that produced by atropine except that visual and tactile hallucinations are a more striking feature. Toxic reactions are dose-dependent and more likely to occur with the 2% solution. Even multiple applications of the 1% concentration may cause adverse reactions, such as drowsiness, hyperexcitability, disorientation, incoherent speech, hallucinations, ataxia, and seizures. Adverse systemic reactions have rarely been seen with use of the 0.5% concentration in children. The treatment of systemic cyclopentolate poisoning is the same as for atropine poisoning (see the discussion of treatment in the comment on atropine).

Tropicamide (Mydriacyl)

PREPARATION. Solution, 0.5% and 1%.

DOSAGE FOR CYCLOPLEGIA. One drop in each eye; repeat once in 5 minutes.

ONSET AND DURATION OF ACTION. Minimal and transient cycloplegic action in infants and children make this drug useful only as a mydriatic. Maximal cycloplegia occurs within 20 to 35 minutes after instillation, with a duration of only 10 to 40 minutes. Cycloplegic refraction therefore must be performed within a short time frame.

CONTRAINDICATIONS. Tropicamide is a safe drug; CNS disturbances are rarely encountered. The drug may be used safely at any age as a mydriatic agent.

COMMENT. Tropicamide combined with phenylephrine (2.5%) eyedrops produces wide pupillary dilation for ophthalmoscopy in all ages, and in darkly pigmented as well as blue irides. Tropicamide may enhance the cycloplegic effect of cyclopentolate (Miranda, 1972). It generally is not effective as a sole cycloplegic agent in patients less than 40 years of age. Dapiprazole (Rev-Eyes) helps to reverse the decreased amplitude of accommodation produced by tropicamide (Nyman and reich, 1993).

Cross-Cylinder Technique for Subjective Refraction

Indications: To determine the amount and axis of astigmatism

Contraindications: Patients unable to communicate and those with significant vision loss or other abnormality that limits their ability to perceive difference

Pre-procedure evaluation: visual acuity, retinoscopy and lensometry (old eyeglasses if available)

Instrumentation and technique

A. Phoropter or trial frame with lens set is used: Starting refraction can be current prescription or determined with retinoscopy, autorefraction or wavefront refraction
B. Sphere is adjusted first
C. The Jackson Cross cylinder is a compound lens with spherical equivalent of zero. It has minus power in one meridian and equal plus power in the other meridian.
D. Cylinder axis is determined prior to axis power: Axis is determined based on subjective responses of patient to flipping of the lens aligned 45 degrees from the principal meridian of the correcting cylinder.
E. After axis is determined, power is determined based on subjective responses of patients to flipping of lens with cross-cylinder aligned along same axis as principal meridian of correcting cylinder.
F. The spherical equivalent is maintained and then refined

Considerations in interpretation of this diagnostic procedure

A. Subjective test
B. Attention to appropriate power of cross cylinder, i.e., larger powers for poorer vision (AAO, 2010-2011).

Refraction: manifest and cycloplegic

The indications: to measure the refractive error ; when the refraction is performed in the natural state, it is known as a manifest reaction. A cycloplegic refraction is typically used to ensure that accommodation is suspended, especially important in younger or hyperopic patients. Measurement of vertex distance is important

The pre-procedure evaluation

A. Medical and ophthalmic history
B. Visual acuity without correction
C. Retinoscopy to obtain refraction for starting point
D. Lensometry (old eyeglasses if available)
E. Autorefraction or wavefront can be used to obtain refraction for starting point

The alternatives to this procedure

A. No real substitute. Autorefraction and wavefront measurements provide similar information and can be used to confirm general accuracy of manifest

The instrumentation and technique

A. The patient is placed at the phoropter or in trial frames
B. Usually a preliminary refractive error can be determined using old eyeglasses, an autorefraction or retinoscopy
C. Then, the patient is offered a series of choices to correct the spherical component of the refractive error until the best vision is achieved with the least amount of minus prescription (or most plus if this be the case)
D. The cylinder component of the refractive error is then determined using the cross-cylinder method (See Cross-cylinder technique for subjective refraction)
E. For manifest refraction, the endpoint should be verified
   1. Fogging: to minimize chance of accommodation
   2. Red/green test: to verify accuracy of spherical correction
   3. Visual acuity: healthy eyes should read 20/20
F. The refraction is cycloplegic if the patient has received cycloplegic eyedrops to paralyze the accommodative mechanism prior to the refraction

The considerations in interpretation of this diagnostic procedure

A. Test is subjective
B. Careful attention must be paid to the accommodative mechanism, particularly in the manifest refraction
C. The usual cause of a disparity between the manifest and cycloplegic refraction is accommodation where the cycloplegic sphere will have less minus power than the manifest sphere (AAO, 2007-2008; Mayer et al. 2001; Hofmeister et al., 2005.

References

American Academy of Ophthalmology (AAO). Basic and Clinical Science Course. Section 3: Optics, Refraction, and Contact Lenses, 2010-2011.

American Academy of Ophthalmology Refractive Management/Intervention Panel Refractive Errors & Refractive Surgery. American Academy of Ophthalmology Preferred Practice Pattern. San Francisco, CA: American Academy of Ophthalmology, 2007, 4th Printing, 2009. Available at:http://www.aao.org/ppp.

Apt L, Gaffney WL. Cycloplegic refraction. In Tasman W, Jaeger EA (eds): Duane's Foundations of Clinical Ophthalmology, Chapter 41.Software/Data, online, 2006 CD-Rom edition. Philadelphia: *JB Lippincott Williams & Wilkins,* 2006.

Apt L, Gaffney WL. Toxic effects of topical eye medication in infants and children. In Tasman W, Jaeger EA (eds): Duane's Foundations of Clinical Ophthalmology, p 4. Philadelphia: *JB Lippincott,* 1990.

Apt L. Pharmacology. In Isenberg SJ (ed). The Eye in Infancy, p 90. 2nd ed. Chicago: Year Book, 1995.

Bartlett JD, Ghormley NR, Jaanus SD et al. Ophthalmic Drug Facts, p 50. St. Louis: Facts and Comparisons, 1998.

Bartlett JD, Jaanus SD. Clinical Ocular Pharmacology, p 171. 3rd ed. Boston: *Butterworth-Heinemann,* 1995.

Ellis PP. Ocular Therapeutics and Pharmacology, p 312. 7th ed. St. Louis: *CV Mosby,* 1985.

Ferris FL III, Kassoff A, Bresnick GH, Balley I. New visual acuity charts for clinical research. *Am J Ophthalmol* 1982;94:91-96.

Gilman AG, Rall TW, Nies AS, Taylor P. Goodman and Gilman's The Pharmacological Basis of Therapeutics, p 150. 8th ed. New York: *Pergamon Press,* 1990.

Havener WH. Ocular Pharmacology. 5th ed. St. Louis: *CV Mosby,* 1983.

Hofmeister EM, Kaupp SE, Schallhorn SC. Comparison of tropicamide and cyclopentolate for cycloplegic refractions in myopic adult refractive surgery patients. *J Cataract Refract Surg* 2005;31:694-700

Holladay JT. Proper method for calculating average visual acuity. *J Refract Surg* 1997;13:388-391.

Ingram RM, Barr A. Refraction of 1-year-old children after cycloplegia with 1% cyclopentolate: Comparison with findings after atropinisation. *Br J Ophthalmol* 1979; 63:348-352.

Jackson E. A trial set of small lenses and a modified trial size frame. *Trans Am Ophthalmol Soc* 1887;4:595.

Jones LW, Hodes DT. Possible allergic reactions to cyclopentolate hydrochloride: Case reports with literature review of uses and adverse reactions. *Ophthalmic Physiol Opt* 1991; 11:16-21.

Jose JG, Polse KA, Holden EK. Optometric Pharmacology, p 101. Orlando: Grune and Stratton, 1984.

Kaimbo Wa Kaimbo D. Astigmatism- Definition, etiology, classification, diagnosis and non-surgical treatment. Chapter 4. In Goggin M (ed). Astigmatism. Optics, physiology and management. Pp59-74. *InTech, Rijeka* 2012.308p.

Kaufman JH. Subjective refraction: fogging and use of the astigmatic dials. In Tasman W, Jaeger EA (eds). Duane's Ophthalmology, 2006 edition.Philadelphia*: Lippicott Williams & Wilkins.*

Keller JT, Chang FW. An evaluation of the use of topical anesthetics and low concentrations of phenylephrine HCL for mydriasis. *J Am Optom Assoc* 1976 47:752-754.

Mayer DL, Hansen RM, Moore BD, et al. Cycloplegic refractions in healthy children aged 1 through 48 months. *Arch Ophthalmol* 2001;119:1625-1628.

Miranda MN. Residual accommodation: A comparison between cyclopentolate 1% and a combination of cyclopentolate 1% and tropicamide 1%. *Arch Ophthalmol* 1972; 87:515-517.

Mordi JA, Lyle WM, Mousa GY. Does prior instillation of a topical anesthetic enhance the effect of tropicamide? *Am J Optom Physiol Opt* 1986; 63:290-293.

Nelso ME, Orton DBO. Counteracting the effects of mydriatics. *Arch Ophthalmol* 1987; 105:486-489.

Nyman N, Reich L. The effect of dapiprazole on accommodative amplitude in eyes dilated with 0.5% tropicamide. *J Am Optom Assoc* 1993; 64:625-628.

Regan DJ, Boeder P. Refraction: Basic optics and clinical technique. Am Acad Ophthalmol Otolaryngol, Instruction Section, 1958

Michaels DD. Accommodation: Clinical aspects. In Smith RE (ed): Focal Points 1987: Clinical Modules for Ophthalmologists 5, Module 1:1. San Francisco: American Academy of Ophthalmology, 1987

Regan J, Regan DJ. Refraction: Its practical aspects and aids in the difficult problems. *Am Acad Ophthalmol Otolaryngol,* Instruction Section, 1955

Spencer JB, Mets MB. Refraction abnormalities in childhood. *Ophthalmol Clin North Am* 1990; 3:265

Varssano D. Etiology and clinical presentation of astigmatism. Chapter 2. In Goggin M (ed). Astigmatism. Optics, physiology and management. Pp15-32. *InTech, Rijeka* 2012.308p.

Wesr D, Somers WW. Binocular balance validity: a comparison of five common subjective techniques. *Ophthalmic Physiol Opt 1984*;4(2):155-159.

Wirstschafter JD, Schwartz GS. Retinoscopy.Tasman W, Jaeger EA (ed). Chapter 3. In Duane's Ophthalmology, 2006 ed. Philadelphia: *Lippincott Williams & Wilkins.*

Chapter IX

Myopia and Associations

1. Myopia and Myelinated Retinal Nerve Fibers

First described by Virchow in 1856 (Virchow, 1856), myelinated nerve fibers of the retina appear as white or graywhite striated patches with frayed borders in a configuration coincident with the distribution of retinal nerve fibers (Straatsma and Foos, 1981). They are usually discovered incidentally during the course of ocular examinations, but have been linked to some disorders, such as vitreoretinopathy with skeletal malformations (Traboulsi et al., 1993), neurofibromatosis, craniofacial abnormalities, and Gorlin syndrome (De Jong et al., 1985). Patients with myelinated retinal nerve fibers (MRNF) may be completely asymptomatic or may have significant visual defects, especially in those with marked axial myopia and amblyopia in the affected eye. Despite refractive correction and occlusion therapy, many such patients do not respond well to treatment (Tarabishy et al., 2007).

In a series of 3,968 consecutive autopsy cases, Straatsma and colleagues reported that MRNF were present in 0.98% of patients and in 0.54% of eyes examined, with bilateral involvement in 7.7% of patients. Multiple distinct lesions were found in the same eye in 12% of specimens. There was no statistical difference between males and females in the study by Straatsma and colleagues, although older studies have reported male predominance (Straatsma and Foos, 1981). Though rare, familial cases of isolated MRNF have been reported (Funnell et al., 2003), in addition to an autosomal dominant syndrome of MRNF, vitreoretinal degeneration, and skeletal abnormalities (Traboulsi et al., 1993).

The pathogenesis of MRNF has not been fully elucidated. Oligodendrocytes are one of the major glial cells in the central nervous system and are responsible for the myelination of neurons in the CNS, which insulate and accelerate conduction of signals along axons. During the prenatal period, these cells actively proliferate and produce myelin under the influence of neuro-hormonal signals (Coman et al., 2005). Normal myelination of optic nerve axons occurs through the migration of oligodendrocyte progenitors along long axons. These progenitors then generate oligodendrocytes, which produce myelin for surrounding axons. In humans, myelination along the optic nerve ceases at the lamina cribrosa, possibly due the dense aggregation of astrocytes that can act as a barrier to prevent oligodendrocytes from migrating to the retina (Hunter and Leavit, 1992).

MRNF can be considered as a developmental anomaly, a consequence of an acquired insult to the functional integrity of the lamina cribrosa. Patients with MRNF and myopia often demonstrate axial myopia as opposed to refractive myopia (Straatsma et al., 1979). Widespread myelination of retinal nerve fibers is associated with increased degrees of myopia (Scmidt et al., 1996). Ellis and colleagues postulated that MRNF interfere with vision and stimulate axial enlargement, leading to the association of MRNF with axial myopia (Ellis et al., 1987). This theory is strengthened by work that shows that the morphology of the eye is influenced by the nature of specific visual experiences (Wallman and Tarkel, 1978), and that axial myopia occurs after visual deprivation in humans and animals (Hoyt et al., 1981; Raviola and Wiesel, 1978). The amblyopia that develops in association with MRNF and myopia may be caused by form deprivation secondary to myelinated patches obscuring vision, or by optical defocus due to the high degrees of myopia that is often seen in association with extensive MRNF. In addition to the association of MRNF with myopia, it should be noted the MRNF may also be seen in emmetropic and hyperopic individuals (Tarabishy et al., 2007).

Myelinated retinal nerve fibers appear as white to gray-white striated patches with feathery edges often distributed around or contiguous with the optic disk and surrounding the vascular arcades. In previous studies, MRNF have been most commonly located in the superior peripapillary region (Straatsma and Foos, 1981).

These retinal lesions are commonly asymptomatic. The effect that MRNF have on visual function is highly variable and is influenced by the location and area of the plaque and by coexisting visual pathology. Visual function may be affected if the myelination plaques are extensive or if the macula is involved. Patients with extensive myelination may also demonstrate pronounced axial myopia, along with amblyopia that is frequently resistant to therapy. Although macula involvement has been rarely reported, severe photophobia has been described in a patient with extensive MRNF involving the macula (Kreidl et al., 2003). MRNF may also present with leukocoria, mimicking retinoblastoma (Straatsma and Foos, 1981). MRNF are generally isolated ocular findings; however, they have also been associated with a variety of other ocular and systemic abnormalities. Ocular and systemic abnormalities may include (Tarabishy et al., 2007):

Retinal vascular abnormalities

- Retinal telangiectasia (Leys et al., 1996; Mehta et al., 2003)
- Neovascularization (Leys et al., 1996; Minning and Davidorf, 1983; Silvestri et al., 1996)
- Branch retinal artery or vein occlusion (Leys et al., 1996))
- Vitreous hemorrhage (Leys et al., 1996; Silvestri et al., 1996)

Retinal membrane abnormalities

- Epiretinal membranes (Karadimas et al., 2003)
- Retinal breaks (Eide, 1986)
- Vitreoretinal traction (Hubbard et al., 2002)

Ocular developmental abnormalities

- Myelinated retinal nerve fibres, myopia, and amblyopia (Kee and Hwang, 2005; Kaimbo et al., 1999)
- Coloboma (Straatsma and Foos, 1981)
- Keratoconus (Straatsma and Foos, 1981)
- Polycoria (Straatsma and Foos, 1981)

Craniocephalic abnormalities

- Craniosynostosis (Straatsma and Foos, 1981)
- Hydrocephalus (Ali et al., 1994)

Hamartoneoplastic disorder

- Von Recklinghausen disease (neurofibromatosis type 1) (Parulekar and Elston, 2002)
- Gorlin's syndrome (basal cell nevus syndrome) (De Jong et al., 1985)

Familial disorders

- Myelinated retinal nerve fibers, vitreoretinal degeneration and skeletal abnormalities (Funnell et al., 2003)
- Familial myelinated retinal nerve fibers (Funnell et al., 2003)

Retinal vascular abnormalities may occur in areas of myelinated retinal nerve fibers and can result in neovascularization and vitreous hemorrhage or branch artery or vein occlusion (Leys et al., 1996; Mehta et al., 2003; Minning and Davidorf, 1983). Epiretinal membranes (Karadimas et al., 2003), vitreomacular traction (Hubbard et al., 2002), and retinal breaks also have been found in the region of MRNF (Eide, 1986). MRNF can also be seen in patients with a number of systemic hamartoneoplastic disorders, such as neurofibromatosis type 1 (NF1, von Recklinghausen disease) (Parulekar and Elston, 2002), or multiple basal cell nevi syndrome (Gorlin's syndrome) (De Jong et al., 1985). MRNF may also occur in patients with severe ocular or craniocephalic developmental abnormalities such as coloboma, polycoria, keratoconus, oxycephalia, and different forms of dyscrania (Straatsma and Foos, 1981). MRNF are typically static lesions; however, reports of progression or even disappearance of involved areas have been described. Disappearance of MRNF may be caused by damage to the retinal ganglion cell layer or de novo demyelination. The latter mechanism is thought to be involved in loss of MRNF that can occur following a bout of optic neuritis (Sharpe and Sanders, 1975). Damage to the retinal ganglion cell layer and MRNF disappearance may be due to mitochondrial respiratory insufficiency, such as in Leber hereditary optic neuropathy (Gicquel et al., 2003), or to decreased oxygen delivery that can occur with certain types of vasculopathy resulting in local ischemia. Several disorders sharing this common potential pathophysiologic feature have been described in association with loss of MRNF such as anterior ischemic optic neuropathy (Schachat and Miller, 1981), branch retinal artery occlusion (Teich, 1987), radiation retinopathy following plaque radiotherapy for choroidal melanoma (Mashayekhi et al., 2003), progressive diabetic retinopathy (Gentile et al., 2002), and following laser photocoagulation of diabetic retinopathy (Zweng et al., 1972). MRNF have been reported to disappear in a patient with Behcet syndrome with recurrent episodes of papillitis and vitritis (Chavis and Tabbara, 1998). Disappearance of MRNF has also been described in chronic glaucoma (Lopez Sanchez et al., 2002), and in a patient following resection of a pituitary adenoma (Gupta et al., 1990). Acquired and progressive MRNF have also been described in both adults and in children and may result in progressive vision loss (Aaby and Kushner, 1985; Ali et al., 1994; Baarsma, 1980; Rosen et al., 1999).

2. Myopia and Tilted Optic Disks (Witmer et al., 2010)

Definition of Tilted Optic Disk

The entity known as tilted disk includes two geometric relationships between the optic nerve head and its point of entry through the sclera. The first and principal component of the anomaly is the apparent angle at which the optic nerve enters the eye, an angle that is inferred by the three dimensional appearance of the optic nerve head clinically. One indirect measure of this entry angle is the disparity between the maximum and minimal surface elevation of the disk. The greater the difference in these two levels, the greater the presumed degree of ''tilt.'' If one considers the disk as a single structural unit, when one edge of the disk tilts up, the other must angle down. Because the angle between the surface maximum and minimum of the disk cannot be measured directly, the amount of tilt is usually estimated by the amount of disk ''ovality.'' When viewed along the visual axis of the eye, the further off the perpendicular that the optic nerve enters the globe because of ''tilt,'' the greater its elliptical appearance. The second geometric variable in tilted disks is rotation about the sagittal axis of the optic nerve. This variable has been referred to in the literature as optic disk torsion (How et al.,2009; Vongphanit et al., 2002). Normal optic disks are minimally oval with the vertical diameter slightly longer than the horizontal. Optic disk torsion can be viewed and measured in two-dimensional space. The longest diameter usually falls within 15 degrees of the vertical meridian; axes beyond 15 degrees are, by definition, torted. As will be discussed later, most tilted disks appear to rotate excessively about the sagittal axis of the optic nerve, such that the longest diameter of the disk falls outside this 30-degree boundary (How et al., 2009; Vongphanit et al., 2002). This apparent rotation is often accentuated by the orientation of retinal vessels that seem to turn in a direction to compensate for the ''twisted''position of the optic disk. Optic disk tilt in three dimensions, as defined previously, and rotation of the disk about the sagittal axis of the optic nerve (i.e., torsion) fully describe the tilted disk anomaly. The vast majority of reports in the literature, however, do not make the distinction between optic disk tilt and the tilt and torsional components of the anomaly. The degree of tilt of an optic nerve is a subjective interpretation.

Tilted discs are not very common in the general population (1.6% in the Blue Mountain Eye Study (Vongphanit et al., 2002)).

In tilted disc syndrome, the field defects usually do not respect the vertical or horizontal midline, whereas in glaucoma, field defects tend to respect horizontal midlines at first.

Usually, a key difference for a myopic defect is that it is minimally progressive and may be surrounded by a normal peripheral field.

Patients with tilted optic disks have an increased prevalence of myopia and astigmatism (Vongphanit et al., 2002; You et al., 2008; Kaimbo Wa Kaimbo, 2010). A comparative study between eyes with tilted and non tilted disks revealed that myopia was present in 66.2% of eyes with tilted disks and in 12.4% of eyes with normal disks (Vongphanit et al., 2002). In the Tanjong Pagar Study, there was a significant association with myopia and tilted disk compared to normal (odds ratio: 2.77; $p < 0.001$) (How et al., 2009). The difference in mean spherical refraction among eyes with tilted disks was also different from disks that were only torted (-5.53 D vs -0.39 D) (How et al., 2009).

Several studies have shown a positive association between tilted disks and long axial lengths (Chihara and Chihara, 1994; Lim et al., 2008; Tay et al., 2005). The severity of myopia and the axial length of the eye have been correlated with the degree of optic disk tilt (Tay et al., 2005). The relationship between optic disk tilt and myopia has also been demonstrated in childhood (Lim et al., 2008). Schoolchildren with tilted disks have significantly longer axial lengths and greater myopic refractive errors than age-matched normal (Lim et al., 2008). Tong et al. found that 48.6% of 142 school-aged children with tilted disks in Singapore had more than 3 D of myopia, and only 8.5% had less than 0.5 D. By comparison, 24.1% of comparably aged children had greater than 3D myopia and 42.5% had less than 0.5 D. In a study of corneal thickness, 61 eyes with tilted disk syndrome showed no difference in mean spherical refraction compared to an equal number of normal control eyes (Ornek and Ozdemir, 2008). Both groups were myopic: -3.06D±1.86 D for tilted disk syndrome eyes and -2.88 D±1.3 7D for control eyes. The amount of refractive error with tilted disk (compared to controls) varies from study to study, which might be expected considering the complex epidemiology of refractive error itself (Sperduto et al., 1983; Weale, 2003). Because refractive error is a function of genetic influences, age, sex, level of education, and occupation, it is difficult to determine the contribution of a single variable such as tilted disk without controlling simultaneously for other independent variables. Although tilted disk is associated with myopia across different populations, the overlapping morphology of myopic and tilted disk may explain some of the variation reported in the literature.

Tilted disks are common anatomical anomalies that need to be distinguished from disorders causing progressive vision loss. The clinical features of tilted disk overlap with other conditions, particularly myopic disk.

3. Myopia and Major Age-Related Eye Diseases

Myopia is a common ocular condition affecting approximately 1.6 billion people worldwide. An increasing trend of myopia has been observed throughout the world, and the prevalence of myopia is expected to increase to 2.5 billion by the year 2020 (Kempen et al., 2004).

Age-related macular degeneration (AMD), diabetic retinopathy (DR), age-related cataract, and primary open-angle glaucoma (POAG) are 4 of the most common age-related eye diseases that lead to visual impairment and blindness.

An important clinical and public health question is whether myopia is associated with these age-related eye diseases. Previous studies have assessed the associations of refractive errors with some of these ocular diseases, but the findings to date have been inconsistent. The US Beaver Dam Eye Study of adults aged 43 to 84 years reported the cross-sectional association between myopia and nuclear cataract (odds ratio (OR), 1.67; 95% confidence interval (CI), 1.23–2.27), but provided no evidence of a relationship between myopia and 5-year incident cataract (Wong et al., 2001). The study by Wong et al. (Wong et al., 2012) also reported an association between myopia and prevalent POAG (Wong et al., 2003) (OR, 1.6; 95% CI, 1.1-2.3), but no association was found between myopia and incident AMD (Wong et al., 2002). The Australian Blue Mountains Eye Study of adults aged >49 years reported that low (OR, 2.1; 95% CI, 1.4 -3.5), moderate (OR, 3.1; 95% CI, 1.6 -5.7), and high (OR, 5.5; 95% CI, 2.8- 10.9) myopia were associated with posterior subcapsular cataract (PSC), but only high myopia was associated with all 3 types of age-related cataract (Lim et al., 1999). Myopia also was found to be associated with a higher risk of POAG (Mitchell et al., 1999) (OR, 2.4; 95% CI, 1.5- 4.0), whereas hyperopia was weakly related to prevalent AMD (Wang et al.,1998) (OR, 1.3; 95% CI, 0.9 -1.9) but not incident AMD (Wang et al., 2004). In Asian studies, where the prevalence of myopia is higher, a study on Malays aged 40 to 80 years in Singapore reported that moderate myopia is positively associated with POAG (Perera et al., 2010) but inversely associated with DR (Lim et al., 2010) and AMD (Lavanya et al., 2010).

The Singapore Indian Eye Study (Pan et al., 2013), a population-based data on the associations of myopia and AL with major eye diseases in ethnic Indian persons showed the associations of myopia and AL with 4 major vision threatening eye diseases (AMD, DR, age-related cataract, and POAG) in a population-based study of ethnic Indians aged 40 to 84 years living in Singapore. The Singapore Indian Eye Study (Pan et al., 2013) found that myopic eyes were less likely to have AMD and DR, but more likely to have nuclear cataract, PSC, and POAG. In addition, The Singapore Indian Eye Study showed that variation in AL explained most of the associations of refractive error with AMD, DR, or POAG, but not the associations with age-related nuclear cataract, which results from changes in the refractive power of the lens associated with nuclear cataract. The Singapore Indian Eye Study population-based study of Singapore Indians shows that myopic eyes seem to be less susceptible to AMD and DR but more susceptible to PSC and POAG. The refractive associations with AMD, DR, and POAG are mostly explained by longer AL. In contrast, the association between myopia and nuclear cataract is explained by lens refraction but not AL.

4. Myopia and Age-Related Macular Degeneration (AMD)

The Singapore Indian Eye Study (Pan et al., 2013) found that myopia was inversely associated with AMD, whereas hyperopia did not confer any increased odds. When any myopia was categorized into mild, moderate, and high myopia, only mild myopia was significantly correlated with AMD. The nonsignificant correlation between moderate and high myopia with AMD may be explained by the small numbers of AMD in moderate and high myopia, leading to a reduction in statistical power. Results from several other population-based studies have shown an inconsistent association between refractive errors and AMD. The Singapore Prospective Study on multiethnic Asian cohorts reported that myopia was protective for AMD in men (OR, 0.45; 95% CI, 0.28–0.70) but not in women (OR, 0.45; 95% CI, 0.28–0.70) (Cheung et al., 2012). The baseline reports of the Blue Mountains Eye Study (Wang et al., 1998), Rotterdam Study (Ikram et al., 2003), and Singapore Malay Eye Study (Lavanya et al., 2010) showed that early AMD was more prevalent in hyperopic eyes. The Beaver Dam Eye Study and the Blue Mountains Eye Study found nonsignificant associations between baseline refractive errors and incident AMD (Wong et al., 2002; Wang et al., 2004). The biological plausibility of refractive error and AMD is not elucidated. One possible explanation is that the use of spectacles in myopic persons may reduce ultraviolet exposure in sunlight, which is known to be a risk factor of AMD (Cruickshanks et al., 1993). However, this assumption was not supported by The Singapore Indian Eye Study (Pan et al., 2013). In The Singapore Indian Eye Study (Pan et al., 2013), only 26.3% of myopic participants and 12.0% of hyperopic participants did not wear glasses. Additional adjustment for glass wear did not alter the significant inverse association between myopia and AMD. In addition, a lower level of vascular endothelial growth factors has been found in myopic eyes, which may protect eyes against AMD (Jonas et al., 2010). Myopic eyes with longer AL were observed to have less rigid and compact sclera compared with hyperopic eyes (Boker et al., 1993). Previous studies have found that increased ocular sclcral rigidity, which impairs the transfer of oxygen and nutrients, may be a significant risk factor for the development of AMD (Pallikaris et al., 2006).

5. Myopia and Diabetic Retinopathy (DR)

The association between refractive error and DR is less well studied. In population-based studies, the Visual Impairment Project did not find any significant association between prevalent DR and myopia (McKay et al., 2000). The Singapore Malay Eye Study showed that myopic refraction was associated with a lower prevalence of DR, particularly VTDR (Lim et al., 2010). In a longitudinal study, myopia was associated with a lower risk of progression to PDR in younger-onset diabetes (Moss et al., 1994). The Singapore Indian Eye Study (Pan et al., 2013) demonstrated that myopia was associated with a lower prevalence of DR, consistent with the findings from the Singapore Malay Eye Study. However, we did not observe a significant association between myopia and VTDR, which differs from the findings of the Singapore Malay Eye Study. The mechanisms underlying the protective effect of myopia on DR currently are unclear. The retinal and choroidal thickness in myopic eyes were observed to be thinner than in hyperopic eyes (Luo et al., 2006; Li et al., 2011). Thus, the myopic retina may be linked with a lower oxygen and nutrient demand compared with hyperopic retina, which may underline the protective effect of myopia on DR. Another explanation may be relatively narrower retinal arterioles in myopic eyes. Myopic eyes with a longer AL were observed to have narrower retinal arterioles than nonmyopic eyes (Lim et al., 2011). Recent studies also support that widening of retinal vascular caliber is associated with increasing risk of DR (Kifley et al., 2007; Klein et al., 2003; Klein et al., 2004). The mechanisms behind the relationship may involve the impairment of vascular autoregulation and hyperperfusion, tissue hypoxia and ischemia, and aggravating DR risk factors such as hypertension (Ciulla et al., 2002; Kohner et al., 1995; Lorenzi and Gerardinger, 2001). Finally, Quigley and Cohen

(Quigley and Cohen, 1999) attributed the pressure attenuation in retinal arterioles in myopic eyes to the observed association between myopia and DR. They believed that myopia results in blood flowing through a longer arteriolar tree in the retina on its course to the capillary bed, the site of disease in clinical DR (Quigley, 2010).

6. Myopia and Age-Related Cataract

Cataract is one of the leading causes of visual impairment in the world (Xu et al., 2006; Congdon et al., 2004; Maberley et al., 2007; Maberley et al., 2006; Duerksen et al., 2003; Dunzhu et al., 2003; Zheng et al., 2011; Thulasiraj et al., 2003; Murthy et al., 2001; Zhao et al., 2010; Hyman et al., 2001; Varma et al., 2004). With longer life expectancies and an aging population, the burden and impact of age-related cataract are expected to increase. Therefore, understanding risk factors and mechanisms for cataract is important to allow further research to enable the eventual prevention of this eye condition. It has been well documented in population-based studies that cataract, especially nuclear cataract, may lead to a myopic shift in refraction in the elderly.

Many studies have cited myopia as a risk factor for cataract (Leske et al., 2002; Lim et al., 1999). There has been much discussion about the amount of myopia and the onset of myopia in relation to cataract association, but the general consensus has been that long-standing myopia (onset before age 20) is a risk factor for age-related cataract and, in particular, posterior subcapsular cataract (Lim et al., 1999).

The cross-sectional association between nuclear cataract and myopia has been demonstrated in several population-based studies (Krishnaiah et al., 2009; Saw et al., 2008; Wensor et al., 1999; Wong et al., 2000; Wu et al., 1999). This association is believed to reflect increasing nuclear sclerosis of the lens with age, leading to a myopic shift in refraction. In longitudinal cohort studies, the Barbados Eye Study (Leske et al., 2002) also revealed an associated risk between myopia at baseline and incident nuclear cataract. However, the Beaver Dam Eye Study (Wong et al., 2001) showed no relationship between baseline refraction and 5-year incident nuclear cataract, whereas eyes with severe nuclear sclerosis at baseline were more likely to have a myopic change in refraction after 10 years, compared with a hyperopic change in eyes with only mild nuclear sclerosis. The Singapore Indian Eye Study (Pan et al., 2013) found that nuclear cataract was associated with myopia but not with AL provide evidence to support that nuclear sclerosis increases the refractive index and refractive power of the lens. The Singapore Indian Eye Study (Pan et al., 2013) also supported findings from most previous studies that cortical cataract is not related to refractive errors (Lim et al., 1999; McCarty et al., 1999; Wong et al., 2003) but contradicts the Visual Impairment Project (Mukesh et al., 2006), in which myopia was found to be associated with cortical cataract. The relationship between myopia and PSC is significant in our study. The Blue Mountains Eye Study (Lim et al., 1999) found that early onset of myopia, defined as a history of wearing spectacles for distance before the age of 20 years, may be a risk factor for the development of PSC. It is argued that the observed association between myopia and PSC has been confounded by difficulty in grading PSC in the presence of advanced nuclear cataract (Lim et al., 1999). The Singapore Indian Eye Study (Pan et al., 2013) suggested that PSC is related not only to myopia but also to longer AL, indicating that the refractive component of myopia is independently associated with PSC because AL is not associated with nuclear cataract. However, AL accounted for only 27.6% of the associations between refractive error and PSC in our study. Another ocular biometric component, rather than AL (e.g., lens thickness), may be the main biometric constituent that explains the observed association. The Singapore Indian Eye Study (Pan et al., 2013) further demonstrated that only high myopia was significantly associated with nuclear cataract and PSC, indicating that there may be a threshold effect in the refractive association with age-related cataract.

It is unclear whether myopia predisposes to cataract formation or the other way around. In the Visual Impairment Project, myopia was related to the development of cortical cataract (Mukesh et al., 2006), whereas this association was not observed in other population-based cohort studies (Younan et al., 2002; Wong et al., 2001). It was also reported that early-onset myopia (defined as self-reported history of distance spectacle use before the age of 20 years) was related to posterior subcapsular (PSC) cataract (Lim et al., 1999; Chang et al., 2005), whereas nonsignificant association was found between baseline refraction and incident PSC cataract (Younan et al., 2002; Wong et al., 2001). In the Tanjong Pagar Study (Wong et al., 2003), no correlation was found between any cataract subtype and AL. However, Kubo et al. (Kubo et al., 2006) reported that an increased severity of nuclear cataract was associated with a longer AL, whereas Lin et al. (Lin et al., 2005) suggested that a longer AL was a risk factor for progression of lenticular opacity.

The Singapore Malay Eye Study (SiMES) (Pan et al., 2013), a population-based study of Malays aged 40 to 80 years, found that myopic refraction was associated with an increased prevalence of both nuclear and PSC cataracts while AL was not associated with any cataract subtypes. The cross-sectional association of myopia with nuclear cataract is most likely to be explained by lens refraction rather than AL. A threshold effect may exist for PSC cataract; that is, the risk of PSC cataract may increase dramatically when refraction is less than -5.0 D. The SiMES (Pan et al., 2013) confirmed the cross-sectional association between myopia and nuclear cataract reported in previous studies (Lim et al., 1999; Wong et al., 2000; Dandona et al., 1999; Wu et al., 1999; Wensor et al., 1999). This cross-sectional association can mainly be explained by myopic shift in refraction in eyes with nuclear cataract. Because myopic shift associated with nuclear cataract usually occurs after the age of 70 years (Panchapakesan et al., 2003), it is possible that myopia could also promote the early onset and development of nuclear cataract, as this association was also observed in adults younger than 70 years in SiMES. In addition, the SimES showed that the mean ages of nuclear cataract cases in persons with and without myopia were 70.3 and 71.1 years, respectively. This appears to suggest that myopia does not lead to a much earlier onset of nuclear cataract, and even if myopia affects nuclear cataract development, the effect would be very weak. On the other hand, nuclear cataract is well known to be a risk factor for myopia. The Blue Mountains Eye Study reported a hyperopic shift in persons younger than 65 years and a myopic shift thereafter, and this myopic refractive change was strongly associated with baseline nuclear cataract at both (Murthy et al., 2001) and 10 years (Guzowski et al., 2003; Fotedar et al., 2008). The Beaver Dam Eye Study also reported similar trends (Lee et al., 2002; Lee et al., 1999) and found that persons with greater severity of nuclear sclerosis at baseline tended to have myopic changes as well.

Previous studies have also demonstrated a clear crosssectional association of myopia with PSC cataract (Lim et al., 1999; Wong et al., 2003). The Tanjong Pagar Survey reported that PSC cataract was related to myopia, as well as a deeper anterior chamber, thinner lens, and longer vitreous chamber (Wong et al., 2003). The Blue Mountains Eye Study reported a weak association between myopia and nuclear cataract, but a strong association between myopia and PSC cataract, especially in eyes with early-onset myopia (defined as having a history of wearing spectacles for distance before the age of 20 years) (Lim et al., 1999). The SiMES indicated that the prevalence of PSC cataract increased dramatically when myopia was defined as less than -5.0 D. Authors in the SiMES though that myopia, especially high myopia, might lead to PSC cataract. The insignificant associations observed in previous cohort studies may be due to a small number of cases, short follow-up period, or inaccurate estimation due to cataract surgery between study visits. PSC cataract affects vision more severely and thus leads to surgery sooner than other types of cataract. Previous studies on the relationship between myopia and cortical cataract have reported conflicting trends. The Tanjong Pagar Survey reported no association between myopia and cortical cataract (Lim et al., 1999; Wong et al.,2003), whereas the Blue Mountains Eye Study demonstrated that high myopia was associated with cortical cataract (Lim et al.,1999). The Beaver Dam Eye Study reported that incident cortical cataract was associated with hyperopia (Wong et al., 2001). The SiMES found no association of myopia with cortical cataract. Whether AL is associated with aged-related cataract remains unclear. Kubo et al. (Kubo et al., 2006) reported that an increased severity of nuclear cataract was associated with a longer AL, whereas Lin et al. (Lin et al., 2005) suggested that a longer AL was a risk factor for lenticular progressive myopia. A possible hypothesis is that a decreased diffusion of nutrients to the lens occurs due to a longer vitreous cavity (Kubo et al., 2006). The Tanjong Pagar Study reported no correlation between any cataract subtype and AL (Wong et al., 2003). The SiMES found similar results to the Tanjong Pagar Study, where axial length was not significantly related to any cataract subtypes. It is likely that factors other than AL are related to cataract development, and previous studies that found an apparent association between the two may have been limited by small samples (198 eyes in the Kubo et al. study (Kubo et al., 2006) and 47 in the Lin et al. study (Lin et al., 2005)). In conclusion, The SiMES shows that myopia was associated with an increased prevalence of both nuclear and PSC cataract. However, the lack of associations with AL suggests that the association between myopia and nuclear cataract is explained by lens refraction rather than AL. The prevalence of PSC cataract increased dramatically when myopia is defined as SE of less than -5.0 D.

7. Myopia and Primary Open-Angle Glaucoma (POAG)

It has been well documented that myopia is a significant risk factor for glaucoma (Wong et al., 2003; Suzuki et al., 2006).The Meiktila Eye study concluded that primary open angle glaucoma was associated with axial myopia (Casson et al., 2007). The amount of myopia has an impact on the risk factor, with higher prescriptions leading to greater incidence of glaucoma (odds ratios have been quoted as 1.85–2.3 for low myopes, -3.00 D and 3.3 for moderate myopes, -3.00 D) (Wong et al., 2003; Mitchell et al., 1999).It has been suggested that a refractive error greater than -6.00 D may be a risk factor associated with glaucomatous optic neuropathy (Xu et al., 2007; Jones and Luensmann). The amount of myopia also has an impact on the incidence of visual field loss progression associated with glaucoma, with lower prescriptions having a lower incidence than higher prescriptions (Lee et al., 2008).

The association of myopia, especially high myopia, with POAG has been confirmed by a systematic review and meta-analysis of 13 population-based studies (Marcus et al., 2011). The Singapore Indian Eye Study (Pan et al., 2013) provides additional insights into this association by showing that AL explained 64.7% of the association between refractive error and POAG. Many hypotheses have attempted to explain the association between myopia or increased AL and glaucoma. One explanation is that increased CDR found in myopic persons may increase risk for damage to ganglion cell axons (Jonas and Dichtl, 1997). In addition, alterations in connective tissue and sclera rigidity, as well as exaggerated shearing forces across the lamina cribrosa found in myopic eyes, may lead to the greater susceptibility of the optic nerve (Cahane and Bartov, 1992).

Glaucoma, the leading cause of irreversible blindness worldwide (Quigley and Broman, 2006), can adversely impact quality of life for patients with visual field defects even if they are unaware of their diagnosis (Varma et al., 2011; Nelson et al., 2003; McKean-Cowdin et al., 2008). In many populations, POAG is the most common form of the disease (Tielsch et al., 1991; Mitchell et al., 1996; Klein et al., 1992; Leske et al., 1994; Dielemans et al., 1994). The only known modifiable risk factor for POAG is IOP, and the goal of treatment is to lower this parameter in afflicted individuals. The underlying pathogenesis of glaucoma is not completely understood and is likely influenced by both genetic and environmental factors (Gemenetzi et al., 2012;Pasquale and Kang, 2009; Sacca et al., 2009), so the identification of other risk factors may allow for earlier and more aggressive screening targeted toward susceptible populations as well as shed light on the pathophysiology of this disease (Qiu et al., 2013).

Myopia has become increasingly prevalent worldwide over the past century (Vitale et al., 2009). The association between myopia and POAG has been recognized for decades (Knapp, 1926, Muller, 1948; Fong et al., 1990) and has been documented in many case series (Podos et al., 1966; Perkins and Phelps, 1982; Phelps, 1982; Lotufo et al., 1989; Mastropasqua et al., 1992; Chihara et al.,1997) and case-control studies (Daubs and Crick, 1981). The underlying hypothesis explaining this association is that individuals with axial myopia have weaker scleral support at the optic nerve, and this contributes to a greater susceptibility of the optic nerve to glaucomatous damage (AAO, Preferred Practice Pattern Guidelines, 2010). More recently, large cross-sectional epidemiologic studies in Australia, China, Japan, India, and the Netherlands also suggest that individuals with myopia have a higher prevalence of open-angle glaucoma than those without myopia (Mitchell et al., 1999; Xu et al.,2007; Suzuki et al., 2006; Ramakrishnan et al., 2003; Czudowska et al., 2010). In the United States (US), there have been similar studies about the association between myopia and glaucoma (Jiang et al., 2012; Centers for Disease Control and Prevention, 2005; Qiu et al., 2013). The study of a population-based sample of adults in the US aged 40 years and older from the National Health and Nutrition Examination Survey (NHANES) (Centers for Disease Control and Prevention, 2005), a large population-based survey conducted annually in the US (Qiu et al., 2013).found an association between myopia and visual field defects, but failed to find an association between myopia and self-reported glaucoma or vertical cup-to disc ratio. In subjects with mild, moderate, and severe myopia, the odds of having any visual field defect were increased approximately 2-fold, 3-fold, and 14-fold, respectively, compared with subjects with emmetropia. This pattern suggests an exponential rather than a linear relationship between myopia and visual field defects. In addition, when visual field defects were further categorized into early, moderate, and severe, a pattern emerged suggesting an exponentially increasing proportion of worse visual field defects among subjects with greater myopia.

Similar results were found in previous large population-based studies on myopia and glaucoma. The BMES in Australia found an association between all categories of myopia and glaucoma diagnosed by the presence of matching optic disc cupping with rim thinning (cup to-disc ratio > 0.7, or cupto-disc asymmetry > 0.3) and characteristic visual field loss on automated perimetry (Xu et al., 2007). The Aravind Comprehensive Eye Survey in India and the Tajimi Study in Japan also found an association between myopia greater than -1 D and POAG diagnosed by a comprehensive ophthalmologic exam (Suzuki et al., 2006; Ramakrishnan et al., 2003). The BES in China found an association between severe myopia greater than -6 D and glaucomatous optic nerve appearance, visual field defects, and elevated IOP (Xu et al., 2007). The Rotterdam Eye Study in the Netherlands found an association between high myopia greater than -4 D and glaucomatous visual field loss (Czudowska et al., 2010). The Los Angeles Latino Eye Study of a Latino population in the US found an association between axial myopia and open angle glaucoma defined by the presence of an open angle and a glaucomatous visual field abnormality and/or evidence of glaucomatous optic nerve damage in at least one eye, particularly in individuals with elevated IOP (Jiang et al., 2012). The study (Qiu et al., 2013) of a representative sample of the entire US population also found an association between myopia and visual field defects, but not between myopia and self-reported glaucoma or vertical cup to disc ratio greater than or equal to 0.7 with the latter being a possible surrogate for glaucomatous disease.

Myopia and OAG (Marcus et al., 2011)

Myopia has long been identified as a risk factor for open-angle glaucoma (OAG) (Knapp, 1925; Daubs and Crick, 1981; Perkins and Phelps, 1982; Mastropasqua et al., 1992). Open-angle glaucoma is an irreversible eye disease responsible for approximately 12% of global blindness, which is second to cataract (Resnikoff et al., 2004). It is largely unknown why myopia increases the risk of OAG. Myopic eyes have longer axial lengths and vitreous chamber depths (Scott and Grosvenor, 1993), and eyes with an increased axial length seem to have a greater deformability of the lamina cribrosa. This might contribute to a higher susceptibility to glaucomatous optic disc changes (Scott and Grosvenor, 1993; Fong et al., 1990).There is conflicting evidence concerning the range of refractive error important for OAG. Although some studies have reported an association with any myopia (Drance et al., 1973; Grødum et al., 2001; Leighton and Tomlinson, 1973; Orzalesi et al.,2007), others have found the relationship only in individuals with high myopia (Podos et al., 1966; Chihara et al., 1997; Mayama et al., 2002; Lee et al., 2008).

The findings from a meta-analysis (Marcus et al., 2011) indicate that individuals with myopia have an approximately doubled risk of developing OAG in comparison with individuals without myopia. The pooled ORs were 2.46 (95% CI, 1.93–3.15) for high myopia and 1.77 (95% CI, 1.41–2.23) for low myopia, with a cutoff value of -3 D. Although the point estimate of the pooled OR of high myopia was larger than that of low myopia, the difference was small. A more pronounced dose-response relationship would have reinforced the association between myopia and OAG. The apparent absence of a clear dose-response relationship might be the consequence of the population-based design of the included studies. Myopia greater than, for example, -10 D is seen on a regular basis in a clinical setting. In a population-based sample, however, most participants with high myopia have a refractive error between -3 and -4 D, and values -5 D are rare (Strömberg, 1936; Xu et al., 2005; Katz et al., 1997). The observed heterogeneity among the included crosssectional studies was explained by the Andhra Pradesh (Garudadri et al., 2010) and Beijing studies (Xu et al., 2007). Although these studies, in contrast with the majority of the included studies, were conducted in Asia and included both urban and rural cohorts, the disparate results of these 2 studies in this meta-analysis remain unclear. Two studies, by Ponte et al. (Ponte et al., 1994) and Czudowska et al. (Czudowska et al., 2010) were omitted beforehand because of different study designs, confirmed the presence of an association between myopia and OAG. In their case-control study, Ponte et al. (Ponte et al., 1994) reported an association between myopia (-1.5 D myopic) and OAG with an OR of 5.56 (95% CI, 1.85–16.67). In their population-based cohort study, Czudowska et al. (Czudowska et al., 2010) reported an association between high myopia and incident OAG with an HR of 2 (Wong et al.,2003). (95% CI, 1.19–4.49); the association between low myopia and incident OAG was not significant (HR 1.16; 95% CI, 0.72–1.88).

Visual field defects and anomalous appearing optic discs have been reported in persons with myopia (Brazitikos et al., 1990; Jonas et al., 1988; Jonas and Dichtl, 1997).

Future research is warranted to determine the association between myopia and OAG in severe myopia (which is rare in population-based samples) and to elucidate the pathophysiologic mechanism underlying the association between myopia and OAG.

High Myopia and Glaucoma Susceptibility

In the Barbados Eye Study and the Blue Mountains Eye Study, myopic subjects compared with hyperopic subjects showed a significantly higher prevalence of glaucomatous optic nerve damage (Leske et al., 1995; Mitchell et al., 1999). In The Beijing Eye Study (Xu et al., 2007) the prevalence of glaucomatous optic nerve damage was significantly higher in the eyes with a myopic refractive error exceeding -6 diopters than in the remaining eyes. In the hyperopic eyes, the emmetropic eyes and the eyes with low to moderate myopia (myopic refractive up to -6 diopters or less), the frequency of glaucoma did not vary significantly. It suggests a higher glaucoma susceptibility in eyes with marked to high myopia. It may fit with the finding of a thinner lamina cribrosa in combination with a secondary enlargement of the optic nerve head in highly myopic eyes and with the pathophysiologic role the lamina cribrosa may play in glaucoma (Jonas and Budde, 2005; Jonas et al., 1988; Jonas et al., 2004; Morgan et al., 1995;Bellezza et al., 2000; Jonas et al., 2003).

These observations were in agreement with hospital-based studies in which axial myopia was reported to be a risk factor for glaucomatous optic neuropathy (Podos et al., 1966; Greve and Furuno, 1980; Daubs and Crick, 1981; Phelps, 1982; Perkins and Phelps, 1982; David et al., 1987;Chihara et al., 1997; Quigley, 1993; Jonas and Budde, 2005). Randomized clinical trials have revealed varying results suggesting that myopia may or may not be a risk factor or predictive factor for the development and progression of glaucomatous optic nerve damage (Drance et al., 2001; Grødum and Heijl, 2001; Gordon et al., 2002; The Advanced Glaucoma

Intervention Study (AGIS), 2002; Leske et al., 2003). These studies did not differentiate between marked to high myopia and low to moderate myopia.

Clinical studies and histomorphometric investigations showed, however, that the optic nerve head appearance varies between subjects with high marked to high myopia and subjects with low to moderate myopia (Jonas et al., 1988; Jonas and Dichtl, 1997; Dichtl et al., 1998; Jonas et al., 2004).

The Beijing Eye Study agreed with preceding hospital based studies that have also suggested an association between glaucomatous optic nerve damage and marked to high myopia, and with epidemiologic studies on non-Chinese populations (Leske et al., 1995; Mitchell et al., 1999; Podos et al., 1966; Greve and Furuno, 1980; Daubs and Crick, 1981; Phelps, 1982; Perkins and Phelps, 1982; David et al., 1987;Chihara et al., 1997; Quigley, 1993; Jonas and Budde, 2005). The Blue Mountains Eye Study reported prevalence figures of glaucoma that ranged from 1.5% in emmetropes to 4.4% in moderate to high myopes (Mitchell et al., 1999). The Barbados Eye Study found that myopia increased the odds of having glaucoma whereas hyperopia reduced the odds of having glaucoma in black participants (Leske et al.,1995). The Beijing Eye Study also was in agreement with a Malmö eye survey, which was performed on > 30 000 individuals as preparation of the Early Manifest Glaucoma Trial (Grødum et al., 2001; Leske et al., 2003). In the Malmö eye survey, the prevalence of glaucoma increased with increasing myopia, and the association between myopia and glaucoma was strong at lower intraocular pressure levels, and weakened gradually with increasing intraocular pressure (Grødum et al., 2001). The results of the Beijing Eye Study might further elucidate the discrepancies between some of the previous studies in which myopia was, or was not, a predictive factor for glaucoma (Jonas et al., 2002). If myopia is differentiated into marked or high myopia beyond a myopic refractive error of -6 diopters and into low to moderate myopia, marked to high myopia may be a risk factor for glaucoma, and low to moderate myopia may not play a pronounced role for glaucoma. Correspondingly, the low to moderate myopic group, the emmetropic group and the hyperopic group did not vary significantly in the prevalence of glaucoma in the Beijing Eye Study.

Highly myopic eyes usually show a characteristic appearance of the optic nerve head with an enlarged macrodisc, shallow cupping, a large myopic crescent, and a bright fundus pigmentation.

The figures in the Beijing Eye Study were similar or even lower instead of being higher than in other epidemiologic studies (Leske et al., 1995; Mitchell et al., 1999; Dielmans et al., 1994; Leske et al., 1994; Quigley et al.,2001; Varma et al., 2004; Aung et al., 2005; He et al., 2006).

High Myopia and Glaucoma

Myopia is a common cause of visual impairment worldwide, and its prevalence has been increasing rapidly within recent decades, notably in Asian countries (Morgan and Rose, 2005; Lin et al., 2004). Theories for the increasing myopia prevalence include more time spent studying and performing near-work, less time spent outdoors, higher education levels, and genetic factors (Pan et al., 2012; Morgan et al., 2012). High myopia (-6 D) has been associated with a number of ocular pathologies, including cataracts, retinal detachment, and glaucoma (Saw et al., 2005). The association between myopia and glaucoma has been reported in studies in the United States (Wong et al., 1995; Qiu et al., 2013; Jiang et al., 2012), The Netherlands (Czudowska et al., 2010), Sweden (Grødum et al., 2001), Australia (Mitchell et al., 1999), Barbados (Wu et al., 1999), India (Ramakrishnan et al., 2003), Japan (Suzuki et al., 2006), China (Xu et al., 2007), and Singapore (Perera et al., 2013) and in Korea (Chon et al., 2013). In Asian population, in the Beijing Eye Study (Xu et al., 2007), glaucoma susceptibility was higher in those with worse than -6 D of myopia. Though the frequency of glaucoma increased with more severe myopia, the relationship was not significant for refractive errors less severe than -6 D.

In the Handan Eye Study (Liang et al., 2011), groups with -3 D to-6 D of myopia had a 4.7 (1.6–13.5, 95% CI) greater odds of having POAG, though not statistically significant at other levels of refractive error. In the Tajimi Study (Suzuki et al.,2006), individuals with-1 to -3 D of myopia had a 1.85 (1.03–3.31) times greater odds of glaucoma and individuals with less than-3 D had a 2.60 (1.56– 4.35) times greater odds of glaucoma.

In the Singapore Malay Eye Study (Perera et al., 2013), refractive error of less than -4 D was associated with a 2.80 (1.07–7.37) greater odds of glaucoma. Similar findings have been shown in American studies of a predominantly Caucasian population in the Beaver Dam Eye Study (Wong et al., 1995), in Latinos in the Los Angeles Latino Eye Study (LALES) (Jiang et al., 2012), and in a nationally representative sample of the United States (Qiu et al., 2013). Similar findings have also been reported in other countries including The Netherlands (Czudowska et al., 2010), Sweden (Grødum et al., 2001), Australia (Mitchell et al., 1999), Barbados (Wu et al., 1999), and India (Ramakrishnan et al., 2003).

The Pathogenesis of the Epidemiological Association between Myopia and Glaucoma

Researchers have proposed that (1) thinner peripapillary sclera and different lamina cribrosa biomechanical properties in myopia could play a role (Cahane and Bartov, 1992); (2) longer AL could be associated with thinner corneal thickness (conflicting literature) (Perera and Aung, 2010); (3) myopia may lead to higher IOP (albeit a small difference) (Perera and Aung, 2010); and (4) myopia could be influencing optic nerve head susceptibility or ocular blood flow through larger disc size which may be associated with thinner scleral/laminar tissue and steeper translaminar pressure gradients (Fong et al., 1990; Perera and Aung, 2010; Burgoyne, 2004). There is a lot of literature on myopic field defects and how tilted discs may mimic false visual field progression (Brazitikos et al., 1990; Vuori et al., 2008; Witmer et al., 2010). Some of the more common characteristic myopic field defects include enlarged blind spot and atypical temporal or cecocentral nerve fiber layer bundle defects (Greve and Furuno, 1980).

8. Myopia and Visual Function

Recent research has focused on describing the negative effect that uncorrected refractive error (URE) has on vision-specific quality of life (Lamoureux et al., 2009; Broman et al., 2002; Coleman et al., 2006; Qwsley et al., 2007).

Uncorrected refractive error is known to be associated with decreased quality of life and visual function difficulty. This association has been demonstrated in a variety of populations using a variety of function assessment tools, including the NEI VFQ-25 (Lamoureux et al., 2009; Broman et al., 2002; Coleman et al., 2006; Qwsley et al., 2007). The National Eye Institute 25-item Visual Function Questionnaire (NEI VFQ-25) is a tool that quantifies the degree to which an individual's visual impairment results in functional difficulty (Mangione et al., 1998; Mangione et al., 2001). Previous studies have used this tool and other questionnaires to demonstrate that URE has a negative impact on vision-specific quality of life. Few studies have examined the effects of different types of refractive error (RE), namely, myopia, hyperopia, and astigmatism, on visual function. (Sandhu et al., 2012). RE correction was associated with higher function scores among subjects with myopic RE, but not among those with hyperopic RE (Sandhu et al., 2012). Persons with corrected myopia reported better distance vision than did those with uncorrected myopia, and persons with corrected hyperopia reported better near vision than did those with uncorrected hyperopia. Unexpectedly, any type of RE, either corrected or uncorrected, was associated with significantly worse distance vision function compared with those without RE (Sandhu et al., 2012).

References

Aaby AA, Kushner BJ. Acquired and progressive myelinated nerve fibers. *Arch Ophthalmol* 1985; 103:542-4.

AGIS Investigators. The Advanced Glaucoma Intervention Study (AGIS): 12. Baseline risk factors for sustained loss of visual field and visual acuity in patients with advanced glaucoma. *Am J Ophthalmol* 2002;134:499 -512.

Ali BH, Logani S, Kozlov KL, et al. Progression of retinal nerve fiber myelination in childhood. *Am J Ophthalmol* 1994;118:515-7.

American Academy of Ophthalmology Glaucoma Panel. Preferred Practice Pattern Guidelines. Primary Open-Angle Glaucoma. San Francisco, CA: American Academy of Ophthalmology; 2010. Available at: www.aao.org/ppp. Accessed September 1, 2012.

American Academy of Ophthalmology Glaucoma Panel. Preferred Practice Pattern Guidelines. Primary Open-Angle Glaucoma. San Francisco, CA: American Academy of Ophthalmology; 2010.

American Academy of Ophthalmology Glaucoma Panel. Preferred practice patternt guidelines. Primary open-angle glaucoma suspect. *Am Acad Ophthalmol.* Available at: www. aao.org/ppp. Accessed July 11, 2013.

American Diabetes Association. Diagnosis and classification of diabetes mellitus. *Diabetes Care* 2010;33(Suppl):S62-9.

Aung T, Nolan WP, Machin D, et al. Anterior chamber depth and the risk of primary angle closure in 2 East Asian populations. *Arch Ophthalmol* 2005;123:527-32.

Baarsma GS. Acquired medullated nerve fibers. *Br J Ophthalmol* 1980; 64:651.

Bellezza AJ, Hart RT, Burgoyne CF. The optic nerve head as a biomechanical structure: initial finite element modeling. *Invest Ophthalmol Vis Sci* 2000;41:2991-3000.

Boker T, Fang T, Steinmetz R. Refractive error and choroidal perfusion characteristics in patients with choroidal neovascularization and age-related macular degeneration. *Ger J Ophthalmol* 1993;2:10 -3.

Brazitikos PD, Safran AB, Simona F, Zulauf M. Threshold perimetry in tilted disc syndrome. *Arch Ophthalmol* 1990;108: 1698–700.

Burgoyne C. Myopic eyes and glaucoma. *J Glaucoma.* 2004;13:85–86.

Cahane M, Bartov E. Axial length and scleral thickness effect on susceptibility to glaucomatous damage: a theoretical model implementing Laplace's law. *Ophthalmic Res* 1992;24:280–284.

Casson RJ, Gupta A, Newland HS, et al. Risk factors for primary open-angle glaucoma in a Burmese population: the Meiktila Eye Study. *Clin Exp Ophthalmol* 2007;35:739-744.

Centers for Disease Control and Prevention (CDC), National Center for Health Statistics (NCHS). National Health and Nutrition Examination Survey Data. Hyattsville, MD: U.S. Department of Health and Human Services, Centers for Disease Control and Prevention. 2005. Available at: http://www.cdc.gov/nchs/nhanes/nhanes_questionnaires.htm. Accessed March 19, 2012.

Chang MA, Congdon NG, Bykhovskaya I, Munoz B, West SK. The association between myopia and various subtypes of lens opacity: SEE (Salisbury Eye Evaluation) project. *Ophthalmology* 2005;112:1395–1401.

Chavis PS, Tabbara KF: Demyelination of retinal myelinated nerve fibers in Behcet's disease. *Doc Ophthalmol* 1998;95:157-64.

Cheung CM, Tai ES, Kawasaki R, et al. Prevalence of and risk factors for age-related macular degeneration in a multiethnic Asian cohort. *Arch Ophthalmol* 2012;130:480-6.

Chihara E, Chihara K. Covariation of optic disc measurements and ocular parameters in the healthy eye. *Graefes Arch Clin Exp Ophthalmol* 1994;232(5):265-71.

Chihara E, Liu X, Dong J, et al. Severe myopia as a risk factor for progressive visual field loss in primary open-angle glaucoma. *Ophthalmologica* 1997;211:66–71.

Chon B, Qiu M, Lin SC. Myopia and glaucoma in the South Korean population. *Invest Ophthalmol Vis Sci* 2013;54:6570–6577. DOI:10.1167/iovs.13-12173.

Ciulla TA, Harris A, Latkany P, et al. Ocular perfusion abnormalities in diabetes. *Acta Ophthalmol Scand* 2002;80: 468-77.

Coman I, Barbin G, Charles P, et al: Axonal signals in central nervous system myelination, demyelination, and remyelination. *J Neurol Sci* 2005; 233:67-71.

Congdon N, O'Colmain B, Klaver CC, et al. Causes and prevalence of visual impairment among adults in the United States. *Arch Ophthalmol* 2004;122:477-485.

Cruickshanks KJ, Klein R, Klein BE. Sunlight and age-related macular degeneration: the Beaver Dam Eye Study. *Arch Ophthalmol* 1993;111:514-8.

Czudowska MA, Ramdas WD, Wolfs RC, et al. Incidence of glaucomatous visual field loss: a ten-year follow-up from the Rotterdam Study. *Ophthalmology.* 2010;117:1705–1712.

Dandona R, Dandona L, Naduvilath TJ, Srinivas M, McCarty CA, Rao GN. Refractive errors in an urban population in Southern India: the Andhra Pradesh Eye Disease Study. *Invest Ophthalmol Vis Sci.* 1999;40:2810–2818.

Daubs JG, Crick RP. Effect of refractive error on the risk of ocular hypertension and open angle glaucoma. Trans Ophthalmol Soc U K. 1981;101:121–126.

David R, Zangwill L, Stone D, Yassur Y. Epidemiology of intraocular pressure in a population screened for glaucoma. *Br J Ophthalmol* 1987;71:766 -71.

De Jong PT, Bistervels B, Cosgrove J, et al: Medullated nerve fibers: a sign of multiple basal cell nevi (Gorlin's) syndrome. *Arch Ophthalmol* 1985;103:1833-6.

Dichtl A, Jonas JB, Naumann GO. Histomorphometry of the optic disc in highly myopic eyes with absolute secondary angle closure glaucoma. *Br J Ophthalmol* 1998;82:286 -9.

Dielemans I, Vingerline JR, Wolfs RCW, Hofman A, Grobbee DE, De Jong PT. The prevalence of primary open-angle glaucoma in a population-based study in The Netherlands: the Rotterdam Study. *Ophthalmology. 1994*;101:1851–1855.

Drance S, Anderson DR, Schulzer M, Collaborative Normal-Tension Glaucoma Study Group. Risk factors for progression of visual field abnormalities in normal-tension glaucoma. *Am J Ophthalmol* 2001;131:699 -708.

Drance SM, Sweeney VP, Morgan RW, Feldman F. Studies of factors involved in the production of low tension glaucoma. *Arch Ophthalmol* 1973;89:457– 65.

Duerksen R, Limburg H, Carron JE, Foster A. Cataract blindness in Paraguay—results of a national survey. *Ophthalmic Epidemiol.* 2003;10:349–357.

Dunzhu S, Wang FS, Courtright P, et al. Blindness and eye diseases in Tibet: findings from a randomised, population based survey. *Br J Ophthalmol.* 2003;87:1443–1448.

Eide N: Retinal break in an area with medullated nerve fibers. *Acta Ophthalmol* (Cophenh) 1986 ;64:271-3.

Ellis GS, Frey T, Gouterman RZ. Myelinated nerve fibers, axial myopia, and refractory amblyopia: an organic disease. *J Pediatr Ophthalmol Strabismus* 1987; 24:111-9.

Eye Diseases Prevalence Research Group. The prevalence of refractive errors among adults in the United States, Western Europe, and Australia. *Arch Ophthalmol* 2004;122:495–505.

Fong DS, Epstein DL, Allingham RR. Glaucoma and myopia: are they related? *Int Ophthalmol Clin* 1990;30:215–218.

Fotedar R, Mitchell P, Burlutsky G, Wang JJ. Relationship of 10- year change in refraction to nuclear cataract and axial length findings from an older population. *Ophthalmology.* 2008;115: 1273–1278.

Funnell CL, George ND, Pai V. Familial myelinated retinal nerve fibres. *Eye* 2003; 17:96—7.

Garudadri C, Senthil S, Khanna RC, et al. Prevalence and risk factors for primary glaucomas in adult urban and rural populations in the Andhra Pradesh Eye Disease Study. *Ophthalmology* 2010;117:1352–9.

Gemenetzi M, Yang Y, Lotery AJ. Current concepts on primary open-angle glaucoma genetics: a contribution to disease pathophysiology and future treatment. *Eye* (Lond). 2012;26:355–369.

Gentile RC, Torqueti-Costa L, Bertolucci A. Loss of myelinated retinal nerve fibres in diabetic retinopathy. *Br J Ophthalmol* 2002; 86:1447.

Gicquel JJ, Salama B, Mercie M, et al: Myelinated retinal nerve fibres loss in Leber's hereditary optic neuropathy. *Acta Ophthalmol Scand* 2003;83:517-8.

Gordon MO, Beiser JA, Brandt JD, et al. The Ocular Hypertension Treatment Study: baseline factors that predict the onset of primary open-angle glaucoma. *Arch Ophthalmol* 2002;120:714 -20.

Greve EL, Furuno F. Myopia and glaucoma. *Graefes Arch Clin Exp Ophthalmol.* 1980; 213:33–41.

Grødum K, Heijl A, Bengtsson B. Refractive error and glaucoma. *Acta Ophthalmol Scand.* 2001;79:560–566.

Gupta A, Khandalavala B, Bansal RK, et al: Atrophy of myelinated nerve fibers fibers in pituitary adenoma. *J Clin Neuroophthalmol* 1990;10:100-2.

Guzowski M, Wang JJ, Rochtchina E, Rose KA, Mitchell P. Fiveyear refractive changes in an older population: the Blue Mountains Eye Study. *Ophthalmology.* 2003;110:1364–1370.

He M, Foster PJ, Ge J, et al. Prevalence and clinical characteristics of glaucoma in adult Chinese: a populationbased study in Liwan District, Guangzhou. *Invest Ophthalmol Vis Sci.* 2006;47:2782–2788.

How AC, Tan GS, Chan YH, et al. Population prevalence of tilted and torted optic discs among an adult Chinese population in Singapore: the Tanjong Pagar Study. *Arch Ophthalmol.* 2009;127(7):894-9.

Hoyt CS, Stone RD, Fromer C: Monocular axial myopia associated with neonatal eyelid closure in human infants. *Am J Ophthalmol* 1981;91:197-200.

Hubbard GB, Thomas MA, Grossniklaus HE: Vitreomacular traction syndrome with extensively myelinated nerve fibers. *Arch Ophthalmol* 2002;120:670-1.

Hunter SF, Leavitt JA, Rodriguez M: Direct observation of myelination in vivo in the mature human central nervous system. *Brain* 1992;120:2071-82.

Hyman L, Wu SY, Connell AM, et al. Prevalence and causes of visual impairment in the Barbados Eye Study. *Ophthalmology.* 2001;108:1751–1756.

Ikram MK, van Leeuwen R, Vingerling JR, et al. Relationship between refraction and prevalent as well as incident agerelated maculopathy: the Rotterdam Study. *Invest Ophthalmol Vis Sci* 2003;44:3778-82.

Jiang X, Varma R, Wu S, et al. Baseline risk factors that predict the development of open-angle glaucoma in a population: the Los Angeles Latino Eye Study. *Ophthalmology.* 2012;119: 2245–2253.

Jiang X, Varma R, Wu S, et al. Baseline risk factors that predict the development of open-angle glaucoma: the Los Angeles Latino Eye Study. *Ophthalmology.* 2012;119:2245–2253.

Jonas JB, Berenshtein E, Holbach L. Anatomic relationship between lamina cribrosa, intraocular space, and cerebrospinal fluid space. *Invest Ophthalmol Vis Sci* 2003;44:5189 95.

Jonas JB, Berenshtein E, Holbach L. Lamina cribrosa thickness and spatial relationships between intraocular space and cerebrospinal fluid space in highly myopic eyes. *Invest Ophthalmol Vis Sci* 2004;45:2660 -5.

Jonas JB, Dichtl A. Optic disc morphology in myopic primary open-angle glaucoma. *Graefes Arch Clin Exp Ophthalmol.* 1997;235:627–633.

Jonas JB, Gusek GC, Naumann GO. Optic disc, cup and neuroretinal rim size, configuration, and correlations in normal eyes. *Invest Ophthalmol Vis Sci* 1988;29:1151-8.

Jonas JB, Gusek GC, Naumann GO. Optic disk morphometry in high myopia. Graefes Arch Clin Exp Ophthalmol 1988;226: 587–90.

Jonas JB, Martus P, Budde WM. Anisometropia and degree of optic nerve damage in chronic open-angle glaucoma. *Am J Ophthalmol* 2002;134:547-51.

Jonas JB, Tao Y, Neumaier M, Findeisen P. VEGF and refractive error [letter]. *Ophthalmology* 2010;117:2234.

Jones D, Luensmann D. Prevalence and Impact of High Myopia. *Eye & Contact Lens* 2012; 38(3): 191-1.

Kaimbo wa Kaimbo D, Mwilambwe wa Mwilambwe A, Leys A, Missotten L. Les fibres à myéline chez les patients Zaïrois [Myelinated retinal nerve fibers in Zairian patients]. *Bull Soc Belge Ophtalmol* 1995; 259:127-131.

Kaimbo Wa Kaimbo D. Tilted disc syndrome in Congolese patients. *J Fr Ophtalmol* 2010;33:174-177.

Karadimas P, Kapetanios A, Panayotidhou E, Bouzas EA: Epiretinalmembrane occurring with myelinated retinal nerve fibers and vascular abnormalities. *Retina* 2003; 23:880-1.

Katz J, Tielsch JM, Sommer A. Prevalence and risk factors for refractive errors in an adult inner city population. *Invest Ophthalmol Vis Sci* 1997;38:334–40.

Kee C, Hwang JM: Visual prognosis of amblyopia associated with myelinated retinal nerve fibers. *Am J Ophthalmol* 2005;139: 259-65.

Kempen JH, Mitchell P, Lee KE, et al., Eye Diseases Prevalence Research Group. The prevalence of refractive errors among adults in the United States, Western Europe, and Australia. *Arch Ophthalmol* 2004;122:495-505.

Kifley A, Wang JJ, Cugati S, et al. Retinal vascular caliber, diabetes, and retinopathy. *Am J Ophthalmol* 2007;143: 1024-6.

Klein BE, Klein R, Sponsel WE, et al. Prevalence of glaucoma: the Beaver Dam Eye Study. *Ophthalmology.* 1992;99:1499–1504.

Klein R, Klein BE, Moss SE, et al. Retinal vascular abnormalities in persons with type 1 diabetes: the Wisconsin Epidemiologic Study of Diabetic Retinopathy: XVIII. *Ophthalmology* 2003;110:2118 -25.

Klein R, Klein BE, Moss SE, et al. The relation of retinal vessel caliber to the incidence and progression of diabetic retinopathy: XIX: the Wisconsin Epidemiologic Study of Diabetic Retinopathy. *Arch Ophthalmol* 2004;122:76-83.

Knapp A. Glaucoma in myopic eyes. *Arch Ophthalmol.* 1926;55:35–37.

Knapp A. Glaucoma in myopic eyes. *Trans Am Ophthalmol Soc* 1925;23:61–70.

Kohner EM, Patel V, Rassam SM. Role of blood flow and impaired autoregulation in the pathogenesis of diabetic retinopathy. *Diabetes* 1995;44:603-7.

Kreidl KO, Lin DY, Egbert JE: Myelination of the macula associated with disabling photophobia. *Arch Ophthalmol* 2003;121:1204-5.

Krishnaiah S, Srinivas M, Khanna RC, Rao GN. Prevalence and risk factors for refractive errors in the South Indian adult population: the Andhra Pradesh Eye disease study. *Clin Ophthalmol* 2009;3:17-27.

Kubo E, Kumamoto Y, Tsuzuki S, Akagi Y. Axial length, myopia, and the severity of lens opacity at the time of cataract surgery. *Arch Ophthalmol.* 2006;124:1586–1590.

Lavanya R, Kawasaki R, Tay WT, et al. Hyperopic refractive error and shorter axial length are associated with age-related macular degeneration: the Singapore Malay Eye Study. *Invest Ophthalmol Vis Sci* 2010;51:6247-52.

Lee KE, Klein BE, Klein R, Wong TY. Changes in refraction over 10 years in an adult population: the Beaver Dam Eye study. *Invest Ophthalmol Vis Sci.* 2002;43:2566–2571.

Lee KE, Klein BE, Klein R. Changes in refractive error over a 5- year interval in the Beaver Dam Eye Study. *Invest Ophthalmol Vis Sci.* 1999;40:1645–1649.

Lee YA, Shih YF, Lin LL, et al. Association between high myopia and progression of visual field loss in primary open-angle glaucoma. *J Formos Med Assoc* 2008;107:952-957.

Leighton DA, Tomlinson A. Ocular tension and axial length of the eyeball in open-angle glaucoma and low tension glaucoma. *Br J Ophthalmol* 1973;57:499 –502.

Leske MC, Connell AM, Wu SY, et al. Risk factors for open-angle glaucoma: the Barbados Eye Study. *Arch Ophthalmol* 1995;113:918 -24.

Leske MC, Connell AMS, Schachat AP, Hyman L. The Barbados Eye Study: prevalence of open angle glaucoma. *Arch Ophthalmol.* 1994;112:821–829.

Leske MC, Heijl A, Hussein M, et al. Factors for glaucoma progression and the effect of treatment: the Early Manifest Glaucoma Trial. *Arch Ophthalmol* 2003;121:48 -56.

Leske MC, Wu SY, Nemesure B, et al. Risk factors for incident nuclear opacities. *Ophthalmology* 2002;109:1303-1308.

Leys AM, Leys MJ, Mooymans JM, et al: Myelinated nerve fibers and retinal vascular abnormalities. *Retina* 1996;16:89-96.

Li XQ, Larsen M, Munch IC. Subfoveal choroidal thickness in relation to sex and axial length in 93 Danish university students. *Invest Ophthalmol Vis Sci* 2011;52:8438-41.

Liang YB, Friedman DS, Zhou Q, et al. Prevalence of primary open angle glaucoma in a rural adult Chinese population: the Handan Eye Study. *Invest Ophthalmol Vis Sci.* 2011;52:8250–8257.

Lim L, Gazzard G, Chan YH, et al. Corneal biomechanics, thickness and optic disc morphology in children with optic disc tilt. *Br J Ophthalmol.* 2008;92(11):1461-6.

Lim LS, Cheung CY, Lin X, et al. Influence of refractive error and axial length on retinal vessel geometric characteristics. *Invest Ophthalmol Vis Sci* 2011;52:669 -78.

Lim LS, Lamoureux E, Saw SM, et al. Are myopic eyes less likely to have diabetic retinopathy? *Ophthalmology* 2010;117: 524-30.

Lim R, Mitchell P, Cumming RG. Refractive associations with cataract: the Blue Mountains Eye Study. *Invest Ophthalmol Vis Sci* 1999;40:3021-3026.

Lin HY, Chang CW, Wang HZ, Tsai RK. Relation between the axial length and lenticular progressive myopia. *Eye.* 2005;19: 899–905.

Lin LLK, Shih YF, Hsiao CK, Chen CJ. Prevalence of myopia in Taiwanese schoolchildren: 1983 to 2000. *Ann Acad Med Singapore.* 2004;33:27–33.

Lopez Sanchez E, et al: A case of loss of retinal myelinated nerve fibers in a chronic glaucoma [Spanish]. *Archivos de la Sociedad Espanola de Oftalmologia* 2002 ; 77:39-42.

Lorenzi M, Gerhardinger C. Early cellular and molecular changes induced by diabetes in the retina. *Diabetologia* 2001; 44:791—804.

Lotufo D, Ritch R, Szmyd L Jr, Burris JE. Juvenile glaucoma, race, and refraction. *JAMA.* 1989;261:249–252.

Luo HD, Gazzard G, Fong A, et al. Myopia, axial length, and OCT characteristics of the macula in Singaporean children. *Invest Ophthalmol Vis Sci* 2006;47;2773- 81.

Maberley DA, Hollands H, Chang A, et al. The prevalence of low vision and blindness in a Canadian inner city. *Eye* (Lond) 2007;21:528-533.

Maberley DA, Hollands H, Chuo J, et al. The prevalence of low vision and blindness in Canada. *Eye* (Lond) 2006; 20:341-346.

Marcus MW, de Vries MM, Montolio FGJ, Jansonius NM. Myopia as a Risk Factor for Open-Angle Glaucoma: A Systematic Review and Meta-Analysis. *Ophthalmology* 2011;118:1989–1994.

Mashayekhi A, Shields CL, Shields JA: Disappearance of retinal myelilnated nerve fibers after plaque radiotherapy for choroidal melanoma. *Retina* 2003;23:572-3.

Mastropasqua L, Lobefalo L, Mancini A, et al. Prevalence of myopia in open angle glaucoma. *Eur J Ophthalmol.* 1992;2:33–35.

Mayama C, Suzuki Y, Araie M, et al. Myopia and advanced- stage open-angle glaucoma. *Ophthalmology* 2002; 109:2072–7.

McCarty CA, Mukesh BN, Fu CL, Taylor HR. The epidemiology of cataract in Australia. *Am J Ophthalmol* 1999;128: 446-65.

McKay R, McCarty CA, Taylor HR. Diabetic retinopathy in Victoria, Australia: the Visual Impairment Project. *Br J Ophthalmol* 2000;84:865-70.

McKean-Cowdin R, Wang Y, Wu J, Azen SP, Varma R. Impact of visual field loss on health-related quality of life in glaucoma: the Los Angeles Latino Eye Study. *Ophthalmology.* 2008;115: 941–948.e1.

Mehta JS, Raman J, Gupta N, Sinha A: Retinal vascular anomalies in acquired myelinated nerve fibers. *Acta Ophthalmol Scand* 2003;81:311-2.

Minning CA Jr, Davidorf FH: Neovascularization associated with myelinated nerve fibers: a case report. *Ann Ophthalmol* 1983;15:1142-4.

Mitchell P, Hourihan F, Sandbach J, Wang JJ. The relationship between glaucoma and myopia: the Blue Mountains Eye Study. *Ophthalmology.* 1999;106:2010–2015.

Mitchell P, Smith W, Attebo K, Healey PR. Prevalence of openangle glaucoma in Australia: the Blue Mountains Eye Study. *Ophthalmology.* 1996;103:1661–1669.

Moller HU. Excessive myopia and glaucoma. *Acta Ophthalmol.*1948;26:185–93.

Morgan I, Rose K. How genetic is school myopia? *Progr Retin Eye Res.* 2005;24:1–38.

Morgan IG, Ohno-matsui K, Saw S-M. Myopia. *Lance*t. 2012;379:1739–1748.

Morgan WH, Yu DY, Cooper RL, et al. The influence of cerebrospinal fluid pressure on the lamina cribrosa tissue pressure gradient. *Invest Ophthalmol Vis Sci* 1995;36: 1163-72.

Moss SE, Klein R, Klein BE. Ocular factors in the incidence and progression of diabetic retinopathy. *Ophthalmology* 1994; 101:77—83.

Mukesh BN, Le A, Dimitrov PN, Ahmed S, Taylor HR, McCarty CA. Development of cataract and associated risk factors: the Visual Impairment Project. *Arch Ophthalmol.* 2006;124:79–85.

Murthy GV, Gupta S, Ellwein LB, Munoz SR, Bachani D, Dada VK. A population-based eye survey of older adults in a rural district of Rajasthan: I. Central vision impairment, blindness, and cataract surgery. *Ophthalmology.* 2001;108:679–685.

Nelson P, Aspinall P, Papasouliotis O, Worton B, O'Brien C. Quality of life in glaucoma and its relationship with visual function. *J Glaucoma.* 2003;12:139–150.

Ornek K, Ozdemir M. Central corneal thickness in tilted disc syndrome. *Optom Vis Sci.* 2008;85(5):E350-2.

Orzalesi N, Rossetti L, Omboni S, OPTIME Study Group (Osservatorio sulla Patologia glaucomatosa, Indagine Medico Epidemiologica), CONPROSO (Collegio Nazionale dei Professori Ordinari di Scienze Oftalmologiche). Vascular risk factors in glaucoma: the results of a national survey. *Graefes Arch Clin Exp Ophthalmol* 2007;245:795– 802.

Pallikaris IG, Kymionis GD, Ginis HS, et al. Ocular rigidity in patients with age-related macular degeneration. *Am J Ophthalmol* 2006;141:611-5.

Pan C-W, Boey PY, Cheng C-Y, Saw S-M, Tay TW, Wang JJ, Tan AG, Mitchell P, Wong TY. Myopia, Axial Length, and Age-Related Cataract: The Singapore Malay Eye Study. *Invest Ophthalmol Vis Sci* 2013;54:4498–4502. DOI:10.1167/iovs.13-1227

Pan CW, Cheung CY, Aung T, Cheung CM, Zheng YF, Wu RY, Mitchell P, Lavanya R, Baskaran M, Wang JJ, Wong TY, Saw SM. Differential Associations of Myopia with Major Age-related Eye Diseases. The Singapore Indian Eye Study. *Ophthalmology* 2013;120:284–291.

Pan C-W, Ramamurthy D, Saw S-M. Worldwide prevalence and risk factors for myopia. *Ophthalmic Physiol Opt.* 2012;32:3–16.

Panchapakesan J, Rochtchina E, Mitchell P. Myopic refractive shift caused by incident cataract: the Blue Mountains Eye Study. *Ophthalmic Epidemiol.* 2003;10:241–247.

Parulekar MV, Elston JS: Acquired retinal myelination in neurofibromatosis. *Arch Ophthalmol* 2002;120:659-61.

Pasquale LR, Kang JH. Lifestyle, nutrition, and glaucoma. *J Glaucoma.* 2009;18:423–428.

Perera SA, Aung T. Myopia and glaucoma. In: Beuerman R, Mei SS, Tan DT, eds. Myopia: Animal Models to Clinical Trials. Singapore: *World Scientific;* 2010:121–133.

Perera SA, Wong TY, Tay WT, et al. Refractive error, axial dimensions, and primary open-angle glaucoma: the Singapore Malay Eye Study. *Arch Ophthalmol* 2010;128:900 -5.

Perera SA, Wong TY, Tay W-T, Foster PJ, Saw S-M, Aung T. Refractive error, axial dimensions, and primary open-angle glaucoma: the Singapore Malay Eye Study. *Arch Ophthalmol.* 2013;128:900–905.

Perkins ES, Phelps CD. Open angle glaucoma, ocular hypertension, low-tension glaucoma, and refraction. *Arch Ophthalmol.* 1982;100:1464–1467.

Phelps CD. Effect of myopia on prognosis in treated primary open-angle glaucoma. *Am J Ophthalmol.* 1982;93:622–628.

Podos SM, Becker B, Morton WR. High myopia and primary open-angle glaucoma. *Am J Ophthalmol.* 1966;62:1038–1043.

Ponte F, Giuffré G, Giammanco R, Dardanoni G. Risk factors of ocular hypertension and glaucoma: the Casteldaccia Eye Study. *Doc Ophthalmol* 1994;85:203–10.

Qiu M, Wang SY, Singh K, Lin SC. Association between Myopia and Glaucoma in the United States Population. *Invest Ophthalmol Vis Sci* 2013;54:830–835.DOI:10.1167/iovs.12-11158.

Quigley HA, Broman AT. The number of people with glaucoma worldwide in 2010 and 2020. *Br J Ophthalmol.* 2006;90:262–267.

Quigley HA, West SK, Rodriguez J, et al. The prevalence of glaucoma in a population-based study of Hispanic subjects: Proyecto VER. *Arch Ophthalmol* 2001;119:1819 -26.

Quigley HA. Open-angle glaucoma. *N Engl J Med* 1993;328: 1097-106.

Quigley M, Cohen S. A new pressure attenuation index to evaluate retinal circulation. A link to protective factors in diabetic retinopathy. *Arch Ophthalmol* 1999;117:84 –9.

Quigley M. Myopia and diabetic retinopathy [letter]. *Ophthalmology* 2010;117:2040.

Ramakrishnan R, Nirmalan PK, Krishnadas R, et al. Glaucoma in a rural population of southern India: the Aravind comprehensive eye survey. *Ophthalmology.* 2003;110:1484–1490.

Raviola E, Wiesel TN: Effect of dark-rearing on experimental myopia in monkeys. *Invest Ophthalmol Vis Sci* 1978;17:485-8.

Resnikoff S, Pascolini D, Etya'ale D, et al. Global data on visual impairment in the year 2002. *Bull World Health Organ* 2004;82:844 –51.

Rosen B, Barry C, Constable IJ: Progression of myelinated retinal nerve fibers. *Am J Ophthalmol* 1999;127:471-3.

Sacca SC, Bolognesi C, Battistella A, Bagnis A, Izzotti A. Geneenvironment interactions in ocular diseases. *Mutat Res.* 2009; 667:98–117.

Sandhu RK, Munoz BE, Swenor BK, West SK. Refractive error and visual function difficulty in a Latino population. *Ophthalmology* 2012;119:1731-1736.

Saw SM, Chan YH, Wong WL, et al. Prevalence and risk factors for refractive errors in the Singapore Malay Eye Survey. *Ophthalmology.* 2008;115:1713–1719.

Saw S-M, Gazzard G, Shih-Yen EC, Chua W-H. Myopia and associated pathological complications. *Ophthalmic Physiol Opt.* 2005;25:381–391.

Schachat AP, Miller NR: Atrophy of myelinated retinal nerve fibers after acute optic neuropathy. *Am J Ophthalmol* 1981; 92: 854-6.

Scott R, Grosvenor T. Structural model for emmetropic and myopic eyes. *Ophthalmic Physiol Opt* 1993;13:41–7.

Sharpe JA, Sanders MD: Atrophy of myelinated nerve fibres in the retina in optic neuritis. *Br J Ophthalmol* 1975;59:229-32.

Silvestri G, Sehmi K, Hamilton P: Retinal vascular abnormalities. A rare complication of myelinated nerve fibers? *Retina* 1996;16:214-8.

Sperduto RD, Seigel D, Roberts J, et al. Prevalence of myopia in the United States. *Arch Ophthalmol.* 1983; 101(3):405-7.

Straatsma BR, Foos BY, Heckenlively JR, Taylor GN: Myelinated retinal nerve fibers. *Am J Ophthalmol* 1981;91:25- 38.

Straatsma BR, Heckenlively JR, Foos RY, Shahinian JK: Myelinated retinal nerve fibers associated with ipsilateral myopia, amblyopia, and strabismus. *Am J Ophthalmol* 1979; 88: 506-10.

Strömberg E. On axial length and refraction of the human eye [in German]. *Acta Ophthalmol* (Copenh) 1936;14:281–97.

Suzuki Y, Iwase A, Araie M, et al., Tajimi Study Group. Risk factors for open-angle glaucoma in a Japanese population: the Tajimi Study. *Ophthalmology* 2006;113:1613–7.

Suzuki Y, Iwase A, Araie M, et al. Risk factors for open-angle glaucoma in a Japanese population: the Tajimi Study. *Ophthalmology* 2006;113:1613-1617.

Tarabishy AB, Alexandrou TJ, Traboulsi EI. Syndrome of myelinated retinal nerve fibers, myopia, and amblyopia : a review. *Surv Ophthalmol* 2007; 52:588-596.

Tay E, Seah SK, Chan SP, et al. Optic disk ovality as an index of tilt and its relationship to myopia and perimetry. *Am J Ophthalmol.* 2005;139(2):247-52.

Teich SA: Disappearance of myelinated retinal nerve fibers after a branch retinal artery occlusion. *Am J Ophthalmol* 1987; 103:835-7.

Thulasiraj RD, Nirmalan PK, Ramakrishnan R, et al. Blindness and vision impairment in a rural south Indian population: the Aravind Comprehensive Eye Survey. *Ophthalmology.* 2003; 110:1491–1498.

Tielsch JM, Sommer A, Katz J, et al. Racial variations in the prevalence of primary open angle glaucoma: the Baltimore Eye Survey. *JAMA.* 1991;266:369–374.

Traboulsi EI, Lim JI, Pyeritz R, et al: A new syndrome of myelinated nerve fibers, vitreoretinopathy, and skeletal malformations. *Arch Ophthalmol* 1993; 111:1543-5.

Varma R, Lee PP, Goldberg I, Kotak S. An assessment of the health and economic burdens of glaucoma. *Am J Ophthalmol.* 2011;152:515–522.

Varma R, Ying-Lai M, Francis BA, et al. Prevalence of open-angle glaucoma and ocular hypertension in Latinos. The Los Angeles Latino Eye Study. *Ophthalmology* 2004;111: 1439-48.

Varma R, Ying-Lai M, Klein R, Azen SP. Prevalence and risk indicators of visual impairment and blindness in Latinos: the Los Angeles Latino Eye Study. *Ophthalmology.* 2004;111: 1132–1140.

Virchow VR: Zur pathologischen anatomic der netzaut und des scherven. *Virchows Arch Pathol Anat* 1856;10:170-93.

Vitale S, Sperduto RD, Ferris FL III. Increased prevalence of myopia in the United States between 1971–1972 and 1999–2004. *Arch Ophthalmol.* 2009;127:1632–1639.

Vongphanit J, Mitchell P, Wang JJ. Population prevalence of tilted optic disks and the relationship of this sign to refractive error. *Am J Ophthalmol.* 2002;133(5): 679-85.

Vuori M-L, M¨antyj¨arvi M. Tilted disc syndrome may mimic false visual field deterioration. *Acta Ophthalmol.* 2008;86:622–625.

Wallman J, Turkel J: Extreme myopia produced by modest change in early visual experience. *Science* 1978;201:1249-51.

Wang JJ, Jakobsen KB, Smith W, Mitchell P. Refractive status and the 5-year incidence of age-related maculopathy: the Blue Mountains Eye Study. *Clin Experiment Ophthalmol* 2004;32: 255-8.

Wang JJ, Mitchell P, Smith W. Refractive error and agerelated maculopathy: the Blue Mountains Eye Study. *Invest Ophthalmol Vis Sci* 1998;39:2167-71.

Weale RA. Epidemiology of refractive errors and presbyopia. *Surv Ophthalmol.* 2003;48(5):515-43.

Wensor M, McCarty CA, Taylor HR. Prevalence and risk factors of myopia in Victoria, Australia. *Arch Ophthalmol.* 1999;117: 658–663.

Witmer MT, Margo CE, Drucker M. Tilted optic disks. *Surv Ophthalmol.* 2010;55:403–428. [Epub July 10, 2010].

Wong TY, Foster PJ, Hee J, et al. Prevalence and risk factors for refractive errors in adult Chinese in Singapore. *Invest Ophthalmol Vis Sci.* 2000;41:2486–2494.

Wong TY, Foster PJ, Johnson GJ, Seah SK. Refractive errors, axial ocular dimensions, and age-related cataracts: the Tanjong Pagar survey. *Invest Ophthalmol Vis Sci.* 2003;44:1479–1485.

Wong TY, Klein BE, Klein R, et al. Refractive errors and incident cataracts: the Beaver Dam Eye Study. *Invest Ophthalmol Vis Sci* 2001;42:1449 -54.

Wong TY, Klein BE, Klein R, et al. Refractive errors, intraocular pressure, and glaucoma in a white population. *Ophthalmology* 2003;110:211-217.

Wong TY, Klein BE, Klein R, Tomany SC, Lee KE. Refractive errors and incident cataracts: the Beaver Dam Eye Study. *Invest Ophthalmol Vis Sci.* 2001;42:1449–1454.

Wong TY, Klein BEK, Klein R, Knudtson M, Lee KE. Refractive errors, intraocular pressure, and glaucoma in a white population. *Ophthalmology.* 1995;110:211–217.

Wong TY, Klein R, Klein BE, Tomany SC. Refractive errors and 10-year incidence of age-related maculopathy. *Invest Ophthalmol Vis Sci* 2002;43:2869 -73.

Wu SY, Nemesure B, Leske MC. Refractive errors in a Black adult population: the Barbados Eye Study. *Invest Ophthalmol Vis Sci.* 1999;40:2179–2184.

You QS, Xu L, Jonas JB. Tilted optic discs: the Beijing Eye Study. *Eye.* 2008;22:728–729.

Younan C, Mitchell P, Cumming RG, Rochtchina E, Wang JJ. Myopia and incident cataract and cataract surgery: the Blue Mountains Eye Study. *Invest Ophthalmol Vis Sci.* 2002;43: 3625–3632.

Zhao J, Ellwein LB, Cui H, et al. Prevalence of vision impairment in older adults in rural China: the China Nine-Province Survey. *Ophthalmology.* 2010;117:409–416.

Zheng Y, Lavanya R, Wu R, et al. Prevalence and causes of visual impairment and blindness in an urban Indian population: the Singapore Indian Eye Study. *Ophthalmology.* 2011; 118:1798–1804.

Zweng HC, Little HL, Peabody RR: Further observations on argon laser photocoagulation of diabetic retinopathy. *Trans Am Acad Ophthalmol Otolaryngol* 1972; 76:990-1004.

Chapter X

Pathologic Complications Associated with Increasing Myopia

Abstract

Myopia is associated with a number of ocular pathologic complications, which usually occur in patients with a higher degree of myopia, also termed "pathologic myopia,""degenerative myopia," and "malignant myopia."

Most pathologic complications are assumed to be related to increased axial length. Most researchers have considered high myopia to describe refractive errors in excess of -6.00 D although some have considered refractive errors higher than -8.00 to be of more significance.

Pathologic complications associated with high myopia are common. Most studies to date have concentrated on the adult population, while specific studies looking at the impact of myopia on children are not common. Published studies suggest that pathologic complications associated with myopia are less common in children, suggesting that prolonged mechanical stretching of the ocular structures and/or aging has an impact on the presence of complications (Kobayashi et al., 2005). It has been suggested that only 8% of children in the United Kingdom presenting with high myopia (greater than -6 D) have simple myopia with no systemic or ocular complications. Indeed 38% demonstrated ocular complications with no other systemic association (Marr et al., 2001).

This chapter describes ocular pathologic complications that can be found in myopia.

1. Fundus Changes, Myopic Retinopathy

Definition

Myopic retinopathy describes changes to the retina that can be attributed to the presence of myopia. Central retinal changes occurring in macular region are given the term myopic maculopathy. Peripheral retinal changes include lattice and paving stone degeneration, retinal tears and pigmentary degenerations. Myopic retinopathy is characterized by changes in the macular region, including staphylomata, lacquer cracks, Fuchs' spot, chorioretinal atrophy, and secondary defects in Bruch's membrane (Curtin, 1977; Klein and Curtin, 1975; Steidl and

Pruett, 1997; Vongphant et al., 2002). Myopic retinopathy could be defined as the presence of at least one of the following lesions according to the classification by Hayashi et al. (Hayashi et al., 2010): diffuse chorioretinal atrophy at the posterior pole, patchy chorioretinal atrophy, lacquer cracks, or macular atrophy (Asakuma et al., 2012). It has been documented that increasing amounts of myopia lead to a higher prevalence of myopic retinopathy (Vongphanit et al.,2002). It has been recognized as one of the leading causes of irreversible visual impairment and blindness worldwide. It was the second most common cause of low vision and blindness in the Handan Eye Study and Beijing Eye Study in mainland China and in the Shihpai Eye Study in Taiwan, and the second most common cause of blindness and third most common cause of low vision in the Tajimi Study in Japan (Xu et al., 2006; Liang et al., 2008; Hsu et al., 2004; Iwase et al., 2006). In white populations in Western countries and in Hispanics, myopic retinopathy was the second to fourth most frequent cause of blindness (Klaver et al., 1988; Cedrone et al., 2003; Buch et al., 2004; Cotter et al., 2006).

2. Myopic Maculopathy

Myopic maculopathy describes a spectrum of clinical changes that comprise the main cause of visual loss among highly myopic individuals (Zambarakji et al., 2011). Typical events that are associated with myopia include lacquer cracks, chorioretinal atrophy, macular atrophy, and choroidal neovascularization. Patients who exhibit signs of myopic maculopathy demonstrate a significant reduction in acuity over a period of time compared with equivalent myopic patients without myopathy. A 10-year study found that over 50% of Taiwanese people over the age of 40 with myopic maculopathy exhibited a 2 or more line decrease in acuity over a 10-year period compared with 3% of subjects without maculopathy (Shih et al., 2006). In an adult Chinese myopic population, it was found that almost 90% of eyes with a refractive error of -10.00 D or greater demonstrated myopic maculopathy compared with less than 4% in patients with prescriptions under -4.00 D (Liu et al., 2010). This finding confirms that the prevalence of retinopathy increases significantly with increasing myopic error.

The Beijing Eye Study 2011 (You et al., 2014) included 3468 subjects with an age of 50 years or more and examined the features of myopia-related optical coherence tomography (OCT) findings in a population-based setting. The frequency of OCT abnormalities in the macular region of highly myopic eyes, defined as a myopic refractive error of more than - 6 diopters (D) or an axial length of more than 26.5 mm, and examined their associations with other ocular and systemic parameters. The most common change in the macula was a maculoschisis, found in 54 eyes (0.8% of the entire study population), followed by an incomplete posterior vitreous detachment in 46 eyes (0.7%), disruption of the photoreceptor inner segment/outer segment interface in 39 eyes (0.6%), epiretinal membranes in 38 eyes (0.6%), macular defects in Bruch's membrane in 24 eyes (0.3%), clumping of the retinal pigment epithelium in 11 eyes (0.2%), vitreofoveal adhesion in 10 eyes (0.2%), and macular holes in 2 eyes (0.1%;). Prevalence of any myopic maculopathy per eye was 112 cases in 6530 eyes, or 1.71±0.16% (95% CI,1.40-2.03). Within the highly myopic group, the prevalence of any maculopathy per eye was 112 cases in 164 eyes, or 68.3±3.6 cases (95% CI, 61.5-75.9), with the highest prevalences for maculoschisis (32.9%), incomplete posterior vitreous detachment (28.0%), and disruption of the photoreceptor inner segment/outer segment interface (23.8%). In binary regression analysis, presence of any myopic maculopathy was associated significantly with longer axial length ($P<0.001$) and more myopic refractive error ($P = 0.001$). After adjustment for axial length and refractive error, it was statistically independent of age, sex, body height, weight, body mass index, arterial blood pressure, diabetes mellitus, biochemical blood examination results, central corneal thickness, ocular biometric measures (except axial length), subfoveal choroidal thickness, retinal vein occlusion, and intraocular pressure. The most important macular changes with a negative effect on best-corrected visual acuity were a disruption of the photoreceptor inner segment/outer segment interface and epiretinal membranes (You et al., 2014). Similar findings were found in previous investigations in which the same morphologic elements of myopic maculopathy were described (Ohno-Matsu et al., 2012; Maruko et al., 2012; Ohno-Matsui et al., 2012; Leveziel et al., 2013; Wang et al., 2013). The results of the Beijing Eye Study 2011 (You et al., 2014) also confirmed a histologic study in which macular defects of Bruch's membrane were reported (Jonas et al., 2013). In that investigation, the regions with macular Bruch's membrane defects were free of retinal pigment epithelium cells and choriocapillaris, with the photoreceptor layer markedly diminished or rudimentary and the remaining choroid containing only few large choroidal vessels. The globe in these regions consisted of a markedly thinned sclera, some melanin-bearing cells on the inner surface of the sclera (lamina fusca sclerae), and remnants of the middle and inner layers of the retina. As in the study by You et al. (You et al., 2013), the presence of a macular Bruch's membrane defect was associated strongly with axial length. The macular Bruch's membrane defect in the highly myopic macula may be regarded as a second hole in Bruch's membrane, which has a primary or physiologic hole in the region of the optic nerve head.

The macular Bruch's membrane defect as described in the Beijing Eye Study 2011 (You et al., 2014) and in the histologic study may be added to the panoply of the features of myopic retinopathy. As recently pointed out, these include the myopic Fuchs' spot; scleral staphylomata and lacquer cracks in the macular region, beta zone, and alpha zone of the parapapillary region; a secondarily enlarged macrodisc; and a marked stretching and thinning of the lamina cribrosa in association with increased susceptibility for glaucomatous optic neuropathy (Jonas et al., 2013). The marked changes in Bruch's membrane in the highly myopic eyes show the involvement of the choroid in the development of high myopia. Because choroidal thickness as the distance between Bruch's membrane and the sclera decreases with increasing myopia, one may postulate that the changes in Bruch's membrane are more marked than the changes in the sclera because otherwise the distance between the sclera and Bruch's membrane would have enlarged (You et al., 2014). It theoretically could point to an active role of the growth and elongation of Bruch's membrane in the process of emmetropization and development of myopia, as was discussed recently (Jonas et al., 2013).

3. Choroidal Neovascularization

Choroidal neovascularization (CNV) is a common complication of high myopia and has a devastating impact on visual acuity. It has been shown that approximately 10% of patients with myopic macular fundus changes will progress to choroidal neovascularization. Patients with choroidal neovascularization have a poor visual prognosis (Hayashi et al., 2010).

Patients with a refractive error of at least -8.00 D were followed for a 10-year period and most showed a drop in visual acuity to 20/200 or less within a 5- to 10-year period after the onset of choroidal neovascularization (Yoshida et al., 2003).

Clinical Findings in Myopic CNV (Silva, 2012)

The biomicroscopic findings of CNV associated with high myopia typically show a small (< 1 disk area), flat, grayish subretinal membrane with hyperpigmented borders. These membranes are typically less than 1,000 μm in diameter (Hampton et al., 1983). They are located in the subretinal space, as opposed to the sub-RPE space in age-related macular degeneration (AMD) and subretinal or sub-RPE fluid, hemorrhage or exudates are uncommon (Gass, 1997). The location of CNV was reported to be subfoveal in 58% of the cases, juxtafoveal in 23% and extrafoveal in 19% (Hampton et al., 1983).

Fluorescein angiography (FA) and ICG angiography are both useful for studying degenerative changes associated with myopic CNV. In all randomized clinical trials for evaluating whether any therapy is indicated for CNV due to pathological myopia almost 90% of myopic CNV demonstrates mild hyperfluorescence confined to the early phase of the fluorescein angiography. Most membranes will hyperfluoresce in the transit phase, but contrasting with AMD, only a minimal leakage beyond the borders of the lesion is observed in the late phases (Soubrane, 2008).

Some membranes may be inactive and stain only in the late frames. Avila et al. (Avila et al., 1984) found that less than 10% of myopic CNV leak beyond the borders in the late phases. This finding was associated with worse prognosis. The visualization of myopic CNV may be complicated by several factors, including reduced leakage, presence of staining associated with lacquer cracks, and subretinal hemorrhage (Soubrane, 2008). ICG angiography may better identify the CNV as a faint hyperfluorescence spot or area often surrounded by a hypopigmented halo. ICG also allows a better definition of lacquer cracks than FA (Brancato et al., 1996; Ohno-Matssui et al., 1998). This was confirmed by Axer-Siegel et al. (Axer-Siegel et al., 2004) showing that ICG angiography was able to identify lacquer cracks in 89% of eyes with pathological myopia, compared with 28% using FA. ICG may also allow a more precise CNV localization and feeder vessel detection (Ohno-Matsui et al., 1998; Axer-Siegel et al., 2004; Liu et al., 2004). Both FA and ICG angiography may complement the study of myopic CNV allied to optical coherent tomography (OCT). OCT appears to be useful in evaluating the stage and activity of myopic CNV. Baba et al. (Baba et al., 2002) described the morphological changes in different stages. In the active stage, time domain OCT clearly displayed a neovascular membrane as a highly reflective dome-like elevation above the RPE with no apparent subretinal fluid accumulation around the CNV. In the scar stage, only the surface of the CNV showed high reflectivity, which was markedly attenuated below the surface. In the atrophic stage the CNV became totally flat and chorioretinal atrophy around the regressed CNV showed high reflectivity (Baba et al., 2002). OCT can provide supplementary information while making treatment decisions by demonstrating various stages and activities of myopic CNV (Baba et al., 2002). SD-OCT is a powerful modality for investigating the retinal/choroidal structure of highly myopic eyes (Sayanagi et al., 2008). It is extremely useful for evaluating the CNV but also associated features like posterior staphyloma, retinoschisis, thinned choroid, posterior vitreous detachment, macular atrophy, macular hemorrhage, retinal traction or macular hole formation. A thinned choroid is a common feature in highly myopic eyes. It was described in histological studies (Grossniklaus and Green, 1992) and in animal models of myopia (Hirata and Negi, 1998). 'In vivo' studies using ICG angiography (Quaranta et al., 1996; Moriyama et al., 2007) and color Doppler ultrasonography (Akyol et al., 1996) also have shown that choroidal circulation is decreased in myopic eyes. But a thinned choroid was also described using SD-OCT (Ikuno and Tano, 2009).

Myopic CNV appears in SD-OCT as a type 2 (subretinal) neovascular membrane associated with a very thin choroid (Vance et al., 2011). A method called 'enhanced depth imaging' SD-OCT has been developed that enables in vivo cross-sectional imaging of the choroid (Spaide et al., 2008). Using this method, choroidal thickness was studied in normal eyes and was shown to be thickest underneath the fovea and to be inversely proportional to age (Margolis and Spaide, 2009). The enhanced depth imaging SD-OCT has demonstrated that the choroid in highly myopic eyes is very thin and undergoes further thinning with increasing age and degree of myopia (Fujiwara et al., 2009). The chorioretinal atrophy adjacent to a myopic CNV can be well documented with SD-OCT. It increases the risk of developing a macular hole, and a periodic OCT is recommended (Shimada et al., 2006). Choroidal thinning seems to be a hallmark of high myopia. Ikuno et al. (Ikuno et al., 2010) found that choroidal thinning is more prominent in eyes with myopic CNV when compared with myopic eyes without CNV. It is unknown how choroidal thinning is associated with the development of myopic CNV. One mechanism is that the choroidal vessels supply retinal oxygen to the outer retina. The outer retina is believed to be a major source of VEGF, and the choroidal thinning at the fovea may lead to outer retinal hypoxic changes via factors such as hypoxia-inducible factor, resulting in VEGF secretion at the fovea (Ikuno et al., 2010).

SD-OCT is also recommended for the evaluation of posterior staphyloma. Ikuno et al. (Ikuno et al., 2010) reported that the absolute value of the nasal posterior staphyloma height from the fovea was significantly greater in eyes with myopic CNV than in myopic eyes without CNV.

4. Peripheral Retinal Complications

Peripheral retinal complications are often present in myopic patients and have been shown to increase with higher levels of myopia in adults and children (Lai et al., 2008; Bansal, 2010).

Lattice degeneration is one of the most common findings, which has been reported to occur in up to 33% of eyes with high myopia (>- 6.00 D) (Lai et al., 2008; Celorio et al., 1991). Children aged 10 years and younger with high myopia (>- 6.00 D) have been shown to exhibit lattice degeneration and other peripheral retinal lesions. The incidence rates seem to be similar to the adult population (Bansal et al., 2010).

It has been demonstrated that lattice degeneration is more prevalent in eyes that have an overall increase in axial length rather than just a posterior increase in axial length (posterior staphyloma), thereby demonstrating that the type of axial elongation can in fluence the retinal complications that are present (Yura, 1998).

5. Retinal Detachment

Myopia has been cited as the principal risk factor for retinal detachment in the pediatric population, with increasing amounts of myopia leading to increased risk of detachment, as in the adult population (Wang et al., 2009; Wang et al., 2005; Mitry et al., 2010; Austin et al., 1990). It has been suggested that a refractive error range of - 1.00 to - 3.00 D results in a 4 times increased risk of retinal detachment compared with that of a nonmyopic eye, whereas a refractive error over - 3.00 D results in an almost 10 times greater risk (The Eye Disease Case-Control Study Group, 1993). This increased risk with increasing refractive error has been quoted as an odds ratio of 1.33 times per diopter of myopia in the adult Taiwanese population (Chou et al., 2007).

Retinal detachment is often a secondary complication of a macular hole. Macular holes in themselves can be devastating to visual acuity. Patients who have macular holes and are highly myopic have a high risk of retinal detachment. The incidence of macular holes in patients without myopia has been found to be close to 1% as opposed to almost 98% in patients with high myopia (Morita et al., 1991; Akiba et al., 1999).

6. Posterior Staphyloma

A posterior staphyloma is a protrusion of the posterior shell of the eye globe that frequently is found in highly myopic eyes and is considered to be a hallmark lesion of high myopia; it is present in up to 90% of the population with myopia over -8.00 D (Hsiang et al., 2008). The prevalence is known to increase with increasing axial length and therefore (by definition) increasing myopia. Prevalence also increases with advancing age. An eye with a posterior staphyloma is more at risk of developing other myopic lesions such as macular holes, choroidal neovascularization, and chorioretinal atrophy (Curtin and Karlin, 1970; Curtin, 1977). The scleral shell of highly myopic eyes has increased elasticity and a tendency to expand gradually and to thin. The collagen fibers in these eyes are pathologic (Curtin and Teng, 1958; Curtin et al., 1979); the fibers are smaller in diameter, appear histologically immature, and may have fewer cross-linkages than those in emmetropic eyes (McBrien and Norton, 1994).

The development of a posterior staphyloma is accompanied by a stretching of the posterior fundus, resulting in various kinds of myopic lesions, for example, chorioretinal atrophy, choroidal neovascularization (CNV), macular retinoschisis, and macular holes. It is known that highly myopic eyes with a posterior staphyloma have a higher probability of having visual disturbances (Pruett, 1998). The most detailed study of posterior staphyloma was probably that carried out by Curtin 30 years ago (Curtin, 1977).

The posterior staphylomas are classified into different types and different grades. The type of posterior staphyloma is determined by the location, size, and severity (Curtin, 1977) and is classified by binocular stereoscopic ophthalmoscopy. The staphylomas are classified into 10 types: types I through V are primary staphylomas, and types IV through X are compound staphylomas (Curtin, 1977). The grade of the posterior staphyloma is determined from the B-scan and A-scan ultrasonographic images based on the criteria of Steidl and Pruett (Steidl and Pruett, 1997). The staphylomas are graded from zero to four based on the depth of the staphyloma measured on A-scan and B-scan ultrasonographic images obtained by Ultrascan. The depth of the staphyloma is measured on a horizontal B-scan image across the optic nerve head as the distance from the inner surface of the optic nerve head to the deepest part of the staphyloma. To ensure that the B-scan passes through the deepest part of the staphyloma, B scans are performed until five well-defined images are obtained from each eye. Because the variance of the depth of the staphyloma of each eye is small, the average distance from the optic nerve head to the deepest part of the staphyloma is selected for the grading. An elongated eye with a smooth scleral contour is graded as zero. A grade 1 staphyloma has a depth of 2 mm or less, a grade 2 staphyloma has a depth of more than 2 mm but less than 4 mm, a grade 3 staphyloma has a depth of more than 4 mm but less than 6 mm, and a grade 4 staphyloma has a depth of more than 6 mm.

The degree of myopic chorioretinal changes is categorized according to the criteria of Avila and associates (Avila et al., 1984). The myopic fundus changes (M) are graded on a scale of increasing severity from zero to five: grade M0, normal-appearing posterior pole; grade M1, choroidal pallor and tessellation; grade M2, choroidal pallor and tessellation, with posterior staphyloma; grade M3, choroidal pallor and tessellation, with posterior staphyloma and lacquer cracks; grade M4, choroidal pallor and tessellation, with posterior staphyloma, lacquer cracks, and focal areas of deep choroidal atrophy; and grade M5, posterior pole with large geographic areas of deep choroidal atrophy (so-called bare sclera).

Although there is no agreed clinical grading for myopic maculopathy, several authors have used a practical classification originally devised by Avila et al. to describe the natural history (Shih et al., 2006; Avila et al., 1984). With this method, a scale of increasing severity from 0 to 5 is used to describe the maculopathy as follows: M0: normal appearing posterior pole, M1: tessellation and choroidal pallor pattern in macular area, M2: M1 and a posterior pole ectasia, M3: M2 and lacquer cracks in Bruch's membrane and posterior staphyloma, M4: M3 and focal areas of deep choroidal atrophy, and M5: M4 and geographic areas of atrophy and choroidal neovascularisation (CNV). Recent studies have suggested modifications to this classification: Hayashi et al. conducted a comprehensive natural history study of myopic maculopathy, and indicated that lacquer cracks should be classified as an independent lesion, due to the likelihood of progression to CNV as well as diffuse atrophy. The authors also highlight the presence of a posterior staphyloma as an important factor leading to the progression of maculopathy (Hayashi et al., 2010). In the Blue Mountains Eye Study, myopic retinopathy was defined to include: staphyloma, lacquer cracks, Fuchs' spot and myopic chorioretinal thinning or atrophy (Vongphanit et al., 2002).

Higher grades of staphyloma are associated with more severe myopic retinal degeneration (Curtin and Karlin, 1971; Stiedl and Pruett, 1997). Curtin and Karlin also reported a strong correlation between axial length and myopic chorioretinal atrophy, although the correlation between the myopic chorioretinopathy and posterior staphyloma was not reported (Curtin and Karlin, 1971).

7. Myopic Macular Schisis

With the advent of OCT, it is now possible to evaluate vitreoretinal disorders of the macula in highly myopic eyes (Coppé and Ripandelli, 2003). One of these is the phenomenon of retinal splitting or schisis that not uncommonly occurs in highly myopic eyes with posterior staphylomas (Baba et al., 2003; Benhamou et al., 2002; Takano and Kishi, 1999). Schisis can rarely have a stellate foveal appearance (Menchini et al., 2000), but more commonly it is difficult to discern biomicroscopically (Baba et al., 2003). Benhamou et al. described the OCT characteristics and evolution of macular retinoschisis in high myopia. This retrospective observational study evaluated 21 high myopes with an average refraction of -15.2 D who presented with macular thickening but without macular hole, in the setting of a staphyloma. The authors described two patterns of schisis. In outer schisis, the retina is split into a thick inner layer and thin outer layer by a wide hyporeflective space. In some cases linear bridging elements were seen traversing the hyporeflective space. In eyes with inner schisis, the splitting of the retina divides a thin inner layer from a thick outer layer. Most eyes demonstrated predominantly outer schisis, with variable components of inner schisis, macular detachment, and lamellar or full-thickness macular hole formation. In four of the 21 patients, the perifoveal posterior hyaloid was seen to be detached with residual vitreomacular adhesion causing traction (Mirza et al., 2007).

Three of these eyes underwent vitrectomy. The vision did not improve in two of these. The third case evolved into a FTMH following surgery. The remaining eye was observed and went on to develop a FTMH. Overall, the authors found schisis to be a fairly stable condition with slow progression. They concluded that vitreomacular traction may lead to FTMH formation (Benhamou et al., 2002; Matsumura et al., 2004). A small percent of highly myopic eyes may develop FTMH asymptomatically. These correlate with the presence of epiretinal tissue, younger age, and degree of myopia (Coppé et al., 2005). In a more recent study, Panozzo and Mercanti conducted an observational case series on 218 eyes with high myopia in order to determine the role of epiretinal traction in myopic maculopathy defined as: schisis, retinal thickening, lamellar macular hole, and posterior neurosensory retinal detachment (Panozzo and Mercanti, 2004). The degree of myopia ranged from -8 to -26 D with a mean axial length of 29.75 mm. Subjects were excluded if they were found to have confounding factors such as other pathologic conditions, active choroidal neovascularization, or diffuse detachment visible on biomicroscopy. A total of 125 eyes were then further analyzed for presence of ERM, VMT, or both ERM and VMT. Traction was found in 46.4% of these eyes. ERM was seen in 24.8%. Retinal damage as defined herein was present in 34.4%. The most frequent form of damage found (20%) was retinoschisis alone or in combination with other lesions. Staphyloma was found in 42.4% of all eyes. When eyes with staphylomas were analyzed further, 16.2% had some form of retinal damage. In contrast, when staphyloma was combined with traction, 83.7% had retinal damage. For this reason, the authors coin the term myopic traction maculopathy (MTM) (Panozzo and Mercanti, 2004) to unify those pathologic features associated with traction in the myopic environment. The authors also discussed the theoretical benefit of vitrectomy and membrane peeling, given the contributing role of traction in the pathogenesis of retinal damage including schisis. Although the precise nature of the traction and its pathogenic importance in this disorder are not completely understood, several reports have documented resolution of myopic schisis following vitrectomy and removal of posterior cortical vitreous with or without internal limiting membrane peeling (Akiba et al., 2000; Hirakata and Hida, 2006; Ichibe et al., 2003; Ikuno et al., 2003; Kobayashi and kishi, 2003; Ratiglia et al., 2005; Ripandelli et al., 2004; Sayanagi et al., 2006). Ikuno and colleagues noted retinal microfolds in eyes with myopic foveoschisis and related this event to insufficient flexibility of sclerotic retinal arterioles during axial length elongation in highly myopic eyes (Ikuno et al., 2005). It was postulated that an inward tractional force on the retina along the arterioles may be related to the pathogenesis of myopic vitreoretinal diseases including retinoschisis and macular hole formation (Ikuno et al., 2005; Sayanagi et al., 2005).

8. Myopic Traction Maculopathy (MTM) (Ouyang, 2012)

The combination of the recent achievements and the broad application of optical coherence tomography (OCT) and vitrectomy has resulted in the conception and classification of myopic traction maculopathy (MTM) (Ouyang, 2012).

In 1999, Takano and Kishi (Takano and Kishi, 1999) identified foveal retinoschisis and retinal detachment without retinal holes in severely myopic eyes by OCT. Others also described similar pathological features of high myopia maculopathy (Benhamou et al., 2002). In 2004, Panozzo and Mercanti(Panozzo and Mercanti, 2007) retrospectively reviewed their medical records and OCT findings for 125 eyes with high myopia. They found cpiretinal traction in 58 eyes (46.4%) and retinal damage in 43 eyes (34.4%), of which 36 had epiretinal traction (83.7%). They were the first to use the term 'myopic traction maculopathy' to refer to these pathologies of the posterior pole in high myopia, such as macular retinoschisis, shallow retinal detachment without retinal holes, lamellar macular holes, and macular holes with or without retinal detachment. Distinguishing these conditions from epiretinal traction syndromes found in eyes without myopia was an important advancement because their distinct features have significantly different clinical effects on retinal tissue and visual function.

In 2007, Panozzo and Mercanti (Panozzo and Mercanti, 2007) suggested that the term 'retinoschisis' used in the literature for high myopic maculopathy was not appropriate as the terms inner or outer retinal schisis suggested a complete separation between the retinal layers that resulted in the irreversible and total loss of retinal function. Since all of the previously published case series of foveal retinoschisis reported good visual improvement without fixed scotoma, this retinal damage is not a schisis but rather due to retinal swelling with the accumulation of fluid. Smiddy (Smiddy et al., 2009) supported this notion and suggested that myopic maculoschisis, foveal schisis, and vitreoschisis in high myopia should all fall under the family of MTM. effects on retinal tissue and visual function

In 2007, Panozzo and Mercanti (Panozzo and Mercanti, 2007) suggested that the term 'retinoschisis' used in the literature for high myopic maculopathy was not appropriate as the terms inner or outer retinal schisis suggested a complete separation between the retinal layers that resulted in the irreversible and total loss of retinal function. Since all of the previously published case series of foveal retinoschisis reported good visual improvement without fixed scotoma, this retinal damage is not a schisis but rather due to retinal swelling with the accumulation of fluid. Smiddy (Smiddy et al., 2009) supported this notion and suggested that myopic maculoschisis, foveal schisis, and vitreoschisis in high myopia should all fall under the family of MTM.

Clinical Features

MTM is more prevalent in populations with high myopia, particularly in females (Panozzo and Mercanti, 2007). Patients usually complain of visual decrease and/or metamorphopsia (Panozzo and Mercanti, 2004), but some harbour no subjective symptoms (Baba et al., 2003). Although there are no specific features in the early stages of MTM that can be identified by routine examinations (Takano and kishi, 1999), OCT can be used to detect retinoschisis, shallow retinal detachment without retinal holes, lamellar macular holes, and other clinical characteristics (Panozzo and mercanti, 2007). Macular holes with or without retinal detachment can only be discovered by an ophthalmoscope at the later stages.

The OCT image features of macular retinoschisis include the significant thickening of the retina at the position of the schisis and the delamination of the neuroretina by a low echo cavum that is separated by an erect columnar microstructure. Macular retinoschisis can be divided into two types: inner and outer retinal schisis. When outer retinal schisis occurs, the neurepithelium layer is divided into two layers. There is a thin layer on the outside and a thick layer on the inside, with the low echo cavum located in the outer part of the neurepithelium layer. When inner retinal schisis occurs, the neurepithelium layer is also divided into two layers. There is a thin layer on the outside and a thick layer on the inside, with the low echo cavum located in the inner part of the neurepithelium layer (Benhamou et al., 2002). The main OCT findings that differentiate macular retinoschisis from retinal detachment are a columnar microstructure and the smooth inner walls of the low echo cavum (Takano and Kishi, 1999). In high myopia, macular retinoschisis is always accompanied by foveal detachment, lamellar macular holes, macular epiretinal membrane, or vitreoretinal traction. In a study of 29 eyes with high myopia and macular retinoschisis, 10 eyes also had foveal detachment (34.5%), 8 had macular epiretinal membrane (27.6%), 5 had vitreoretinal traction, 7 had lamellar macular holes (24.1%), and 4 had two or more of the above lesions (Gaucher et al., 2007).

OCT of eyes with shallow macular detachment accompanied by macular retinoschisis display two walls of limited shallow macular detachment forming the shape of the Chinese character eight (八). At the top is a thin neurepithelium layer and at the bottom is a smooth but strong reflection pigment epithelial layer.

Pathogenesis

The pathogenesis of MTM is complicated (Vanderbeek and Johnson, 2012) and may develop due to several factors relating to the retina itself: preretinal factors, and subretinal factors. The factors relating to the retina itself include: 1) thickening (Bando et al., 2005) and/or stiffening (Kuhn, 2003) of the internal limiting membrane (ILM), which can prevent the retina from adapting to high myopia posterior scleral staphyloma that produce centripetal traction and tangential traction to the retina; 2) choroidal atrophy, which can lead to the shortage in blood supply in the retina that reduces adhesion between the nerve layers; and 3) the retinal pigment epithelium and choroid may succumb to atrophy, thus reducing the adhesion between the retinal pigment epithelium and neuroretina (Cho et al., 2004). Preretinal factors include: 1) incomplete posterior vitreous detachment (Polito et al., 2003) or adhesion(Spaide et al., 2005) between the remaining vitreous and the retina, which can produce centripetal traction and tangential traction to the retina; 2) the Bruch membrane, which can be ruptured, and the pigment epithelium, which can migrate to the front of the retina in high myopia forming an epiretinal membrane whose shrinkage produces tangential traction to the retina(Stirpe and Michels, 1990); and 3) small retinal vessels that can cause traction on the retina (Ikuno et al., 2005). One subretinal factor is the formation of posterior scleral staphyloma fromthe extension of the axis of the eye (Wu et al., 2009), which produces centrifugal traction on the retina.

Some researchers postulate that vitreous traction contributes the most toward MTM pathogenesis (Benhamou et al., 2002; Ishida et al., 2000; Oshima et al., 1998; Kobayashi and Kishi, 2003), others hold the opinion that the extension of the eye axis and the formation of staphyloma may also be major contributing factors(Smiddy et al., 2009; Robichaud et al., 2011). Panozzo and Mercanti (Panozzo and mercanti, 2007) reported that women constituted to 87.5% of MTM patients, suggesting that MTM may be linked to hormonal differences (Panozzo and Mercanti, 2007). Others have shown that high myopia is a polygenic inherited disease. Seven pairs of related genes have been identified, with six located on autosomal chromosomes and one on the X chromosome (Xq28) (Soubrane, 2008). The higher incidence of MTM in women indicates that it may be a sex-linked genetic disease, but further research is needed to confirm this hypothesis.

Development

Panozzo and Mercanti(Panozzo and mercanti, 2007) suggested that high myopia macular holes and macular holes accompanied by retinal detachment occur in the advanced stages of MTM while macular retinoschisis, shallow retinal detachment without holes, and lamellar macular holes occur in the early stages of MTM.

In 1999, Tokano and Kishi speculated that the formation of high myopia macular holes is the result of macular retinoschisis or shallow retinal detachment without holes. This hypothesis has been confirmed by several other groups (Panozzo and Mercanti, 2004; Smiddy et al., 2009; Gaucher et al., 2007; Ikuno and Tano, 2003; Shimada et al., 2006; Matsumura et al., 2004). Although Panozzo and Mercanti (Panozzo and Mercanti, 2004) did not observe the developmental process of MTM, they did study some patients with bilateral high myopia eyes who had stable macular retinoschisis in one eye and a macular hole with posterior retinal detachment in the other eye.

The development of early MTM into macular holes may be related to the following factors: if the central fovea itself is thin (Shimada et al., 2006), the existence of posterior scleral staphyloma (Oie et al., 2005), preretinal traction (macular epiretinal membrane, incomplete posterior vitreous detachment, and the remaining vitreous) (Benhamou et al., 2002; Panozzo and Mercanti, 2004; Gaucher et al., 2007; Shimada et al., 2006; Matsumura et al., 2004), MTM that is accompanied by central foveal detachment (Guacher et al., 2007), and the degree of stiffness of the internal limiting membrane (Kihn, 2003). Gaucher (Guacher et al., 2007) discovered that myopic foveal retinoschisis may not affect vision for several years, but it is more likely to occur if preretinal structures have formed. Therefore, early MTM can be divided into two types: affected vision and unaffected vision. Patients with affected vision may seek medical attention earlier than those with unaffected vision, thus increasing their chances of preventing the illness from reaching a more advanced stage.

Retinal detachment occurs more readily after the formation of high myopia macular holes compared to idiopathic macular holes because of vitreous retinal traction, low adhesion between the pigment epithelial layer and neuroepithelial layer, posterior scleral staphyloma, and obvious liquefaction of the high myopia vitreous (Panozzo and Mercanti, 2004)

9. Myopic Macular Retinoschisis

Myopic macular retinoschisis (MR) is thought to occur in 9–20% of highly myopic eyes with posterior staphyloma. The clinical presence of macular retinoschisis has been demonstrated with optical coherence interferometry (OCT) by Takano and Kishi (Takano and Kishi, 1999). A posterior vitreous detachment (PVD) based on the presence of a Weiss ring is only noted in 7% of patients with MR. The OCT features of MR comprise retinal thickening and splitting of the neurosensory retina into a thin outer outer layer and a thicker reflective inner layer; however, an inner retinoschisis may also be present in some eyes (Benhamou et al., 2002). This can be associated with a foveal cyst, which can be partially de-roofed giving the appearance of a lamellar hole, and in some patients a foveal detachment may be present. Preretinal structures, representing either a thickened posterior hyaloid or epiretinal membrane, may be seen as a hyper-reflective layer indicating the presence of tangential traction. A natural history study of nine eyes with MR without preretinal membranes over at least 1 year demonstrated no significant progression (Benhamou et al., 2002). However, a macular hole may develop spontaneously or possibly after vitreous surgery, as shown in nine of 29 eyes reported by Gaucher et al. (Gaucher et al., 2007).

Myopic Macular Retinoschisis and Progression

Myopic macular retinoschisis was first identified through the use of optical coherence tomography (OCT) by Takano and Kishi in 1999 (Takano and Kishi, 1999), and it was found in 9% to 34% of highly myopic eyes with posterior staphyloma (Takano and Kishi, 1999; Baba et al., 2003). The terminology used in discussing this condition has not been consistent, and Panozzo and associates (Panozzo and Mercanti, 2004) proposed in 2004 to unify all of the pathologic features generated by traction in the myopic environment under the term myopic traction maculopathy. Eyes with myopic traction maculopathy include those with vitreomacular traction, retinal thickening, macular retinoschisis, lamellar macular hole (lamellar MH), and foveal retinal detachment (RD). Recently, Vanderbeek and Johnson (Vanderbeek and Johnson, 2012) reviewed the charts of 6 consecutive patients who had undergone vitreoretinal surgery for myopic traction maculopathy, and they found that the traction mechanisms causing the myopic traction maculopathy were diverse. Surgical repair of myopic traction maculopathy was successful both anatomically and visually when the major traction mechanism was relieved (Vanderbeek and Johnson, 2012; Johnson, 2012). Eyes with myopic traction maculopathy have varying traction mechanisms and degrees of retinal damage, so it is to be expected that the prognoses will vary during the natural course of individual eyes. The natural course of macular retinoschisis has been studied in 8 eyes, 5 eyes (Sun et al., 2010), 21 eyes (Benhamou et al., 2002), 18 eyes (Gaucher et al., 2007), and 54 eyes (Ripandelli et al., 2012). These studies have reported that the eyes with myopic macular retinoschisis can progress to more serious complications such as fullthickness MH and foveal RD during the follow-up period. On the other hand, Polito and associates reported one patient whose foveal RD and macular retinoschisis disappeared after a spontaneous posterior vitreous detachment (PVD) during the follow-up period. The results of these studies suggested the natural course of myopic traction maculopathy varies, and eyes with more extensive macular retinoschisis tend to progress more commonly. A complete resolution of macular retinoschisis can occur after a release of traction on the retina (Shimada et al., 2013).

10. Macular Hole and Associated Retinal Detachment

Macular holes (MH) with associated retinal detachment are rare in the general population. They occur principally in highly myopic eyes, and are thought to be the result of tangential vitreoretinal traction (Wolfensberger and Gonvers, 2000). A foveal detachment often precedes the formation of a MH in highly myopic eyes, and axial elongation, the posterior staphyloma, and a PVD probably all contribute to the formation of a retinal detachment (Gaucher et al., 2007; Morita et al., 1991; Akiba et al., 1999). Whilst the relationship between MR and MH is unknown, it has been reported that MR may be a precursor to MH formation in PM (Takano and kishi, 1999; Gaucher et al., 2007; Kobayashi and Kishi, 2003). The reported closure rates for MH associated with RD and PM are disappointing.

11. Optic Disc Abnormalities

Myopic discs tend to be characteristic in their appearance. There is an increased prevalence of tilted optic discs in patients with myopia, and the prevalence increases with increasing myopia (Vongphanit et al., 2002). Myopic optic discs also have a tendency to be larger in size than the discs of nonmyopic eyes. This enlargement of the disc is associated with thinning of the lamina cribrosa, a possible factor in the development of glaucomatous optic nerve damage (Vongphanit et al., 2002; Xu et al., 2007).

Peripapillary choroidal atrophy is another characteristic sign in myopic eyes. The size of the peripapillary crescent has been shown to increase with increasing amounts of myopia (Kobayashi et al., 2005).

A white sharply defined area on the temporal side of the disc, named myopic crescent, is seen. The crescent is basically caused due to stretching. Due to stretching the choroid terminates some distance from the margin of the disc. As a result of this, one can see the sclera behind, as the choroid is absent and the retina is transparent. Thus, next to the disc the crescent is seen. Another crescent, called choroidal crescent, is present temporal to the myopic crescent. In this crescent, choroidal vessels can be seen. The reason is that here the pigment epithelium is absent, but the choroid is present. This leads to the formation of a choroidal crescent. A temporal nerve fiber loop can also occur.

The characteristic shape of the myopic disc includes a tiltled appearance and temporal crescent (Yamazaki et al., 1999). The disc tilt is mostly from the nasal to the temporal side with the nasal margin elevated relative to the temporal margin (Curtin, 1985). Myopic temporal crescent, which is also called "β-zone parapapillary atrophy" (PPA) (Teng et al.,2010; Jonas et al.,1989; Uchida et al., 1998; See et al., 2009) is white, sharply defined area lying on the temporal side of the optic disc where the inner surface of the sclera is directly seen. Although myopic temporal crescent is usually considered to be acquired, resulting from chorioretinal stretching (Apple et al., 1982; Nakazawa et al., 2008), it is generally thought that the tilted disc results from the oblique insertion of the optic nerve at birth (Apple et al., 1982).

Tilted appearance and temporal crescent are hallmarks of the myopic optic disc. The temporal crescent is considered to be generally acquired and the consequence of scleral stretching (Apple et al., 1982; Nakazawa et al., 2008). In contrast, it has been hypothesized that a tilted disc originates from oblique insertion of the optic nerve at birth (Apple et al., 1982), but the tilted disc also may be acquired. The association with the myopic shift and its occurrence along with development and enlargement of PPA suggest that disc shape change is the result of scleral stretching associated with axial elongation of the eyeball. As the eyeball grows axially, the temporal sclera moves back and becomes flattened. In this process, the optic nerve is pulled toward the temporal direction, which eventually results in an optic disc with a tilted appearance, including nasal elevation and temporal flattening. The course of the optic nerve vessels is also changed. This speculation is consistent with histologic findings in the myopic tilted disc. Apple et al. (Apple et al., 1982) described that the retinal nerve fibers traverse the ONH in an obliquely nasal direction in a myopic individual with a tilted disc, which indicates that the ONH has been dragged temporally (Kim et al., 2012).

The optic nerve head shows a different appearance in highly myopic eyes than in non–highly myopic eyes (Jonas et al., 1988; Xu et al., 2007 a). The features of highly myopic optic nerve heads include a secondary macrodisc with an abnormal, elongated disc shape; a shallow disc cupping; a decreased contrast between the color of the neuroretinal rim and the color of the optic cup; and a marked parapapillary atrophy, which is also called myopic crescent or "conus myopicus" (Dichtl et al., 1998; Jonas and Dichtl, 1997; Xu et al., 2010)."

Histomorphometric study on parapapillary optic nerve head structures in axially highly myopic eyes vs non–highly myopic human globes showed that in all highly myopic eyes with a distance between the optic nerve border and beginning of Bruch membrane of more than 0.5 mm, the parapapillary region consisted of a markedly elongated and thinned sclera with some overlying retinal nerve fiber layer, without Bruch membrane, choroid, retinal pigment epithelium, or retinal photoreceptors interposed between the sclera and the retinal nerve fiber layer. This was in contrast to non– highly myopic eyes, in which, independent of the presence or absence of glaucomatous optic nerve damage, the Bruch membrane extended to the optic nerve border, and in which the scleral flange was significantly shorter and thicker (Jonas et al., 2011).

Since the scleral flange formed the anterior border of the retrobulbar cerebrospinal fluid space, the elongation of the scleral flange in the highly myopic eyes caused an extension of the retrobulbar cerebrospinal fluid space into the parapapillary region in the highly myopic eyes (Jonas et al., 2011).

Peripapillary Atrophy

Peripapillary atrophy (PPA) is a clinical finding associated with chorioretinal thinning and disruption of the retinal pigment epithelium (RPE) in the area surrounding the optic disc. It is non-specific and is seen in a number of different disease states in both benign and pathologic conditions, including glaucoma (Jonas et al., 1999) and high myopia (Xu et al., 2007). Peripapillary atrophy is also considered a normal aging phenomenon (Curcio et al., 2000; Spaide, 2009).

The normal cross-sectional anatomic structure of the peripapillary region of the eye is arranged with all the retinal cell layers organized in a parallel fashion, ending at the edge of the optic disc, with the topmost retinal nerve fiber layer increasing in thickness before diving into the disc. This normal architecture is disrupted with the development of peripapillary atrophy.

Classification of peripapillary atrophy into two zones was first proposed by Jonas, et al. (Jonas et al., 1989): zone beta, a central zone of chorioretinal atrophy with visible large choroidal vessels and sclera, and zone alpha, a more peripheral area of irregular hypo- and hyper-pigmentation, with both types often present side by side in the same eye (Jonas et al., 1989). Histological investigations of peripapillary atrophy describe changes in beta zone atrophy as a complete loss of retinal pigment epithelium cells and photoreceptors, and thinning of the choroid in combination with an almost complete collapse of the choriocapillaris. Alpha zone atrophy has been described as having structural irregularities in the retinal pigment epithelium cells (Jonas et al., 1989; Fantes and Anderson, 1989; Jonas et al., 1992; Kubota et al., 1993; Dichtl et al., 1998).

Retinal changes associated with peripapillary atrophy using high definition OCT(Manjunath et al., 2011): the qualitative findings include RPE and photoreceptor loss. RPE disruption, inner/outer retinal thinning, which have been described previously through histological studies, as well as the novel findings of RNFL, thickening and plaque-like formation, intraretinal cystic changes, and abnormal changes in retinal sloping.

Peripapillary atrophy (PPA), divided into zones β (PPA-β) and α (PPA-α), has been known to be associated with myopia and glaucoma, especially open- angle glaucoma with normal intraocular pressure (Jonas et al., 1989; Jonas and Naumann, 1989; Araie et al., 1994; Jonas et al., 1992; Rockwood and Anderson, 1988; Park et al., 1996; Uchida et al., 1998).

Studies of enucleated eyes have shown that PPA-β represents histologically a complete loss of retinal pigment epithelial (RPE) cells and an incomplete loss of adjacent photoreceptors, and PPA-α correlate with irregularities in the RPE (Jonas et al.,1992; Fantes and Anderson, 1989; Kubota et al., 1993; Curcio et al., 2000). Both PPA-β and –α have been found to be significantly larger in eyes with glaucoma than in normal eyes, whereas the size, shape, and frequency of both PPA zones are not significantly different between normal eyes and eyes with optic neuropathy other than glaucoma (Jonas et al., 1989; Jonas and Naumann, 1989; Araie et al., 1994; Jonas et al., 1992; Rockwood and Anderson, 1988; Park et al., 1996, Uchida et al., 1998; Jonas et al., 1991; Jonas et al., 1993; Lee et al., 2010).

12. Choroidal Thickness Measurement in High Myopia

Pathologic myopia or high myopia is associated with a progressive elongation of the globe, resulting in a variety of fundal changes that lead to visual disturbance (Klein and Curtin, 1975; Curtin, 1982; Hotchkiss and Fine, 1981; Vongphanit et al., 2002; Saw et al., 2005; Lai et al., 2008). Possible causes for visual disturbances include lacquer cracks in Bruch's membrane, choroidal neovascularization, chorioretinal degeneration or atrophy, retinal detachment, myopic macular schisis, and macular hole (Hotchkiss and Fine, 1981; Vongphanit et al., 2002; Saw et al., 2005; Lai et al., 2008; Iwase et al., 2006; Karlin and Curtin, 1976;Curtin and Karlin, 1971; Buch et al., 2004).

Evidence supports the theory that axial elongation of the globe leads to the stretching of retinal tissue and reduced retinal function (Coletta and Watson, 2006; Kitaguchi et al., 2007; Chui et al., 2008; Chui et al., 2008; Chui et al., 2005; Atchison et al., 2006; Morgan, 2003).

The choroid is an integral structure in the eye that accounts for most of the ocular blood flow. Thus, the choroid is of paramount importance to retinal and visual function because it supplies nutrients to retinal pigment epithelial cells and the outer retina. In addition, the choroid also contributes to the blood supply of the prelaminar portion of the optic nerve. Compromised choroidal circulation may account for the retinal dysfunction and vision loss that is observed in highly myopic and glaucomatous patients. However, it is difficult to image the full thickness of the choroid because of pigments in the retinal pigment epithelium (RPE) layer (Povazay, 2007). Its physiochemical nature impedes visualization by ophthalmoscopy, fundus photography, and fluorescein angiography. Direct choroidal layer visualization and measurement could be obtained through enhanced depth imaging (EDI) spectral-domain optical coherence tomography (OCT) (Spaide et al., 2008; Fujiwara et al., 2009; Margolis and Spaide, 2009). The mean subfoveal CT was found to be 118±68 mm standard deviation (Fujiwara et al., 2009; Ho et al., 2013) and was significantly thinner than the subfoveal CT of normal eyes (287 mm) (Margolis and Spaide, 2009; Ho et al., 2013). The mean CT was computed on the basis of the thickness at the subfoveal region and varied significantly at different locations. The CT was inversely correlated with myopic diopters ($r2 = 0.217$, $P = 0.011$) and age (r2 ¼ 0.078, $P = 0.032$). Subfoveal CT correlated negatively with the logMAR visual acuity ($r2 = 0.295$, $P = 0.008$). The CT of 3 mm in the temporal to subfoveal areas also correlates negatively with age ($r2 = 0.168$, $P = 0.005$). The mean subfoveal CT 3 mm nasal to fovea was 94.8±54.3 mm standard deviation, which is significantly thinner than the subfoveal CT. This could be explained by the fact that choroids near to the peripapillary atrophy are extremely thin and difficult to measure (Ho et al., 2013).

13. Choroidal Thickness and Visual Acuity in Highly Myopic Eyes

High myopia is characterized by excessive and progressive elongation of the globe, resulting in a variety of secondary fundus changes that themselves may lead to visual impairment and includes retinal detachment, myopic macular schisis, macular hole, choroidal neovascularization, and zonal areas of chorioretinal atrophy (Curtin and Karlin, 1971; Karlin and Curtin, 1976; Hotchkiss and Fine, 1981; Curtin, 1997; Klayer et al., 1998; Krumpaszky et al., 1999; Liu et al., 2001; Vongphanit et al., 2002; Evans et al., 2004; Buch et al., 2004; Saw et al., 2005; Xu et al., 2006; Iwase et al., 2006; Avisar et al., 2006; Lai et al., 2008; Yamada et al., 2010; You et al., 2011;). Even in eyes with no observable macular pathology, visual function in highly myopic eyes declines with increasing age (Curtin, 1977,Vongphanit et al., 2002; Goldschmidt and Fledelius, 2005; Kora et al., 1998; Luu et al., 2006; Xu et al., 2007). The age-related loss in visual function is not limited to decreased visual acuity but also includes reduced threshold visual field sensitivity (Aung et al., 2001; Ito et al., 2001) and electrooculography (Blach et al., 1966), full-field electroretinography (Blach et al., 1966; Westall et al., 2001, and multifocal electroretinography results (Kawabata and Adachi-Usami, 1997).

Epidemiologty of Pathologic and Myopic Choroidal Neovascularization (Wong et al., 2014)

Myopia is a common eye condition, affecting 20%-40% of adults, which poses a significant public health burden and cost to society (Wong et al., 2000; Morgan et al., 2012). A proportion of people with myopia have pathologic myopia, which is characterized by excessive and progressive elongation of the globe, and is now considered to be an important cause of impaired vision and blindness worldwide. Choroidal neovascularization (CNV) is a frequent complication associated with pathologic myopia that threatens vision, and is characterized by the occurrence of newly formed abnormal blood vessels that grow under the retinal pigment epithelium or retina and can penetrate the Bruch membrane to extend into the subretinal space, with subsequent scarring (Green and Wilson, 1986). The precise pathogenesis of CNV in eyes with pathologic myopia is unclear, and a range of hypotheses were discussed in detail in a recent review (Neelam et al., 2012). CNV is acutely symptomatic, is associated with the occurrence of a central scotoma, and can result in a rapid deterioration of central vision; hence, there is a need for urgent clinical treatment. Data on the epidemiology of pathologic myopia and CNV secondary to pathologic myopia (myopic CNV) in the literature are inconsistent, and the impact of this condition on vision remains unclear; hence, we conducted a systematic review to describe the epidemiology and visual burden of pathologic myopia and myopic CNV.

Pathologic Myopia as a Cause of Blindness or Low Vision (Wong et al., 2014)

Pathologic myopia was the cause of low vision or blindness in 5.8% and 7.8% of eyes with low vision or blindness in European populations (Klaver et al., 1998; Cedrone et al., 2006). The Los Angeles Latino Eye Study (LALES), which examined Latin American residents of Los Angeles, reported pathologic myopia as the cause of blindness or low vision in 4.5% of eyes (Cotter et al., 2006). In contrast, in the 3 large studies performed in China and Japan, pathologic myopia was the cause of blindness or low vision in 12.2%-27.4% of individuals with low vision (Xu et al., 2006; Iwase et al., 2006; Yamada et al., 2010), and in a pilot study performed in Hong Kong, pathologic myopia was the cause of low vision in 31.3% of individuals with low vision (Van Newkirk, 1997). In the 6 studies reporting the contribution of pathologic myopia to blindness, pathologic myopia was the first, second, or third most frequent cause of blindness.

A further 5 studies reported pathologic myopia as a cause of blindness in individuals registered as blind in a particular country or region of a country (MacDonald, 1965; Avisar et al., 1998; Ghafour et al., 1983; Krumpaszky et al., 1999; Wu et al., 2011). Four studies concerned individuals newly registered as blind over a single year (Avisar et al., 1998; Ghafour et al., 1983; Krumpaszky et al., 1999) or over 3 years (Wu et al., 2011), whereas a Canadian study involved all individuals registered blind at the time of the study (MacDonald, 1965). The frequency of pathologic myopia as the cause of blindness was relatively consistent across the 4 studies in white populations (6.0%-9.1%) and was much higher in the Chinese study (26.1%). Pathologic myopia was ranked as the second to fifth most frequent cause of blindness in the studies of white populations, and was the most frequent cause in the Chinese study. Two studies reported the frequency of pathologic myopia as the cause of blindness or low vision in children (Shah et al., 2011; Pi et al., 2012). Pi and associates reported that pathologic myopia was the cause of low vision in 1.3%of visually impaired school-aged children in Western China (Pi et al., 2012), whereas Shah and associates reported that 11.1% of children attending a low-vision clinic in Peshawar, Pakistan, had pathologic myopia as the main cause of visual impairment (Shah et al., 2011). In both studies, pathologic myopia was the third most common cause of visual impairment. Two further studies reported on pathologic myopia as the cause of low vision or blindness in institutionalized elderly people (Sainz-Gomez et al., 2010) in Pamplona, Spain (average age, 82 years), and individuals seen at a tertiary care eye hospital in Hyderabad, India (46%of patientswere less than 30 years of age) (Khan, 2000).

Prevalence and incidence of pathologic myopia and visual impairment attributable to pathologic myopia in general (Wong et al., 2014): The Blue Mountains Eye Study (BMES) (Vongphanit et al., 2002) recorded a prevalence of 1.2% (per individual) for a predominantly white population, whereas 4 studies of Asian populations reported a prevalence of 0.90%-3.1% per individual (Hu, 1987; Liu et al., 2010; Gao et al., 2011; Asakuma et al., 2012). A study in school-aged children in China reported a prevalence of pathologic myopia at 0.19% per eye (Pi et al., 2012). The study by Wang and associates assessed the prevalence and causes of visual field loss (VFL) (Wang et al., 2006) while other studies evaluated vision loss per se. Although the prevalence of pathologic myopia in the general population was not expressly stated in these papers, the prevalence of visual impairment attributable to pathologic myopia was estimated by expressing the number of cases of low vision/blindness caused by pathologic myopia as a percentage of the number of participants examined in the survey. Three studies of European populations yielded an estimated prevalence of 0.11%-0.47% (Klaver et al., 1998; Buch et al., 2001; Cedrone et al., 2006); LALES (Cotter et al., 2006) presented results equating to a prevalence of 0.05%; and 5 studies of Far East Asian populations yielded an estimated prevalence of 0.17%-1.41% (Xu et al., 2006; Iwase et al., 2006; Yamada et al., 2010; Van Newkirk, 1997; Wang et al., 2006). Furthermore, Pi and associates estimated a prevalence of pathologic myopia– related visual impairment in children in China of 0.10% (Pi et al., 2012), and Avisar and associates recorded the prevalence of blindness attributable to pathologic myopia in Israel as 0.02%-0.03% (Avisar et al., 1998). Values of the annual incidence of blindness attributable to pathologic myopia in the general population ranged from 0.77 per 100 000 for Germany (Krumpaszky et al., 1999) to 2.1-4.3 per 100 000 for Israel (Avisar et al., 1998). In China, a 5-year follow-up of the Beijing Eye Study reported an overall pathologic myopia incidence of 0.05% (Liu et al., 2010), while the annual incidence of blindness attributable to pathologic myopia was estimated as 12.6 per 100 000 in Shanghai for the 2007-2009 period (Wu et al., 2011).

Risk Factors for Pathologic Myopia (Wong et al., 2014):

Four studies assessed risk factors for pathologic myopia (Vongphanit et al., 2002; Liu et al., 2010; Gao et al., 2011; Asakuma et al., 2012) and found that greater axial length (3 studies (Liu et al., 2010; Gao et al., 2011; asakuma et al., 2012)) and age (2 studies (Gao et al., 2011; Asakuma et al., 2012)) were found to be significantly associated with pathologic myopia. Other risk factors for pathologic myopia identified by a single study were larger optic disc area (Liu et al., 2010), female sex (Asakuma et al., 2012), myopic refractive error (per -1 diopter) (Asakuma et al., 2012), and family history of myopia (Gao et al., 2011). One study assessed the impact of sex and age on pathologic myopia, though no significant associations were identified (Vongphanit et al., 2002). Two review articles (Montero and ruiz-Moreno, 2010; Young et al., 2007) described evidence for a genetic basis for pathologic myopia. Based on studies in twins and in families with pathologic myopia, 9 loci for pathologic myopia have been identified, including 7 autosomal dominant loci on chromosomes 2, 4, 7, 12, 17, 18, and 21; 1 autosomal recessive locus on chromosome 14; and 1 recessive locus on the X chromosome (Montero and Ruiz-Moreno, 2010). Furthermore, 1 article has identified a novel susceptibility locus at chromosome band 11q24.1 for pathologic myopia in a Japanese Population (Nakanishi et al., 2009). Possible environmental factors associated with pathologic myopia (including annual hours of sunshine, water hardness, selenium levels, and use of fluorinated water) have been reported in 2 US studies (Daubs, 1982; Daubs, 1984) from the 1980s, although the authors state that identified factors were not necessarily causally related to the development of pathologic myopia.

Pathologic Myopia and Pathogenesis

Myopia-related visual impairment affects the productivity, mobility, quality of life and activities of daily living of individuals (Saw, 2006). Although there is no universally agreed definition, pathological or degenerative myopia has been defined in recent studies as a spherical equivalent refractive error of at least −6 dioptres (D) accompanied by characteristic degenerative changes, with complications of pathological myopia being much more common when the refractive error is −8 D or worse (Yamamoto et al., 2007; Tano, 2002; Yoshida et al., 2002). As elongation of the globe is a key feature of pathological myopia (PM), an axial length of ≥26.5 mm has been adopted as a biometric definition in clinical trials (Verteporfin in Photodynamic Therapy Study Group, 2001), with recent studies reporting a mean of 29 mm (range 26.8–31.5 mm) (Yoshida et al., 2002; Yoshida et al., 2003). Pathological myopia is one of the leading causes of visual loss in the world (Grossniklaus and Green, 1992). The prevalence of PM is known to differ between ethnicities. In the adult Asian population, its prevalence is 9–21% (Yamada et al., 2010; Hsu et al., 2004) compared to 2.8–4.6% in the U.S and Australia (Kempen et al., 2004), and the prevalence is thought to be rising globally (Saw, 2006). The pathogenesis of high myopia is unknown. Twin studies have estimated high trait heritabilities, and genetic and environmental susceptibility factors have been demonstrated to play an important role in its development (Hombeak and Young, 2009; Jacobi and Pusch, 2010).

Myopic Maculopathy, Progression and Visual Acuity Loss

Long-term studies suggest that approximately 40% of highly myopic eyes develop progressive maculopathy, and over 10 years more than half of these individuals will lose 2 lines of Snellen acuity (Hayashi et al., 2010; Shih et al., 2006). Although there is no agreed clinical grading for myopic maculopathy, several authors have used a practical classification originally devised by Avila et al. to describe the natural history (Shih et al., 2006; Avila et al., 1984). With this method, a scale of increasing severity from 0 to 5 is used to describe the maculopathy as follows: M0: normalappearing posterior pole, M1: tessellation and choroidal pallor pattern in macular area, M2: M1 and a posterior pole ectasia, M3: M2 and lacquer cracks in Bruch's membrane and posterior staphyloma, M4: M3 and focal areas of deep choroidal atrophy, and M5: M4 and geographic areas of atrophy and choroidal neovascularisation (CNV). Recent studies have suggested modifications to this classification: Hayashi et al. conducted a comprehensive natural history study of myopic maculopathy, and indicated that lacquer cracks should be classified as an independent lesion, due to the likelihood of progression to CNV as well as diffuse atrophy. The authors also highlight the presence of a posterior staphyloma as an important factor leading to the progression of maculopathy (Hayashi et al., 2010). In the Blue Mountains Eye Study, myopic retinopathy was defined to include: staphyloma, lacquer cracks, Fuchs' spot and myopic chorioretinal thinning or atrophy (Vongphanit et al., 2002).

Myopic macular CNV occurs in 4% to 11% of patients with high myopia, and is the most common vision threatening complication of high myopia (Soubrane and Coscas, 1994). It is subfoveal in 58%, and juxtafoveal in 32% of cases, and is the leading aetiology of CNV among patients younger than 50 years of age (Cohen et al., 1996). In its advanced stage, CNV appears as a Fuchs' spot, which is a macular scar with pigment clumping and hyperpigmentation in association with fibrosis and retinal atrophy. Among myopic patients with preexisting CNV, more than 30% will develop CNV in the fellow eye within 8 years (Avila et al., 1984). Although natural history studies of untreated myopic CNV have presented conflicting evidence on visual prognosis, the overall trend suggests that long-term visual prognosis with observation alone is poor. Early studies demonstrated that over a mean follow-up of 3.4 years, 96% of 70 eyes with myopic CNV regressed or stabilized (Avila et al., 1984). More recently, however, patients over 50 years with myopic CNV observed for a mean of 4 years had a final visual acuity (VA) of 20/200 or worse in over two-thirds of cases, and a 10-year follow-up observational study noted that 96% of eyes achieve a final VA of 20/200 or worse (Yoshida et al., 2003). Prognostic factors associated with a poor visual outcome included extensive chorioretinal atrophy, an older age of onset and a larger area of CNV (Hayashi et al., 2005; Kojima et al., 2004).

Myopic Maculopathy and OCT

Degenerative myopia, also called pathologic or high myopia, is defined as a myopic refractive error of more than 6 diopters (D) associated with degenerative fundus changes. The main feature of degenerative myopia is congenital scleral weakness, leading to progressive globe enlargement, axial lengthening, and finally the formation of posterior staphyloma (Forte et al.,2008). Scleral stretching can lead to such degenerative changes as vitreous degeneration, progressive atrophy of the choriocapillaris and choroid, linear ruptures of the Bruch membrane (lacquer cracks), and retinal thinning. The posterior retina can be damaged by traction induced by an epiretinal membrane or residual focal vitreoretinal adhesion. The combination of retinal traction, posterior staphyloma, and progressive global scleral stretching frequently leads to macular holes (Phillips and Dobbie, 1963; Abdel-Latif, 1969), retinoschisis and posterior retinal detachment (Takano and Kishi, 1999), detachment of the internal limiting membrane (ILM) (Sayanagi et al., 2006), peripapillary detachment of the pigment epithelium (PDPM) (Freund et al., 2003; Toranzo et al., 2005; Shimada et al., 2006), vascular traction with retinal microfolds, and paravascular intraretinal cysts (Sayanagi et al., 2005; Ikono et al., 2005; Ohno-Matsui et al., 2006).

Retinal abnormalities associated with high myopia examined with en face optical coherence tomography (OCT) (Forte et al., 2007; Forte et al., 2007; Forte et al., - forthcoming).include posterior retinal detachment (present in 18.5% of eyes) and stretching-related fundus abnormalities, namely, retinoschisis, ILM detachment, and vascular microfolds. Posterior detachment without macular hole was always in the area of the staphyloma, which suggests that the staphyloma could play an important etiologic role in this condition (Forte et al., 2008). All the abnormalities identified seem to be related with the mechanical elongation forces taking place in highly myopic eyes. The stretching of retinochoroidal tissues may result from a combination of vitreoretinal adhesion (Gaucher et al., 2007; Panozzo and mercanti, 2004), posterior staphyloma (Takano and Kishi, 1999; Baba et al., 2003), rigidity of the ILM (Sayanagi et al., 2006), and inflexibility of the retinal vessels (Sayanagi et al., 2005).

Vitreomacular traction has been implicated in the formation of posterior detachment in patients with pathologic myopia, and it has been reported that removal of a thin layer of adherent vitreous led to the resolution of the detachment (Ikuno et al., 2004; Kobayashi and kishi, 2003). On the other hand, all cases of peripapillary retinal detachment or ILM detachment were affected by retinal vascular microfolds, which are thought to be caused by the inflexibility of retinal vessels as opposed to retinal stretching (Sayanagi et al., 2005). These data could suggest that retinal splitting at different depths in high myopia could be attributable to vitreoretinal traction, to the staphyloma, and to the inward forces exerted by the rigid vessels and ILM.No significant correlation between foveal detachment without macular hole and visual impairment was found (Takano and Kishi, 1999; Gaucher et al., 2007; Ichibe et al., 2004; Forte et al., 2008).

Myopia-Related Fundus Changes

The pattern of myopia-related macular and optic disc changes in Singapore adults 40 years and older with high myopia (greater than -6.00 D) identified from population-based studies, the the major pathologic findings were staphyloma (23.0%) and chorioretinal atrophy (19.3%). Lacquer crack (1.8%) and T-sign (1.8%) were present in a few individuals. Fuchs spot (0%) and choroidal neovascularization (0.9%) were relatively rare complications of high myopia (Chang et al., 2013). In the Blue Mountains Eye Study, where the average SE was -6.10 D, and 35 of 67 eyes (52.2%) had staphyloma (Vonghanit et al., 2002 a). Staphyloma increased in prevalence with respect to increasing age, increasing myopic refractive error, and increasing axial length. In a Japanese cohort with myopia greater than -8.00 D or axial length greater than 26.5 mm, staphyloma was identified in 90% of subjects and in 96.7% of those 50 years of age and older (Hsiang et al., 2008). Progression of type II staphyloma to type IX was seen, along with an associated increased incidence of lacquer cracks, supporting the theory of progressive mechanical expansion of the globe (Hsiang et al., 2008). In a cross-sectional study in Hong Kong, highly myopic eyes with the presence of posterior pole lesion were reported to have significantly longer AL (28.84 vs 26.59 mm) and greater degree of myopia (-16.8 D vs -9.4 D) (Lai et al., 2008). In the Shihpai Eye Study in Taiwan, highly myopic eyes with maculopathy had a greater myopic degree (-12.8 vs -7.6 D, P < .001) than those without (Chen et al., 2012). Understanding the associations of myopic refraction and AL with staphyloma is important from a clinical perspective, as vitreoretinal interface pathology in pathologic myopia with posterior staphyloma encompasses a spectrum of conditions whose baseline functionality, prognosis, rate, and amount of progression vary significantly (Ripandelli et al., 2012). Chorioretinal atrophy is an area of well-circumscribed chorioretinal degeneration in the posterior pole. Chorioretinal atrophy was seen in 64 subjects (19.3%) in our study. This number is lower than in the Japanese study, where diffuse chorioretinal atrophy was seen in 491 eyes (60.9%) and patchy chorioretinal atrophy in 163 eyes (20.2%) (Hayashi et al., 2010). The difference is mainly attributable to higher refractive error among the Japanese subjects from a high myopia clinic. Of our subjects with greater than -6.00 D of myopic refractive error, 42.3% had refractive error greater than -8.00 D, and within this subgroup, 39.0% had chorioretinal atrophy. Chorioretinal atrophy is also more prevalent in older adults and in adults with more severe refractive error and longer axial length. In the Beijing Eye Study, increased prevalence of myopic chorioretinopathy was associated with increasing myopic refractive error, and a significant rate of progression was seen even at 5 years (Liu et al., 2010). Posterior staphyloma was reported to be a causative factor for chorioretinal atrophy (Hayashi et al., 2010). However, the correlation between posterior staphyloma and chorioretinal atrophy was not high, possibly because of the small number of cases in our study.

Lacquer cracks were identified in only 6 subjects (1.8%), but more so in those with higher myopic refractive error (P< .001) and longer AL (P = .04) (Chang et al., 2013). This suggests that these breaks in the Bruch membrane are highly associated with advanced myopia and axial elongation.

Peripapillary atrophy was the most common finding associated with the myopic fundus among adults (Chang et al., 2013), observed in 268 subjects (81.2%). Optic disc tilting is thought to be more common in those with astigmatism or high refractive error, particularly myopia (Vongphanit et al., 2002(b)). Disc tilt was observed in 190 subjects (57.4%) among Singapore adults (Chang et al., 2013). A smaller cup-to-disc ratio, another optic disc feature associated with high myopia, was also observed in subjects with higher myopic refractive error (Chang et al., 2013), corroborating findings by Wu and associates (Wu et al., 2011),

Jonas and Dichtl (Jonas and Dichtl, 1997), Xu and associates (Xu et al., 2007), and Nonaka and associates (Nonaka et al., 2011).

References

Abdel-Latif S. Macular hole with central retinal detachment in high myopia with posterior staphyloma. *Br J Ophthalmol* 1969;53:62-63.

Akiba J, Konno S, Sato E, et al: Retinal detachment and retinoschisis detected by optical coherence tomography in a myopic eye with a macular hole. *Ophthalmic Surg Lasers* 2000;31:240-242.

Akiba J, Konno S, Yoshida A. Retinal detachment associated with a macular hole in severely myopic eyes. *Am J Ophthalmol* 1999;128:654–655.

Akyol N, Kukner AS, Ozdemir T, Esmerligil S. Choroidal and retinal blood flow changes in degenerative myopia. *Can J Ophthalmol* 1996; 31: 113–119.

Araie M, Sekine M, Suzuki Y, Koseki N. Factors contributing to the progression of visual field damage in eyes with normal tension glaucoma. *Ophthalmology* 1994;101(8):1440–1444.

Asakuma T, Yasuda M, Ninomiya T, et al. Prevalence and risk factors for myopic retinopathy in a Japanese population: the Hisayama Study. *Ophthalmology* 2012;119(9):1760–1765.

Asakuma T, Yasuda M, Ninomiya T, Noda Y, Arakawa S, Hashimoto S, Ohno-Matsui K, Kiyohara Y, Ishibashi T. d risk factors for myopic retinopathy in a Japanese population. The Hisayama Study. *Ophthalmology* 2012; 119:1760-1765.

Atchison DA, Schmid KL, Pritchard N. Neural and optical limits to visual performance in myopia. *Vision Res* 2006;46: 3707–3722.

Aung T, Foster PJ, Seah SK, et al. Automated static perimetry: the influence of myopia and its method of correction. *Ophthalmology* 2001;108:290–295.

Austin KL, Palmer JR, Seddon JM, et al. Case-control study of idiopathic retinal detachment. *Int J Epidemiol* 1990;19:1045–1050.

Avila MP, Weiter JJ, Jalkh AE, Trempe CL, Pruett RC, Schepens CL. Natural history of choroidal neovascularization in degenerativemyopia. *Ophthalmology* 1984;91(12):1573–1581.

Avisar R, Friling R, Snir M, et al. Estimation of prevalence and incidence rates and causes of blindness in Israel, 1998-2003.*Isr Med Assoc J* 2006;8:880–881.

Axer-Siegel R, Cotlear D, Priel E, Rosen blatt I, Snir M, Weinberger D. Indocyanine green angiography in high myopia. *Ophthalmic Surg Lasers Imaging* 2004; 35: 139–145.

Baba T, Hirose A, Kawazoe Y, et al. Optical coherence tomography for retinal detachment with a macular hole in a highly myopic eye. *Ophthalmic Surg Lasers Imaging* 2003; 34: 483-484.

Baba T, Ohno-Matsui K, Futagami S, et al. Prevalence and characteristics of foveal retinal detachment without macular hole in high myopia. *Am J Ophthalmol* 2003;135:338 -342.

Baba T, Ohno-Matsui K, Futagami S, Yoshida T, Yasuzumi K, Kojima A, Tokoro T, Mochizuki M. Prevalence and characteristics of foveal retinal detachment without macular hole in high myopia. *Am J Ophthalmol* 2003; 135(3): 338-342

Baba T, Ohno-Matsui K, Yoshida T, Yasuzumi K, Futagami S, Tokoro T, et al: Optical coherence tomography of choroidal neovascularization in high myopia. *Acta Ophthalmol Scand* 2002; 80: 82-87.

Bando H, Ikuno Y, Choi JS, Tano Y, Yamanaka I, Ishibashi T. Ultrastructure of internal limiting membrane in myopic foveoschisis. *Am J Ophthalmol* 2005;139(1):197-199

Bansal AS, Hubbard GB, 3rd. Peripheral retinal findings in highly myopic children,or =10 years of age. Retina 2010;30(Suppl.):S15–S19.

Benhamou N, Massin P, Haouchine B, Erginay A, Gaudric A. Macular retinoschisis in highly myopic eyes. *Am J Ophthalmol* 2002;133 (6):794-800

Blach RK, Jay B, Kolb H. Electrical activity of the eye in high myopia. *Br J Ophthalmol* 1966;50:629-641.

Brancato R, Trabucchi G, Introini U, Avanza P, Pece A: Indocyanine green angiography (ICGA) in pathological myopia. *Eur J Ophthalmol* 1996; 6: 39-43.

Buch H, Vinding T, La Cour M, et al. Prevalence and causes of visual impairment and blindness among 9980 Scandinavian adults: the Copenhagen City Eye Study. *Ophthalmology* 2004;111:53-61.

Cedrone C, Culasso F, Cesareo M, et al. Incidence of blindness and low vision in a sample population: the Priverno Eye Study, Italy. *Ophthalmology* 2003;110:584-588.

Cedrone C, Nucci C, Scuderi G, Ricci F, Cerulli A, Culasso F. Prevalence of blindness and low vision in an Italian population: a comparison with other European studies. *Eye* 2006; 20(6):661-667.

Celorio JM, Pruett RC. Prevalence of lattice degeneration and its relation to axial length in severe myopia. *Am J Ophthalmol* 1991;111:20-23.

Chang L, Pan C-W, Ohno-Matsui K, Lin X, Cheung GCM, Gazzard G, Koh V, Hamzah H, Tai ES, Lim SC, Mitchell P, Young TL, Aung T, Wong T-Y, Saw S-M. Myopia-related fundus changes in Singapore adults with high myopia. *Am J Ophthalmol* 2013; 155:991-999.

Chen H, Wen F, Li H, et al. The types and severity of high myopic maculopathy in Chinese patients. *Ophthalmic Physiol Opt* 2012;32(1):60-67.

Chen SJ, Cheng CY, Li AF, et al. Prevalence and associated risk factors of myopic maculopathy in elderly Chinese: the Shihpai eye study. *Invest Ophthalmol Vis Sci* 2012;53(8): 4868-4873.

Cho H, Choi A, Kang SW. Effect of internal limiting membrane removal in treatment of retinal detachment caused by myopic macular hole. *Korean J Ophthalmol* 2004;18(2):141-147

Chou SC, Yang CH, Lee CH, et al. Characteristics of primary rhegmatogenous retinal detachment in Taiwan. *Eye* 2007;21:1056-1061.

Chui TY, Song H, Burns SA. Individual variations in human cone photoreceptor packing density: variations with refractive error. *Invest Ophthalmol Vis Sci* 2008;49:4679-4687.

Chui TY, Yap MK, Chan HH, Thibos LN. Retinal stretching limits peripheral visual acuity in myopia. *Vision Res* 2005;45: 593-605.

Cohen SY, Laroche A, Leguen Y, Soubrane G, Coscas GJ. Etiology of choroidal neovascularization in young patients. *Ophthalmology* 1996; 103:1241-1244.

Coletta NJ, Watson T. Effect of myopia on visual acuity measured with laser interference fringes. *Vision Res* 2006;46: 636-651.

Cotter SA, Varma R, Ying-Lai M, Azen SP, Klein R. Los Angeles Latino Eye Study Group. Causes of low vision and blindness in adult Latinos: the Los Angeles Latino Eye Study. *Ophthalmology* 2006;113(9):1574-1582.

Curcio CA, Saunders PL, Younger PW, Malek G. Peripapillary chorioretinal atrophy: Bruch's membrane changes and photoreceptor loss. *Ophthalmology*. 2000;107:334-343.

Curtin BJ, Iwamoto T, Renaldo DP. Normal and staphylomatous sclera of high myopia: an electron microscopic study. *Arch Ophthalmol* 1979;97:912-915.

Curtin BJ, Karlin DB. Axial length measurements and fundus changes of the myopic eye. I. The posterior fundus. *Trans Am Ophthalmol Soc* 1970;68:312-334.

Curtin BJ, Karlin DB. Axial length measurements and fundus changes of the myopic eye. *Am J Ophthalmol* 1971;71:42-53.

Curtin BJ, Teng CC. Scleral changes in pathological myopia. Trans Am Acad Ophthalmol Otolaryngol 1958;62:777-790.

Daubs J. Environmental factors in the epidemiology of malignant myopia. *Am J Optom Physiol Opt* 1982;59(3):271-277.

Daubs JG. Some geographic, environmental and nutritive concomitants of malignant myopia. *Ophthalmic Physiol Opt* 1984;4(2):143-149.

Dichtl A, Jonas JB, Naumann GO. Histomorphometry of the optic disc in highly myopic eyes with glaucoma. *Br J Ophthalmol* 1998;82(3):286 -289.

Evans JR, Fletcher AE, Wormald RP. MRC Trial of Assessment and Management of Older People in the Community. Causes of visual impairment in people aged 75 years and older in Britain: an add-on study to the MRC Trial of Assessment and Management of Older People in the Community. *Br J Ophthalmol* 2004;88:365-370.

Fantes FE, Anderson DR. Clinical histologic correlation of human peripapillary anatomy. *Ophthalmology* 1989;96:20-25.

Forte R, Pascotto F, Cennamo G, de Crecchio G. Evaluation of peripapillary detachment in pathologic myopia with en face optical coherence tomography. *Eye* (London) 2008; 22(1):158-161.

Forte R, Pascotto F, de Crecchio G. Visualization of vitreomacular tractions with en face optical coherence tomography. *Eye* (London) 2007;21(11):1391-1394.

Forte R, Pascotto F, Napolitano F, Cennamo G, de Crecchio G. En face optical coherence tomography of macular holes in high myopia. *Eye* 2007;21:436-437.

Forte R, Pascotto F, Soreca E, Cusati G, de Crecchio G. Posterior retinal detachment without macular hole in high myopia: visualization with en face optical coherence tomography. *Eye* 2007;21:111-113.

Freund KB, Ciardella AP, Yannuzzi LA, et al. Peripapillary detachment in pathologic myopia. *Arch Ophthalmol* 2003; 121:197-204.

Fujiwara A, Shiragami C, Shirakata Y, et al. Enhanced depth imaging spectral-domain optical coherence tomography of subfoveal choroidal thickness in normal Japanese eyes. *Jpn J Ophthalmol* 2012;56:230-235.

Fujiwara T, Imamura Y, Margolis R, Slakter JS, Spaide RF: Enhanced depth imaging optical coherence tomography of the choroid in highly myopic eyes. *Am J Ophthalmol* 2009; 148: 445-450.

Gao LQ, Liu W, Liang YB, et al. Prevalence and characteristics of myopic retinopathy in a rural Chinese adult population: the Handan Eye Study. *Arch Ophthalmol* 2011;129(9):1199-1204.

Gass JDM (ed). Stereoscopic Atlas of Macular Disease. St Louis, *Mosby* Co, 1997.

Gaucher D, Haouchine B, Tadayoni R, et al. Long-term follow-up of high myopic foveoschisis: natural course and surgical outcome. *Am J Ophthalmol* 2007;143:455- 462.

Ghafour I, Allan D, Foulds W. Common causes of blindness and visual handicap in the west of Scotland. *Br J Ophthalmol* 1986; 67: 209-213.

Ghafour IM, Allan D, Foulds WS. Common causes of blindness and visual handicap in the west of Scotland. Br J Ophthalmol 1983;67:209 -213.

Gimbel HV. The control of myopia with atropine. *Can J Ophthalmol* 1973;8:527-532.

Goldschmidt E, Fledelius HC. High myopia progression and visual impairment in a nonselected group of Danish 14-year-olds followed over 40 years. *Optom Vis Sci* 2005;82:239-243.

Green WR, Wilson DJ. Choroidal neovascularization. *Ophthalmology* 1986;93(9):1169 - 1176.

Grossniklaus H, Green W. Pathologic findings in pathologic myopia. *Retina* 1992; 12: 127-133.

Hampton GR, Kohen D, Bird AC. Visual prognosis of disciform degeneration in myopia. *Ophthalmology* 1983; 90: 923-926.

Hayashi K, Hayashi H. Intravitreal versus retrobulbar injections of triamcinolone for macular edema associated with branch retinal vein occlusion. *Am J Ophthalmol* 2005;139(6):972-982.

Hayashi K, Ohno-Matsui K, Shimada N, Moriyama M, Kojima A, Hayashi W, et al. Long-term pattern of progression of myopic maculopathy: a natural history study. *Ophthalmology* 2010; 117: 1595-1611.

Hayashi K, Ohno-Matsui K, Yoshida T, Kobayashi K, Kojima A, Shimada N, Yasuzumi K, Futagami S, Tokoro T, Mochizuki M. Characteristics of patients with a favorable natural course of myopic choroidal neovascularization. *Graefes Arch Clin Exp Ophthalmol* 2005; 243:13-19.

Hirakata A, Hida T. Vitrectomy for myopic posterior retinoschisis or foveal detachment. Jpn J Ophthalmol 2006; 50: 53-61.

Hirata A, Negi A. Morphological changes of choriocapillaris in experimentally induced chick myopia. *Graefes Arch Clin Exp Ophthalmol* 1998; 236: 132-137.

Ho M, Liu NTL, Chan VCK, Lam DSC. Choroidal thickness measurement in myopic eyes by enhanced depth optical coherence tomography. *Ophthalmology* 2013; 120:1909-1914.

Hotchkiss ML, Fine SL. Pathologic myopia and choroidal neovascularization. *Am J Ophthalmol* 1981;91(2):177-183.

Hsiang HW, Ohno-Matsui K, Shimada N, et al. Clinical characteristics of posterior staphyloma in eyes with pathologic myopia. *Am J Ophthalmol* 2008;146:102-110.

Hsu WM, Cheng CY, Liu JH, Tsai SY, Chou P. Prevalence and causes of visual impairment in an elderly Chinese population in Taiwan: the Shihpai Eye Study. *Ophthalmology* 2004; 111:62-69

Hu DN. Prevalence and mode of inheritance of major genetic eye diseases in China. *J Med Genet* 1987;24(10):584-588.

Hussain A, Hussain N, Nutheti R. Comparison of mean macular thickness using optical coherence tomography and visual acuity in diabetic retinopathy. *Clin Experiment Ophthalmol* 2005; 33:240-245.

Ichibe M, Baba E, Funaki S, Yoshizawa T, Abe H. Retinoschisis in a highly myopic eye without vision impairment. *Retina* 2004;24:331–333.

Ichibe M, Yoshizawa T, Murakami K, et al. Surgical management of retinal detachment associated with myopic macular hole: anatomic and functional status of the macula. *Am J Ophthalmol* 2003;136:277-284.

Ikuno Y, Gomi F, Tano Y. Potent retinal arteriolar traction as a possible cause of myopic foveoschisis. *Am J Ophthalmol* 2005;139(3):462-467

Ikuno Y, Jo Y, Hamasaki T, Tano Y. Ocular risk factors for choroidal neovascularization in pathologic myopia. *Invest Ophthalmol Vis Sci* 2010;51(7):3721-3725.

Ikuno Y, Sayanagi K, Ohji M, et al. Vitrectomy and internal limiting membrane peeling for myopic foveoschisis. *Am J Ophthalmol* 2004;137:719 -724.

Ikuno Y, Sayanagi K, Oshima T, et al. Optical coherence tomographic findings of macular holes and retinal detachment after vitrectomy in highly myopic eyes. *Am J Ophthalmol* 2003; 136:477-481.

Ikuno Y, Tano Y: Retinal and choroidal biometry in highly myopic eyes with spectral-domain optical coherence tomography. *Invest Ophthalmol Vis Sci* 2009; 50: 3876-3880.

Ishida S, Yamazaki K, Shinoda K, Kawashima S, Oguchi Y. Macular hole retinal detachment in highly myopic eyes: ultrastructure of surgically removed epiretinal membrane and clinicopathologic correlation. *Retina* 2000,20(2):176-183

Ito A, Kawabata H, Fujimoto N, Adachi-Usami E. Effect of myopia on frequency-doubling perimetry. *Invest Ophthalmol Vis Sci* 2001;42:1107-1110.

Iwase A, Araie M, Tomidokoro A, et al. Prevalence and causes of low vision and blindness in a Japanese adult population: the Tajimi Study. *Ophthalmology* 2006;113:1354-1362.

Jacobi FK, Pusch CM. A decade in search of myopia genes. *Front Biosci* 2010; 15:359-372

Johnson MW. Myopic traction maculopathy: pathogenic mechanisms and surgical treatment. *Retina* 2012;32(Suppl 2): S205-S210.

Jonas JB, Berenshtein E, Holbach L. Anatomic relationship between lamina cribrosa, intraocular space, and cerebrospinal fluid space. Invest Ophthalmol Vis Sci 2003;44:5189 -5195.

Jonas JB, Budde WM, Panda-Jonas S. Ophthalmoscopic evaluation of the optic nerve head. *Surv Ophthalmol* 1999;43:293-320.

Jonas JB, Dichtl A. Optic disc morphology in myopic primary open-angle glaucoma. *Graefes Arch Clin Exp Ophthalmol* 1997;235(10):627-633.

Jonas JB, Fernandez MC, Naumann GO. Parapapillary atrophy and retinal vessel diameter in non-glaucomatous optic nerve damage. *Invest Ophthalmol Vis Sci* 1991;32:2942-2947.

Jonas JB, Gusek GC, Naumann GO. Optic disk morphometry in high myopia. *Graefes Arch Clin Exp Ophthalmol* 1988;226(6):587–590.

Jonas JB, Konigsreuther KA, Naumann GO. Optic disc histomorphometry in normal eyes and eyes with secondary angle-closure glaucoma. II. Parapapillary region. *Graefes Arch Clin Exp Ophthalmol* 1992;230:134-139. [PubMed: 1577293]

Jonas JB, Naumann GO. Parapapillary chorioretinal atrophy in normal and glaucoma eyes: II, correlations. *Invest Ophthalmol Vis Sci* 1989;30:919-926.

Jonas JB, Nguyen XN, Gusek GC, Naumann GO. Parapapillary chorioretinal atrophy in normal and glaucoma eyes, I: morphometric data. *Invest Ophthalmol Vis Sci* 1989;30:908-918.

Jonas JB, Ohno-Matsui K, Spaide RF, et al. Macular Bruch's membrane defects and axial length: associated with gamma zone and delta zone in parapapillary region. Invest Ophthalmol Vis Sci 2013;54:1295-1302.

Jonas JB, Xu L. Optic disc morphology in eyes after nonarteritic anterior ischemic optic neuropathy. *Invest Ophthalmol Vis Sci* 1993;34:2260-2265.

Jonas SB, Jonas RA, Holbach L, Panda-Jonas S. Histology of the Parapapillary Region in High Myopia. *Am J Ophthalmol* 2011;152:1021-1029.

Karlin DB, Curtin BJ. Peripheral chorioretinal lesions and axial length of the myopic eye. *Am J Ophthalmol* 1976;81:625-635.

Kawabata H, Adachi-Usami E. Multifocal electroretinogram in myopia. *Invest Ophthalmol Vis Sci* 1997;38:2844-2851.

Kempen JH, Mitchell P, Lee KE, Tielsch JM, Broman AT, Taylor HR, Ikram MK, Congdon NG, O'Colmain BJ. The prevalence of refractive errors among adults in the United States, Western Europe, and Australia. Arch Ophthalmol 2004; 122:495-505

Khan SA. A retrospective study of low-vision cases in an Indian tertiary eye-care hospital. *Indian J Ophthalmol* 2000; 48(3):201-207.

Kim TW, Kim M, Weinreb RN, Woo SJ, Park KH, Hwang JM. Optic disc change with incipient myopia of childhood. *Ophthalmology* 2012;119:21-26.

Kitaguchi Y, Bessho K, Yamaguchi T, et al. In vivo measurements of cone photoreceptor spacing in myopic eyes from images obtained by an adaptive optics fundus camera. Jpn J Ophthalmol 2007;51:456-461.

Klaver CC, Wolfs RC, Vingerling JR, et al. Age-specific prevalence and causes of blindness and visual impairment in an older population: the Rotterdam Study. *Arch Ophthalmol* 1988;116:653-658.

Klaver CC, Wolfs RC, Vingerling JR, Hofman A, de Jong PT. Age-specific prevalence and causes of blindness and visual impairment in an older population: the Rotterdam Study. *Arch Ophthalmol* 1998;116(5):653-658.

Klein RM, Curtin BJ. Lacquer crack lesions in pathologic myopia. *Am J Ophthalmol* 1975;79:386-392.

Kobayashi K, Ohno-Matsui K, Kojima A, et al. Fundus characteristics of high myopia in children. *Jpn J Ophthalmol* 2005;49:306-311.

Kojima A, Ohno-Matsui K, Teramukai S, Yoshida T, Ishihara Y, Kobayashi K, Shimada N, Yasuzumi K, Futagami S, Tokoro T, Mochizuki M. Factors associated with the development of chorioretinal atrophy around choroidal neovascularization in pathologic myopia. *Graefes Arch Clin Exp Ophthalmol* 2004; 242:114-119.

Kora Y, Nishimura E, Kitazato T, et al. Analysis of preoperative factors predictive of visual acuity in axial myopia.*J Cataract Refract Surg* 1998;24:834-839.

Krumpaszky HG, Lüdtke R, Mickler A, et al. Blindness incidence in Germany. A population-based study from Württemberg-Hohenzollern. *Ophthalmologica* 1999;213:176-182.

Kubota T, Jonas JB, Naumann GOH. Direct clinico-histological correlation of parapapillary chorioretinal atrophy. *Br J Ophthalmol* 1993;77:103-106.

Kuhn F. Internal limiting membrane removal for macular detachment in highly myopic eyes. *Am J Ophthalmol* 2003;135(4):547-549

Lai TY, Fan DS, Lai WW, Lam DS. Peripheral and posterior pole retinal lesions in association with high myopia: a crosssectional community-based study in Hong Kong. *Eye* (Lond) 2008;22:209-213.

Lee KYC, Tomidokoro A, Sakata R, Konno S, Mayama C, Saito H, Hayash Ki, Iwase A, Araie M. Cross-sectional Anatomic Configurations of Peripapillary Atrophy Evaluated with Spectral Domain-Optical Coherence Tomography. *Invest Ophthalmol Vis Sci* 2010;51:666-671 doi:10.1167/iovs.09-3663

Leveziel N, Caillaux V, Bastuji-Garin S, et al. Angiographic and optical coherence tomography characteristics of recent myopic choroidal neovascularization. *Am J Ophthalmol* 2013;155:913-919.

Liang YB, Friedman DS, Wong TY, et al; Handan Eye Study Group. Prevalence and causes of low vision and blindness in a rural Chinese adult population: the Handan Eye Study. *Ophthalmology* 2008;115:1965-1972.

Liu HH, Xu L, Wang YX, Wang S, You QS, Jonas JB. Prevalence and progression of myopic retinopathy in Chinese adults: the Beijing Eye Study. *Ophthalmology* 2010;117(9):1763-1768.

Luu CD, Lau AM, Lee SY. Multifocal electroretinogram in adults and children with myopia. *Arch Ophthalmol* 2006;124:328-334.

Macdonald AE. Causes of blindness in Canada: an analysis of 24,605 cases registered with the Canadian National Institute for the Blind. *Can Med Assoc J* 1965;92:264-279.

Manjunath V, Shah H, Fujimoto JG, Duker JS. Analysis of peripapillary atrophy using Spectral Domain Optical Coherence Tomography. *Ophthalmology* 2011 March ; 118(3): 531-536. doi:10.1016/j.ophtha.2010.07.013

Margolis R, Spaide RF. A pilot study of enhanced depth imaging optical coherence tomography of the choroid in normal eyes. *Am J Ophthalmol* 2009; 147: 811-815.

Marr JE, Halliwell-Ewen J, Fisher B, et al. Associations of high myopia in childhood. *Eye* (Lond) 2001;15(Pt 1):70-74.

Maruko I, Iida T, Sugano Y, et al. Morphologic analysis in pathologic myopia using high-penetration optical coherence tomography. *Invest Ophthalmol Vis Sci* 2012; 53:3834-3838.

Matsumura N, Ikuno Y, Tano Y. Posterior vitreous detachment and macular hole formation in myopic foveoschisis. *Am J Ophthalmol* 2004; 138(6):1071-1073

McBrien NA, Norton TT. Prevention of collagen crosslinking increases form deprivation myopia in tree shrew. *Exp Eye Res* 1994;59:475- 486.

Menchini U, Brancato R, Virgili G, et al. Unilateral macular retinoschisis with stellate foveal appearance in two females with myopia. *Ophthalmic Surg Lasers* 2000;31:229-232.

Mirza RG, Johnson MW, MD, Jampol LM. Optical coherence tomography use in evaluation of the vitreoretinal interface: a review. *Surv Ophthalmol* 2007; 52:397-421.

Mitry D, Charteris DG, Yorston D, et al. The epidemiology and socio-economic associations of retinal detachment in Scotland: A two-year prospective population-based study. *Invest Ophthalmol Vis Sci* 2010;51:4963-4968.

Mitry D, Zambarakji H. Recent trends in the management of maculopathy secondary to pathological myopia. *Graves Arch Clin Exp Ophthalmol* 2012:250:3-13.

Montero JA, Ruiz-Moreno JM. Treatment of choroidal neovascularization in high myopia. *Curr Drug Targets* 2010; 11(5):630-644.

Morgan IG, Ohno-Matsui K, Saw SM. Myopia. *Lancet* 2012; 379(9827):1739-1748.

Morgan IG. The biological basis of myopic refractive error. Clin Exp Optom 2003;86:276-88.

Morita H, Ideta H, Ito K, Yonemoto J, Sasaki K, Tanaka S. Causative factors of retinal detachment in macular holes. *Retina* 1991; 11:281-284

Moriyama M, Ohno-Matsui K, Futagami S, Yoshida T, Hayashi K, Shimada N, et al: Morphology and long-term changes of choroidal vascular structure in highly myopic eyes with and without posterior staphyloma. *Ophthalmology* 2007; 114: 1755-1762.

Nakanishi H, Yamada R, Gotoh N, et al.Agenome-wide association analysis identified a novel susceptible locus for pathological myopia at 11q24.1. *PLoS Genet* 2009;5(9):e1000660.

Nakazawa M, Kurotaki J, Ruike H. Long-term findings in peripapillary crescent formation in eyes with mild or moderate myopia. *Acta Ophthalmol* 2008;86:626-629.

Neelam K, Cheung CM, Ohno-Matsui K, Lai TY, Wong TY. Choroidal neovascularization in pathological myopia. *Prog Retin Eye Res* 2012;31(5):495-525.

Nonaka A, Hangai M, Akagi T, et al. Biometric features of peripapillary atrophy beta in eyes with high myopia. *Invest Ophthalmol Vis Sci* 2011;52(9):6706-6713.

Ohno H. Electron microscopic studies of myopic retinochoroidal atrophies. 1. Choroidal changes (in Japanese). *Folia Ophthalmol Jpn* 1983; 43: 1244-1253.

Ohno-Matsui K, Akiba M, Modegi T, et al. Association between shape of sclera and myopic retinochoroidal lesions in patients with pathologic myopia. *Invest Ophthalmol Vis Sci* 2012;7(53):6046-6061.

Ohno-Matsui K, Akiba M, Moriyama M, et al. Intrachoroidal cavitation in macular area of eyes with pathologic myopia. *Am J Ophthalmol* 2012;154:382-393.

Ohno-Matsui K, Hayashi K, Tokoro T, Mochizuki M. Detection of paravascular retinal cysts before using OCT in a highly myopic patient. *Graefes Arch Clin Exp Ophthalmol* 2006;244:642-644.

Ohno-Matsui K, Morishima N, Ito M, et al. Indocyanine-green angiographic findings of lacquer cracks in pathologic myopia. *Jpn J Ophthalmol* 1998; 42: 293-299.

Ohno-Matsui K, Yoshida T, Futagami S, et al. Patchy atrophy and lacquer cracks predispose to the development of choroidal neovascularisation in pathological myopia. *Br J Ophthalmol* 2003;87(5):570-573.

Oie Y, Ikuno Y, Fujikado T, Tano Y. Relation of posterior staphyloma in highly myopic eyes with macular hole and retinal detachment. *Jpn J Ophthalmol* 2005;49(6):530-532

Oshima Y, Ikuno Y, Motokura M, Nakae K, Tano Y. Complete epiretinal membrane separation in highly myopic eyes with retinal detachment resulting from a macular hole. *Am J Ophthalmol* 1998;126(5): 669-676

Pan CW, Wong TY, Lavanya R, et al. Prevalence and risk factors for refractive errors in Indians: the Singapore Indian Eye Study (SINDI). *Invest Ophthalmol Vis Sci* 2011;52(6): 3166-3173.

Panozzo G, Mercanti A. Optical coherence tomography findings in myopic traction maculopathy. *Arch Ophthalmol* 2004;122(10):1455-1460

Panozzo G, Mercanti A. Vitrectomy for myopic traction maculopathy. *Arch Ophthalmol* 2007;125(6):767-772

Park KH, Tomita G, Liou SY, Kitazawa Y. Correlation between peripapillary atrophy and optic nerve damage in normal-tension glaucoma. *Ophthalmology* 1996;103:1899-1906.

Phillips CI, Dobbie JG. Posterior staphyloma and retinal detachment. *Am J Ophthalmol* 1963;55:332-335.

Pi LH, Chen L, Liu Q, et al. Prevalence of eye diseases and causes of visual impairment in school-aged children in Western China. *J Epidemiol* 2012;22(1):37-44.

Polito A, Lanzetta P, Del Borrello M, Bandello F. Spontaneous resolution of a shallow detachment of the macula in a highly myopic eye. *Am J Ophthalmol* 2003;135(4):546-547

Povazay B, Hermann B, Unterhuber A, et al. Three-dimensional optical coherence tomography at 1050 nm versus 800 nm in retinal pathologies: enhanced performance and choroidal penetration in cataract patients. *J Biomed Opt* 2007;12: 041211.

Pruett R. Pathologic myopia; in Albert DM, Jakobiec JF (eds): Principles and Practice of Ophthalmology. Philadelphia, *Saunders Co,* 1994, pp 878-889.

Pruett RC. Complications associated with posterior staphyloma. *Curr Opin Ophthalmol* 1998;9:16 -22.

Quaranta M, Arnold J, Coscas G, Francais C, Quentel G, Kuhn D, et al: Indocyanine green angiographic features of pathologic myopia. *Am J Ophthalmol* 1996; 122: 663-671.

Ratiglia R, Osnaghi S, Bindella A, et al. Posterior traction retinal detachment in highly myopic eyes: clinical features and surgical outcome as evaluated by optical coherence tomography. *Retina* 2005;25:473-478.

Ren R, Jonas JB, Tian G, et al. Cerebrospinal fluid pressure in glaucoma: a prospective study. *Ophthalmology* 2010; 117(2):259 -266.

Ripandelli G, Parisi V, Friberg TR, et al. Retinal detachment associated with macular hole in high myopia: using the vitreous anatomy to optimize the surgical approach. *Ophthalmology* 2004; 111:726-731.

Ripandelli G, Rossi T, Scarinci F, Scassa C, Parisi V, Stirpe M. Macular vitreoretinal interface abnormalities in highly myopic eyes with posterior staphyloma: 5-year follow-up. *Retina* 2012;32(8):1531-1538.

Robichaud JL, Besada E, Basler L, Frauens BJ. Spectral domain optical coherence tomography of myopic traction maculopathy. *Ophthalmic Surg Lasers Imaging* 2011;82(10):607-173

Rockwood EJ, Anderson DR. Acquired peripapillary changes and progression in glaucoma. *Graefes Arch Clin Exp Ophthalmol* 1988;226:510-515.

Sainz-Gomez C, Fernandez-Robredo P, Salinas-Alaman A, et al. Prevalence and causes of bilateral blindness and visual impairment among institutionalized elderly people in Pamplona, Spain. *Eur J Ophthalmol* 2010;20(2):442-450.

Saw SM, Gazzard G, Shih-Yen EC, Chua WH. Myopia and associated pathological complications. *Ophthalmic Physiol Opt* 2005;25:381-391.

Saw SM. How blinding is pathological myopia? *Br J Ophthalmol* 2006; 90:525-526

Sayanagi K, Ikuno Y, Gomi F, et al. Retinal vascular microfolds in highly myopic eyes. Am J Ophthalmol 2005; 139: 658-663.

Sayanagi K, Ikuno Y, Gomi F, Tano Y. Retinal vascular microfolds in highly myopic eyes. *Am J Ophthalmol* 2005; 139:658-663.

Sayanagi K, Ikuno Y, Soga K, Tano Y: Photoreceptor inner and outer segment defects in myopic foveoschisis. *Am J Ophthalmol* 2008; 145: 902-908.

Sayanagi K, Ikuno Y, Tano Y. Tractional internal limiting membrane detachment in highly myopic eyes. *Am J Ophthalmol* 2006;142:850-852.

See JL, Nicolela MT, Chauhan BC. Rates of neuroretinal rim and peripapillary atrophy area change: a comparative study of glaucoma patients and normal controls. *Ophthalmology* 2009;116:840-847.

Shah M, Khan M, Khan MT, Khan MY, Saeed N. Causes of visual impairment in children with low vision. *J Coll Physicians Surg Pak* 2011;21(2):88-92.

Shih YF, Ho TC, Hsiao CK, Lin LL. Visual outcomes for high myopic patients with or without myopic maculopathy: a 10 year follow up study. *Br J Ophthalmol* 2006; 90:546-550

Shimada N, Ohno-Matsui K, Baba T, Futagami S, Tokoro T, Mochizuki M. Natural course of macular retinoschisis in highly myopic eyes without macular hole or retinal detachment. *Am J Ophthalmol* 2006;142 (3): 497-500

Shimada N, Ohno-Matsui K, Yoshida T, et al. Characteristics of peripapillary detachment in pathologic myopia. *Arch Ophthalmol* 2006;124:46 -52.

Shimada N, Tanaka Y, Tokoro T, Ohno-Matsui K. Natural course of myopic traction maculopathy and factors associated with progression or resolution. *Am J Ophthalmol* 2013; 156:948-957.

Smiddy WE, Kim SS, Lujan BJ, Gregori G. Myopic traction maculopathy: spectral domain optical coherence tomographic imaging and a hypothesized mechanism.*Ophthalmic Surg Lasers Imaging* 2009;40 (2):169-173

Soubrane G, Coscas GJ. Choroidal neovascular membranes in degenerative myopia. In: Ryan SJ (ed) Retina. *Mosby,* St Louis,1994 pp 1143-1157

Soubrane G. Choroidal neovascularization in pathologic myopia: recent developments in diagnosis and treatment. *Sur Ophthalmol* 2008;53 (2): 121-138

Spaide R, Koizumi H, Pozonni M: Enhanced depth imaging spectral-domain optical coherence tomography. *Am J Ophthalmol* 2008; 146: 496-500.

Spaide RF, Fisher Y. Removal of adherent cortical vitreous plaques without removing the internal limiting membrane in the repair of macular detachments in highly myopic eyes. *Retina* 2005;25(3): 290-295.

Spaide RF. Age-related choroidal atrophy. *Am J Ophthalmol* 2009;147:801-810. [PubMed:19232561]

Sperduto R, Seigel D, Roberts J, et al: Prevalence of myopia in the United States. *Arch Ophthalmol* 1983; 101: 405-407.

Steidl SM, Pruett RC. Macular complications associated with posterior staphyloma. *Am J Ophthalmol* 1997;123:181-187.

Stirpe M, Michels RG. Retinal detachment in highly myopic eyes due to macular holes and epiretinal traction. *Retina* 1990;10(2):113-114

Sun CB, Liu Z, Xue AQ, Yao K. Natural evolution from macular retinoschisis to full-thickness macular hole in highly myopic eyes. *Eye* (Lond) 2010;24(12): 1787-1791.

Takano M, Kishi S. Foveal retinoschisis and retinal detachment in severely myopic eyes with posterior staphyloma. *Am J Ophthalmol* 1999; 128(4):472-476

Tano Y. Pathologic myopia: where are we now? *Am. J Ophthalmol* 2002; 134:645-660

Teng CC, De Moraes CG, Prata TS, et al. Beta-zone parapapillary atrophy and the velocity of glaucoma progression. *Ophthalmolohy* 2010;117:909-915.

The Eye Disease Case-Control Study Group. Risk factors for idiopathic rhegmatogenous retinal detachment. *Am J Epidemiol* 1993;137:749-757.

Toranzo J, Cohen SY, Erginay A, Gaudric A. Peripapillary intrachoroidal cavitation in myopia. *Am J Ophthalmol* 2005;140:731-732.

Van Newkirk MR. The Hong Kong vision study: a pilot assessment of visual impairment in adults. *Trans Am Ophthalmol Soc* 1997;95:715-749.

Vance SK, Khan S, Klancnik JM, Freund KB: Characteristic spectral-domain optical coherence tomography findings of multifocal choroiditis. *Retina* 2011; 31: 717-723.

Vanderbeek BL, Johnson MW. The diversity of traction mechanisms in myopic traction maculopathy. *Am J Ophthalmol* 2012;153(1):93-102

Verteporfin in Photodynamic Therapy Study Group. Photodynamic therapy of subfoveal choroidal neovascularization in pathologic myopia with verteporfin. 1-year results of a randomized clinical trial–VIP report no. 1. *Ophthalmology* 2001; 108:841-852

Vongphanit J, Mitchell P, Wang JJ. Population prevalence of tilted optic disks and the relationship of this sign to refractive error. *Am J Ophthalmol* 2002;133(5):679-685.

Vongphanit J, Mitchell P, Wang JJ. Prevalence and progression of myopic retinopathy in an older population. *Ophthalmology* 2002;109:704-711.

Wang NK, Chen YP, Lai CC, et al. Paediatric retinal detachment: Comparison of high myopia and extreme myopia. *Br J Ophthalmol* 2009;93:650-655.

Wang NK, Lai CC, Chou CL, et al. Choroidal thickness and biometric markers for the screening of lacquer cracks in patients with high myopia. *PLoS One* [serial online] 2013;8:

Wang NK, Tsai CH, Chen YP, et al. Pediatric rhegmatogenous retinal detachment in East Asians. Ophthalmology 2005;112:1890-1895.

Wang Y, Xu L, Jonas JB. Prevalence and causes of visual field loss as determined by frequency doubling perimetry in urban and rural adult Chinese. *Am J Ophthalmol* 2006;141:1078-1086.

Westall CA, Dhaliwal HS, Panton CM, et al. Values of electroretinogram responses according to axial length. *Doc Ophthalmol* 2001;102:115-130.

Wolfensberger TJ, Gonvers M. Surgical treatment of retinal detachment owing to macular hole. *Semin Ophthalmol* 2000; 15:122-127.

Wong TY, Ferreira A, Hughes R, Carter G, Mitchell P. Epidemiology and disease burden of pathologic myopia and myopic choroidal neovascularization: An evidence-based systematic review. *Am J Ophthalmol* 2014;157:9-25.

Wong TY, Foster PJ, Hee J, et al. Prevalence and risk factors for refractive errors in adult Chinese in Singapore. *Invest Ophthalmol Vis Sci* 2000;41(9):2486-2494.

Wu HM, Seet B, Yap EP, et al. Does education explain ethnic differences in myopia prevalence? A population-based study of young adult males in Singapore. *Optom Vis Sci* 2001;78: 234-239.

Wu L, Sun X, Zhou X, Weng C. Causes and 3-year-incidence of blindness in Jing-An District, Shanghai, China 2001-2009. *BMC Ophthalmol* 2011;11:10.

Wu PC, Chen YJ, Chen YH, Chen CH, Shin SJ, Tsai CL, Kuo HK. Factors associated with foveoschisis and foveal detachment without macular hole in high myopia. *Eye (London)* 2009;23(2):356-361

Wu RY, Wong TY, Zheng YF, et al. Influence of refractive error on optic disc topographic parameters: the Singapore Malay eye study. *Am J Ophthalmol* 2011;152(1):81-86.

Yamada M, Hiratsuka Y, Roberts CB, Pezzullo ML, Yates K, Takano S, Miyake K, Taylor HR. Prevalence of visual impairment in the adult Japanese population by cause and severity and future projections. *Ophthalmic Epidemiol* 2010; 17:50-57.

Yamamoto I, Rogers AH, Reichel E, Yates PA, Duker JS. Intravitreal bevacizumab (Avastin) as treatment for subfoveal choroidal neovascularisation secondary to pathological myopia. *Br J Ophthalmol* 2007; 91:157-160.

Yamazaki Y, Yoshikawa K, Kunimatsu S, et al. Influence of myopic disc shape on the diagnostic precision of the Heidelberg Retina Tomograph. *Jpn J Ophthalmol* 1999;43:392-397.

Yoshida T, Ohno-Matsui K, Ohtake Y, Takashima T, Futagami S, Baba T, Yasuzumi K, Tokoro T, Mochizuki M. Long-term visual prognosis of choroidal neovascularization in high myopia: a comparison between age groups. *Ophthalmology* 2002; 109:712-719.

Yoshida T, Ohno-Matsui K, Yasuzumi K, Kojima A, Shimada N, Futagami S, Tokoro T, Mochizuki M. Myopic choroidal neovascularization: a 10-year follow-up. *Ophthalmology* 2003; 110:1297-1305

You QS, Peng XY, Xu L, Chen CX. Myopic maculopathy imaged by optical coherence tomography. The Beijing Eye Study. *Ophthalmology* 2014;121(1):220-224.

You QS, Xu L, Yang H, et al. Five-year incidence of visual impairment and blindness in adult. Chinese: the Beijing eye study. *Ophthalmology* 2011;118:1069-1075. Epub 2011.

Young TL, Metlapally R, Shay AE. Complex trait genetics of refractive error. *Arch Ophthalmol* 2007;125(1):38-48.

Chapter XI

Myopia and Management

Abstract

The purpose of managing a patient with myopia is to improve visual acuity, visual function, and visual comfort by correcting the refractive error when appropriate.

Goals (AAO, 2007)

- Determine the patient's visual needs
- Identify and quantify any amount of refractive errors
- Discuss with the patient the nature of the myopia, appropriate alternatives for correction, and the risks and benefits of each approach
- Inform patients, especially those with high myopia, about the potentially increased incidence of associated pathologic conditions
- Correct symptomatic refractive errors with eyeglasses, contact lenses, or surgery as desired by the informed patient and as deemed appropriate by the physician
- Provide the patient with follow-up care and management of any side effects or complications resulting from the correction provided

Patient Outcome Criteria (AAO, 2007)

Outcome criteria vary depending on the individual's needs, lifestyle, and overall medical condition. The goal is to provide vision that meets the patient's functional needs with minimal and tolerable side effects.

The need to correct refractive errors depends on the patient's symptoms and visual needs. Patients with low refractive errors may not require correction; small changes in refractive corrections in asymptomatic patients are generally not recommended. Correction options include eyeglasses, contact lenses, or refractive surgery. Various occupational and recreational requirements as well as personal preferences affect the specific choices for any individual patient.

1. Eyeglasses

Myopia has been known for more than 2000 years and was first described by the ancient Greeks (Donders, 1866; Hirschberg, 1985). However, despite the recorded use of convex lenses for presbyopia in the late 13th century in Florence, Italy, the correction of myopic refractive error had to await the development of concave lenses in the mid 16th century.

Eyeglasses are the simplest and safest means of correcting a refractive error, therefore eyeglasses should be considered before contact lenses or refractive surgery. A patient's eyeglasses and refraction should be evaluated whenever visual symptoms develop. Optimal eyeglass correction for higher refractive errors requires precision in fitting, especially with respect to the position of the optical center of each lens relative to the pupil. High-index lenses, which reduce the lenses' thickness and weight, are useful in correcting high refractive errors and providing increased comfort and better cosmetic appearance (AAO, 2007; Marcus and Rubin, 2006).

The principles and guidelines for correcting myopia with eyeglasses: individuals with asymptomatic myopia do not need eyeglass correction except for visually demanding activities like driving or school work. Overcorrecting myopic patients will cause excessive accommodation, which may create symptoms. Some patients may become symptomatic from an increased degree of myopia that occurs at low levels of illumination (night myopia), and they may require increased minus correction for clearer vision at night.

Because of the progressive nature of myopia in childhood and adolescence, screening examinations that include visual acuity are recommended every 1 to 2 years.

Difficulties and Complications of Eyeglass Wear

A variety of factors related to lenses and frames may cause difficulties in wearing eyeglasses. These include (AAO, 2007; Marcus and Rubin, 2006):

- Incorrect prescription
- Base curve and location of the cylinder on the front or back surface
- Bifocal power and segment position (height and size)
- Tint
- Anisometropia (if large)
- Prisms or prism effects
- Pantoscopic tilt
- Centration of lenses with respect to the pupil
- Vertex distance
- Size of frame and fit
- Contact sensitivity to frame material
- Change in lens material

In addition, the myopic lenses in the eyeglasses can cause spherical and chromatic aberrations, lens distortions and minification.

(Marcus and Rubin, 2006)

The provision of spectacles to correct vision is based on both science and art. Prescribing appropriate corrective lenses depends on the ability of the patient to adapt to change and the patient-specific relationship between accommodation and vergence (Marcus and Rubin, 2006).

Correction of Myopia with Spectacle Lenses: Basic Optics

The far point plane of the myopic eye is located at a certain distance in front of the eye and determines the degree of myopia. The greater the myopia, the closer the far point will be. A real object placed at that distance (far point plane) will be in sharp focus on the retina. Thus, an uncorrected myope can hold an object at the eye's far point plane and see it clearly. The term *nearsighted* is an accurate description of the myope's visual condition. By measuring the distance at which a nonaccommodating myope holds reading material, one can make a good estimation of the degree of myopia present. For example, if a presbyopic patient holds reading material at 20 cm, he is likely to be a 5D myope (Marcus and Rubin, 2006).

For the myope, all objects located further away than the far point plane will result in blurred retinal imagery. The far point plane for even low degrees of myopia will be relatively near to the patient; 1 meter away for 1D of myopia, 4 meters away for only 0.25D of myopia. This accounts for the difficulty even "low" myopes have in recognizing a friend's face from across the street. To be seen really clearly, the friend must be no further away than the far point plane.

By definition, the lens that corrects a given degree of myopia images an object at the far point plane of the eye. A "minus" lens, a lens that diverges light, is necessary to accomplish this task. From objects at a distance, parallel light rays traveling from left to right will encounter the minus lens, the light rays will be diverged, and a virtual image will be formed to the left of the lens, at the lens' secondary focal point. When that point is located at the far point plane of the eye, that minus lens will "correct" the myopia. Again, minus lenses of different powers can correct this eye as long as each is placed at the necessary vertex distance to keep its secondary focal point precisely positioned at the eye's far point plane. Each will have the same optical effectivity, and therefore, any of them may be used to correct this myopic eye. The closer to the eye the corrective lens is placed, the less divergence power it needs to allow its secondary focal plane to be coincident with the eye's far point plane, therefore necessitating a weaker minus corrective lens. Obviously, a contact lens will not need to be as strong as the corresponding spectacle lens to correct the same degree of myopia. Because of the small difference in power induced by changes in vertex distance in low refractive errors, it is not typically necessary to make corresponding prescriptive changes unless the myopia is 4D or greater (Marcus and Rubin, 2006).

Full Versus Partial Correction of Myopia

To create a truly clear retinal image of a distant object, the full extent of myopia must be corrected. However, several issues need to be considered. First, the length of the examination room is significantly shorter than infinity. So, when refractions are performed without cycloplegia, a slight undercorrection of the full myopia may result, but this is typically no more than 0.25D. This 0.25D discrepancy may be irrelevant, but it depends on the individual's tolerance for blur and his or her visual requirements. Usually for myopes, prescribing the actual refractive findings will be sufficient to improve vision satisfactorily (Marcus and Rubin, 2006).

Another factor is night myopia, which results from a reduction in contrast induced by low illumination. This causes the patient's focus to drift toward a “resting” level of accommodation that is not zero, thus inducing some degree of residual myopia. In such patients, this increase in myopia may be symptomatic, and patients may report blurred vision or halos around lights at night. Symptomatic night myopia requires correction, such as wearing nighttime driving glasses to correct 0.50D to 1.50D more than the degree of myopia you identify during your office refraction (Milder and Rubin, 2004).

Yet another prescribing consideration involves the patient's visual needs. A myope who is bedridden, for example, and infrequently leaves her home may not have a need for clear vision beyond a 10 ft distance. In addition, if the same patient is significantly presbyopic, undercorrecting the myopia may allow her to function comfortably with a bifocal instead of a trifocal or progressive power lens (Marcus and Rubin, 2006).

If a significantly myopic patient has never worn a correction before, prescribing the full correction may result in significant asthenopia. The patient may feel dizzy and uncomfortable and end up rejecting the glasses. In such cases, especially in older patients, partial correction of the myopia will likely dramatically improve vision, yet permit easier adaptation. It is a matter of clinical judgment whether or not to prescribe the full prescription to start with or, alternatively, to prescribe only a partial correction of the myopia. Either choice has the potential to provide a satisfactory visual result for the patient (Marcus and Rubin, 2006).

Myopic Progression and Spectacles

The topics of myopia progression and the effects of corrective lenses on this progression have been, and continue to be, hot topics for the ophthalmic community. Some think that the development of myopia is environmentally induced, and that excessive near work perhaps combined with accommodative or binocular dysfunctions are to blame. Such associations are supported in the literature (Goss, 1990; Parssinen et al., 1989). In such patients, many believe that what starts as accommodative spasm due to nearpoint stress may become imbedded into a permanent myopic condition. If this early stage of myopia is treated with “vision therapy” or orthoptic training instead of full myopic spectacle correction, this “pseudomyopia” might be reversible.

On the other hand, others believe that the development of refractive error is based on a hard-wired inheritance pattern, and that attempted manipulations to alter progression are not indicated. Several recent studies have found heredity to be the most important factor in the development of both juvenile and adult onset myopia (Mutti et al., 2002; Iribarren et al., 2002).

Numerous studies utilizing methods for influencing accommodation (bifocals and/or pharmaceutical agents) have been undertaken in an attempt to address the topic (Marcus and Rubin, 2006).

Effects of Spectacle Prescription on Accommodation

When prescribing spectacles, you should always consider how the refractive correction may affect the accommodative function of each patient, especially those with accommodative dysfunction or those with early or established presbyopia. A careless refractive exam may result in prescribing more minus than is actually needed, an especially common problem in the young, actively accommodating patient. Such overminused prescriptions will necessitate excess accommodative effort, especially during near tasks. Such accommodative stress may lead to asthenopia or even avoidance of near tasks such as reading. Particularly in the pediatric population (but actually important for all patients), a cycloplegic refraction is necessary to suppress accommodation during testing. As patient age increases and accommodative amplitude decreases, the negative impact of myopic overcorrection becomes even more marked. Such faulty prescribing may result in creating early presbyopia that erroneously requires premature prescription of multifocal lenses, much to the dismay of the patient. In fact, when early presbyopia occurs in a myope, we suggest you slightly undercorrect the myopia to delay the need for bifocals or progressives (Marcus and Rubin, 2006).

Presbyopia

Patients with presbyopia have several options for eyeglass correction: bifocals, trifocals, progressive addition lenses, or separate eyeglasses for distance and reading. Individuals with myopia must exert more accommodative effort when using contact lenses, or after refractive surgery, than when using eyeglasses. Individuals with hyperopia must exert more accommodative effort when using eyeglasses than contact lenses.

Effects of Spectacle Prescription on Binocularity

Because accommodation and binocularity are neurologically linked, one cannot regard one without the other. Because spectacles affect accommodation, the prescribing clinician needs to understand the resultant effects on binocularity, especially in patients with esophoria or esotropia. All esophoric and esotropic patients should first have a cycloplegic refraction to uncover any accommodative spasm or latent hyperopia, and then appropriate treatment with lenses should be instituted. Once corrective lenses restore binocularity at distance, additional plus power may need to be prescribed in the form of bifocal lenses to lessen accommodative demand and any induced esotropia at near. Whether uncorrected hyperopia or a high AC/A ratio is at fault in inducing the eso tendency, spectacle lenses are frequently helpful in restoring binocular function (Marcus and Rubin, 2006).

In contrast, inadvertent overcorrection of myopia or undercorrection of hyperopia may result in a significant iatrogenic esophoria. Obviously, this should be avoided.

In exophoria and exotropia, the overcorrection with plus lenses or the undercorrection with minus lenses will likely exacerbate the condition because accommodation is relaxed. Here, prescription of the least plus, or sometimes even an overcorrection with minus lenses, may help to restore proper binocular posture. By inducing a state in which the patient must actively use some amount of accommodation, the linked convergence is activated and may be sufficient to correct the dysphoria or strabismus (Marcus and Rubin, 2006).

Spectacle Design Considerations

The spectacle lens market, like most others, is driven by competition. As such, companies are continuously developing new and more desirable lens and frame materials to satisfy an ever-demanding public. Lens designs are being improved to provide better visual comfort and cosmesis. Newly available lenses and frames are more lightweight and comfortable. Instead of merely prescribing refractive findings, the clinician is in a prime position to recommend the best lens designs and materials (Marcus and Rubin, 2006).

Although lens weight and thickness have never posed a significant problem for patients with low refractive errors, historically those with significant degrees of refractive error have been quite encumbered by the very glasses they depended on. Over the last several decades, new lens materials, including high-index plastics, have emerged that have greatly improved lens appearance. Materials have been designed with protective qualities such as impact resistance and UV protection, allowing the clinician the opportunity to become active in promoting ophthalmic safety (Marcus and Rubin, 2006).

Polycarbonate and Trivex are plastic polymers that are excellent choices for correcting high refractive errors because they are lightweight and can be fabricated to very thin profiles. In addition, these materials have excellent impact resistance and inherent UV absorption, making them fine choices for children, for whom eye safety is a significant concern and who spend significant amounts of time out of doors. Choosing an impact-resistant material is equally important for patients who are monocular and those with hazardous vocations or avocations (Marcus and Rubin, 2006).

Proper lens design can also improve cosmetic and visual comfort. Aspheric lenses made with flatter base curves, thinner edge or center thicknesses, and decreased lens volumes facilitate the fabrication of thinner, lighter finished lenses. Frames are now made increasingly flexible, lightweight, durable, and with hypoallergenic materials, such as titanium and genium (Marcus and Rubin, 2006).

The prescribing clinician can now utilize both the art and science of refraction and choose from an arsenal of ophthalmic materials and designs, to provide a wide variety of products that correct vision both effectively and comfortably.

Prevention and management of traumatic fracture of eyeglasses consists of use of shatter resistant materials.

2. Contact Lenses

A contact lens can correct a wide range of refractive errors by replacing the cornea as the initial refractive surface of the eye. Soft hydrogel or rigid gas-permeable contact lenses are used most commonly, and silicone hydrogel contact lenses with greater oxygen transmissibility are more recently available. Polymethylmethacrylate (PMMA) contact lenses are now rarely used because of their limited oxygen transmissibility. Currently, approximately 36 million individuals in the United States successfully use contact lenses for visual correction (Barr, 2006). Although contact lenses are of great visual benefit, their use does carry some risk of ocular complications.

Indications

Contact lenses are most frequently used by patients who do not wish to wear eyeglasses. Many patients who use contact lenses note better field of vision, greater comfort, and/or an improved quality of vision. Some patients have special occupational needs that cannot be met by eyeglasses, and others prefer their appearance without eyeglasses. Some patients achieve optimal visual function only with contact lenses. These may include patients with high myopia, symptomatic anisometropia or aniseikonia, or an irregular corneal surface or shape.

Relative Contraindications

The use of contact lenses to correct refractive errors may not be advisable when there are significant eyelid, tear film, or ocular surface abnormalities related to keratoconjunctivitis sicca, blepharoconjunctivitis, acne rosacea, conjunctival cicatrization, corneal exposure, neurotrophic keratitis, or other corneal abnormalities. Other relative contraindications include use of topical corticosteroids, inflammation of the anterior segment, presence of a filtering bleb, poor hygiene, certain environmental or work settings (e.g., dust, volatile chemicals), a history of contact-lens-related corneal complications, limited dexterity, or inability to understand the risks and responsibilities involved. The risks of complications associated with contact lenses should be weighed against the protective benefit of eyeglasses for monocular or functionally monocular patients (AAO, 2007).

Complications

The most serious risk of contact lens use is the development of microbial keratitis, which can lead to visual loss even if properly treated (AAO, 2007). Other complications with all types of contact lens use include tarsal papillary conjunctivitis and bulbar conjunctival changes, epithelial keratopathy, corneal neovascularization, nonmicrobial infiltrates, and corneal warpage (Aquavella, 1987; Asbell and Wasserman, 1991; Allansmith et al., 1977; Donshik, 1994; Macsai et al., 1990). Endothelial changes can also occur, including polymegethism, pleomorphism, and, rarely, reduction of endothelial cell density (Macrae et al., 1986; Macrae et al., 1989; Macrae et al., 1994). While transient stromal edema frequently occurs, progressive corneal thinning of the epithelium and stroma during contact lens wear has also been reported (Liu and Pflugfelder, 2000). The clinical significance of these corneal changes is uncertain. The delivery of adequate oxygen to the cornea is of particular concern when contact lenses are used to correct high refractive errors because of increased contact lens thickness and potential contact lens movement problems.

Microbial keratitis is most frequently caused by bacteria, but can also be caused by more unusual organisms that are difficult to diagnose and treat such as *Acanthamoeba* and fungi (Baum and Barza, 1990; Koidou-Tsiligianni, 1989; Cohen et al., 1987; Wilson and Ahearn, 1986; Wilhelmus et al., 1988; Moore et al., 1985; Stehr-Green, 1989). An increase in the incidence of *Acanthamoeba* and fungal keratitis since 2004 has been noted. The etiology of this rise is currently being investigated (Acanthamoeba Keratitis multiple states, 2007; Alfonso et al., 2006; Bernal et al., 2006; Chang et al., 2006; Joslin et al., 2006; Joslin et al., 2007; Khor et al., 2006; Margolis and Whitcher, 2006; Thebpatiphat et al., 2007), but may be associated with limitations in the antimicrobial efficacy of some multipurpose solutions. An outbreak of *Fusarium* keratitis cases among contact lens users was reported in 2006 and was linked to a specific multipurpose contact lens care solution (Saw et al., 2007; Update – Fusarium keratitis, 2006).109,110 Another outbreak of *Acanthamoeba* keratitis was reported in 2007 and was linked to a specific multipurpose contact lens care solution (American Society of Cataract and refractive Surgery, 2007).

After the introduction of soft contact lenses for extended wear in the early 1980s, *Pseudomonas aeruginosa* became a frequently identified pathogen in cases of keratitis in individuals using extended wear contact lenses (Baum and Barza, 1990; Cohen et al., 1987). Investigations into the pathogenesis of *Pseudomonas* keratitis showed that *Pseudomonas aeruginosa* adhered readily to contact lens deposits (Stern et al., 1986). This was of concern since contact lenses develop more deposits with increasing duration of use. Other investigations demonstrated that the relative risk of ulcerative keratitis was 10 to 15 times greater in patients using soft contact lenses on an extended-wear basis compared with those using soft lenses for daily wear (Schein et al., 1989) and that extended-wear soft lens users had an annualized incidence five times that of daily-wear patients (21 vs. 4 per 10,000 persons) (Poggio et al.,1989).

Disposable soft contact lenses for extended wear were introduced in the late 1980s in an attempt to improve the safety of extended wear by allowing more frequent lens replacement. Disposable soft contact lenses for extended wear were eventually found to have the same incidence of ulcerative keratitis as conventional reusable soft lenses for overnight wear (Schein et al., 1994; Nilsson and Montan, 1994). It was the pattern of contact lens wear (overnight vs. daily) rather than the type of contact lens (disposable vs. nondisposable) that appeared to be the overriding risk factor for ulcerative keratitis (Schein et al., 1994; Nilsson and Montan, 1994). Although the incidence of ulcerative keratitis is similar whether disposable or conventional contact lenses are used for overnight wear, disposable lenses are more often associated with relatively benign peripheral infiltrates than with the aggressive central ulcerative keratitis that is common with conventional soft lenses used for overnight wear (Nilsson and Montan, 1994, Poggio and Abelson,1993; Nilsson and Montan, 1994). In cases where infectious keratitis does occur, disposable contact lenses for extended wear are more often associated with gram-positive organisms than with gram-negative organisms (Laibson et al., 1993; Maguen et al., 1991; Maguen et al., 1991; Cohen et al., 1996). Patients using disposable soft contact lenses for overnight wear are also less likely to be symptomatic in terms of discomfort or red eye complaints than patients using conventional reusable lenses for overnight wear (Poggio and Abelson, 1993).

Although disposable contact lenses were initially introduced for extended wear, they have become popular for daily wear as well. Patients who use disposable soft contact lenses on a daily-wear basis tend to be less symptomatic in terms of lens-related complaints when compared with conventional soft daily wear lens users (Poggio and Abelson). Disposable soft contact lenses intended for one day of use only (daily disposables) were introduced in 1995. Their use currently represents the safest method of soft contact lens wear (Suchecki et al., 2000). However, the parameters available for daily disposable contact lenses are somewhat more limited than disposable lenses intended for longer use or conventional reusable soft lenses.

Another important factor in the development of ulcerative keratitis with extended wear of contact lenses is corneal hypoxia. Investigators have shown that contact lenses of lower oxygen transmission are more likely to be associated with corneal epithelial binding of *Pseudomonas aeruginosa* than are higher oxygen transmissible lenses (Imayasu et al., 1994; Ren et al., 1999; Ren et al., 2002; Ladage et al., 2001). Soft silicone hydrogel contact lenses with extremely high gas transmission have now been developed for extended wear. A small percentage of patients who are fitted with these contact lenses developed sterile inflammatory peripheral corneal infiltrates (Nilsson, 2001). A study of patients using silicone hydrogel contact lenses continuously for up to 30 days concluded that the overall rate of microbial keratitis was similar to that of conventional extended wear soft lenses (Schein et al., 2005).

Selection and Fitting

Before contact lens fitting, an ocular history including past contact lens experience should be obtained and a comprehensive medical eye evaluation should be performed (American Academy of Ophthalmolgy Preferred Practice Patterns Committee. Preferred Practice Patterns Guidelines. Comprehensive Adult Medical Eye Evaluation, 2005; American Academy of Ophthalmolgy Preferred Practice Patterns Committee. Preferred Practice Patterns Guidelines. Pediatric Eye Evaluations, 2007). During this examination, particular attention should be directed at evaluating patient hygiene and the patient's ability to follow proper contact lens care as well as ocular parameters such as lid function, lid margins, meibomian glands, tear film, conjunctival surface, and the corneal surface.

Patient Education and Contact Lens Care

The United States Food and Drug Administration (FDA) has made the following recommendations for contact lens wearers regarding proper lens care practices (U.S. Food and Drug Administration, 2006):

- Wash hands with soap and water, and dry (lint-free method) before handling contact lenses.
- Wear and replace contact lenses according to the schedule prescribed by the doctor.
- Follow the specific contact lens cleaning and storage guidelines from the doctor and the solution manufacturer.
- Keep the contact lens case clean and replace every 3 to 6 months.
- Remove the contact lenses and consult your doctor immediately if you experience symptoms such as redness, pain, tearing, increased light sensitivity, blurry vision, discharge, or swelling.

When contact lenses are initially dispensed, patients should understand and practice contact lens insertion and removal. Contact lens cleaning and disinfection should be carefully explained, since improper care may be associated with complications of contact lens wear

(Nilsson and Montan, 1994 ;Bowden et al., 1989). Patients should be instructed to use only sterile products that are commercially prepared specifically for contact lens care and to replace these at the intervals recommended by the manufacturers (Acanthamoeba keratitis associated with contac lenses, 1986). Specifically, patients should be instructed not to rinse contact lenses or lens cases with nonsterile water, e.g., tap water, bottled water. Patients should also be instructed to clean and replace contact lens cases frequently because they can be a source of lens contamination (Bowden et al., 1989; Wilson et al.,1991). Patients should be instructed to replace the solution in contact lens cases each time the lenses are disinfected (i.e., old solution should not be "topped off").

Patients should be made aware that using contact lenses can be associated with the development of ocular problems, including microbial corneal ulcers that may be vision threatening, and that overnight wear of contact lenses is associated with an increased risk of ulcerative

Keratitis (Poggio et al., 1989; Mondino et al., 1986; Stehr-Green et al., 1987). The increased risk of ulcerative keratitis with extended contact lens wear should be discussed with patients who are considering this modality of vision correction (Poggio et al., 1989). If patients choose overnight wear, they should be instructed to use only lenses specifically approved for extended wear.

Swimming with contact lenses has been associated with the development of *Acanthamoeba* keratitis (Stehr-Green et al., 1987). Therefore, patients should be instructed to minimize water contact when wearing contact lenses and informed of the risks of wearing contact lenses while swimming or in a hot tub.

Directions for use of a no-rub solution require that a steady stream of the product be directed at the contact lens for a specific length of time. In general, however, rubbing the contact lenses during cleaning and rinsing with contact lens solution is considered by some experts to be a superior method of cleaning (American Society of Cataract and Refractive Surgery. Acanthamoeba Keratitis, 2007; Butcko et al., 2007).

Follow-Up Examination and Contact Lens Replacement

Initial contact lens fitting should include follow-up examinations to assess visual acuity, comfort, contact lens fit, and the effect of the contact lens health of the ocular surface before the fitting process is considered completed. First-time daily-wear or extended-wear contact lens users should be checked soon after the contact lenses are initially dispensed. Experienced contact lens users should generally be examined annually (AAO, 2007).

After contact lens fitting, follow-up examinations are important to promote safe lens wear. Patients should be questioned about problems such as irritation, redness, itching, discharge, decreased vision, or post-contact lens wear eyeglass blur. The patient's wear schedule and contact lens-care regimen should be reviewed. Visual acuity with the contact lenses should be checked, and the cause of any changes should be determined. The contact lenses themselves should be examined to make certain that they fit and wet well and are free of deposits or defects.

The external eye and cornea should also be evaluated in the follow-up examination. Findings of conjunctival injection, corneal edema, staining, infiltrates, changes at the superior limbus, or tarsal papillary conjunctivitis all indicate possible problems with contact lens wear.

The practitioner should examine patients for signs of corneal hypoxia including epithelial microcysts, epithelial edema, stromal thickening, corneal folds, corneal vascularization, and corneal warpage. If findings of corneal hypoxia are recognized, the contact lens fit, material, or wearing time should be adjusted to allow for better oxygenation of the cornea. Keratometry or corneal topography, and refraction without the contact lenses should be compared to initial readings in patients suspected of having corneal warpage (AAO, 2007).

The length of time a particular pair of contact lenses can be used will vary among individual patients. Rigid gas-permeable contact lenses are generally useful for 18 to 24 months, although the surface quality of these lenses may deteriorate more rapidly in some individuals. Conventional daily-wear soft contact lenses usually require replacement at least annually. Conventional extended-wear soft contact lenses often require replacement more frequently than once a year. Disposable soft contact lenses and silicone hydrogel lenses for daily wear or extended wear should be replaced according to the manufacturers' guidelines, which vary from 1 day to several months. The frequency of contact lens replacement should also be adjusted based on patient symptoms and findings at eye examinations. If a particular contact lens shows excessive deterioration or deposits, it should be replaced regardless of the length of wear (AAO, 2007).

3. Refractive Surgery for Myopia

The term refractive surgery describes various elective procedures that modify the refractive status of the eye. Procedures that involve altering the cornea are collectively referred to as keratorefractive surgery, refractive keratoplasty, or refractive corneal surgery. Other refractive surgery procedures include the placement of an intraocular lens (IOL) implant, either in front of the crystalline lens (phakic IOL) or in place of the crystalline lens (refractive lens exchange). Refractive surgery may be considered when a patient wishes to be less dependent on eyeglasses or contact lenses, or when there are occupational or cosmetic reasons not to wear eyeglasses. Keratorefractive surgery can be applied to a broad range of refractive errors, but in some circumstances, the surgeon may consider an intraocular procedure (AAO, 2007).

The surgical correction of myopia currently includes intraocular and corneal techniques that produce changes in corneal and total ocular refraction. For low myopia, keratorefractive surgeries such as photorefractive keratectomy, LASIK, and laser epithelia keratomileusis currently are the most popular techniques (El-Maghraby et al.,1999; Schallhorn et al.,2008; Sugar et al.,2002; Varley et al., 2004, Du et al., 2012).

Because of the possibility of contact-lens-induced corneal warpage and corneal edema, patients who use contact lenses should discontinue their use before the preoperative examination and procedure (Nourouzi et al., 2006). As a general guideline, spherical soft contact lenses should be discontinued for approximately 1 week (Nourouzi et al., 2006). Toric soft contact lenses and rigid contact lenses should be discontinued for a longer period because they are associated with a greater potential for corneal warpage and refractive instability. Particular attention should be paid to establishing refractive stability for these patients (AAO, 2007).

Corneal topography should be evaluated for evidence of irregular astigmatism, corneal warpage, or abnormalities suggestive of keratoconus or other corneal ectasias, because all may be associated with unpredictable refractive outcomes and the latter with progressive ectasia following surgery (Binder et al., 2005).

When astigmatism determined by subjective refraction differs significantly from astigmatism found by corneal topography, lenticular astigmatism is presumed to be the cause. Caution should be taken to identify early cataract formation in the presence of significant lenticular astigmatism. In this situation, lenticular refractive surgery may be the better option for the patient than corneal refractive surgery (AAO, 2007).

If irregular astigmatism is present, typically detected as reduced best corrected visual acuity (BCVA) using spherocylindrical lenses or identified on corneal topography, a wavefront measurement should be obtained to determine candidacy for a wavefront driven excimer laser ablation.

The central corneal thickness measurement should be obtained during the preoperative evaluation to identify unusually thin corneas and estimate residual stromal bed thickness. Corneas with central corneal thickness values less than 500 μm should be considered potentially abnormal. Photorefractive keratectomy corrections that result in a very thin residual stromal bed are associated with an increased risk for ectasia. In the case of laser in situ keratomileusis (LASIK) procedures, 250 μm has been suggested as a safe residual stromal bed thickness (Seiler et al., 1998), but there is no absolute value that guarantees that ectasia cannot occur. The risk of postoperative ectasia may increase with decreasing stromal bed thickness and may also be influenced by other factors yet to be identified (Pallikaris et al., 2001; Argento et al.,2001). Until risk factors for corneal ectasia following LASIK are better defined, the residual stromal bed thickness should not be less than 250 m.

The importance of pupillometry in the preoperative workup is controversial. Most studies of conventional and wavefront-guided LASIK have not shown a relationship between the diameter of the low light pupil and disturbing visual symptoms postoperatively (Pop and Payette, 2004; Schallhorn et al., 2003; Tuan and Liang, 2006). A benefit of wavefront-guided LASIK relative to conventional LASIK may be found under low light conditions when the pupil is dilated because that is where a reduction, or less induction, of higher order aberrations should be most apparent. Some studies comparing conventional and wavefront-guided LASIK have reported fewer postoperative complaints of glare or halo under mesopic conditions with wavefront-guided procedures (Lee et al., 2006; Farooquin et al., 2006). Irrespective of pupil size, it is important for potential patients to understand that there is a risk for night vision problems after surgery.

Keratorefractive Surgery

The most frequently performed procedures for low to moderate myopia utilize the excimer laser, which was first approved for this purpose by the FDA in 1995. A surface ablation technique, photorefractive keratectomy (PRK), was the first procedure performed; subsequently, LASIK has become the most commonly performed keratorefractive surgery. Other keratorefractive procedures to correct low to moderate myopia include variations of PRK called laser epithelial keratomileusis (LASEK) and epi-LASIK, insertion of intrastromal corneal ring segments (Rapuano et al., 2001) and RK (AAO, 1993).

Intraocular Refractive Surgery

Intraocular refractive surgery is the elective use of an IOL in a phakic eye, or in the case of elective refractive lens exchange, to allow use of a pseudophakic IOL, to achieve a particular refraction. Intraocular refractive surgery can be considered for patients who desire to reduce their dependency on eyeglasses or contact lens wear. Use of a pseudophakic IOL for the sole purpose of correction of refractive error in the absence of visually significant cataract has not been approved by the FDA.

Phakic Intraocular Lens Implantation: Specially designed IOLs may be surgically placed in the anterior chamber, attached to the iris, or placed in the posterior chamber anterior to the crystalline lens in the phakic eye to correct refractive error (Fechner et al., 1989; Landesz et al., 1995; Erturk and Ozcetin, 1995;Sanders et al., 1998; Fechner et al., 1998; Fink et al., 1999). Advantages include rapid visual recovery, stability of achieved correction, and the ability to correct high myopic refractive errors. Potential complications include endophthalmitis, endothelial cell loss, chronic iridocyclitis, cataract formation, iris distortion, pigment dispersion, elevated IOP, glaucoma, and IOL dislocation (Mimouni et al., 1991; Saragoussi et al., 1993). Two styles of PIOLs have been approved by the FDA for use in the United States and other designs are in clinical trials. Prototypes of multifocal PIOLs have demonstrated potential for treatment of presbyopia (Alio and Mulet, 2005; Baikoff et al.,2004).

*Intraocular Lenses:*Posterior chamber lenses are the most frequently used implants and the implant of choice. If there is inadequate capsular or zonular support, a suture-fixated or appropriately sized anterior chamber IOL may be required.

References

Acanthamoeba keratitis associated with contact lenses--United States. *MMWR Morb Mortal Wkly Rep* 1986;35:405-408.

Acanthamoeba keratitis multiple states, 2005-2007. *MMWR Morb Mortal Wkly Rep* 2007;56:532-534.

Alfonso EC, Cantu-Dibildox J, Munir WM, et al. Insurgence of Fusarium keratitis associated with contact lens wear. *Arch Ophthalmol* 2006;124:941-947.

Alio JL, Mulet ME. Presbyopia correction with an anterior chamber phakic multifocal intraocular lens. *Ophthalmology* 2005;112:1368-1374.

Allansmith MR, Korb DR, Greiner JV, et al. Giant papillary conjunctivitis in contact lens wearers. *Am J Ophthalmol* 1977;83:697-708.

American Academy of Ophthalmology and American Society of Cataract and Refractive Surgery Joint Position Statement. Ophthalmic Postoperative Care. San Francisco: American Academy of Ophthalmology, 2000. Available at: http://one.aao.org/CE /PracticeGuidelines/ClinicalStatements.aspx.

American Academy of Ophthalmology Committee on Ophthalmic Procedure Assessment. Ophthalmic Procedure Assessment. Epikeratoplasty. *Ophthalmology* 1996;101:983-991.

American Academy of Ophthalmology Refractive Management/Intervention Panel Refractive Errors & Refractive Surgery. San Farncisco, CA: American Academy of Ophthalmology, 2007. Available at: http://www.aao.org/ppp.

American Academy of Ophthalmology, American Society of Ophthalmic Registered Nurses, and American Association of Eye and Ear Hospitals. Joint Patient Safety Bulletin. Eliminating Wrong Site Surgery. San Francisco, CA: American Academy of Ophthalmology; 2001. Available at: http://one.aao.org/CE/PracticeGuidelines/Patient.aspx. Accessed August 16, 2007.

American Academy of Ophthalmology. Policy Statement. An Ophthalmologist's Duties Concerning Postoperative Care. San Francisco, CA: American Academy of Ophthalmology; 2006. Available at: http://one.aao.org/CE/PracticeGuidelines/Clinical Statements.aspx.

American Academy of Ophthalmology. Policy Statement. Pretreatment Assessment: Responsibilities of the Ophthalmologist. San Francisco, CA: American Academy of Ophthalmology; 2006. Available at: http://one.aao.org/CE/PracticeGuidelines/Clinical Statements.aspx.

American Academy of Ophthalmology. Radial keratotomy for myopia. American Academy of Ophthalmology. *Ophthalmology* 1993;100(7):1103-1115.

American Society of Cataract and Refractive Surgery. Acanthamoeba Keratitis: ASCRS Infectious Disease Task Force report and recommendations. Available at: http://www.ascrs.org/press_releases/Acanthamoeba-Keratitis-ASCRS-Report.cfm. Accessed August 16, 2007.

Aquavella JV, Rao GN, eds. Contact Lenses. Philadelphia: JB Lippincott Co., 1987; 211-225.

Argento C, Cosentino MJ, Tytiun A, et al. Corneal ectasia after laser in situ keratomileusis. *J Cataract Refract Surg* 2001;27:1440-1448.

Asbell PA, Wasserman D. Contact lens-induced corneal warpage. *Int Ophthalmol Clin* 1991;31:121-126.

Baikoff G, Matach G, Fontaine A, et al. Correction of presbyopia with refractive multifocal phakic intraocular lenses. *J Cataract Refract Surg* 2004;30:1454-1460.

Barr JT. Annual report: Contact lenses 2005. Contact Lens Spectrum January 2006. Available at: http://www.clspectrum.com/article.aspx?article=12913.

Baum J, Barza M. Pseudomonas keratitis and extended-wear soft contact lenses. *Arch Ophthalmol* 1990;108:663-664.

Bernal MD, Acharya NR, Lietman TM, et al. Outbreak of Fusarium keratitis in soft contact lens wearers in San Francisco. *Arch Ophthalmol* 2006;124:1051-1053.

Binder PS, Lindstrom RL, Stulting RD, et al. Keratoconus and corneal ectasia after LASIK. *J Cataract Refract Surg* 2005;31:2035-2038.

Bowden FW, III, Cohen EJ, Arentsen JJ, Laibson PR. Patterns of lens care practices and lens product contamination in contact lens associated microbial keratitis. *CLAO J* 1989;15:49-54.

Butcko V, McMahon TT, Joslin CE, Jones L. Microbial keratitis and the role of rub and rinsing. *Eye Contact Lens* 2007;33:421-3; discussion 424-425.

Chang DC, Grant GB, O'Donnell K, et al. Multistate outbreak of Fusarium keratitis associated with use of a contact lens solution. *JAMA* 2006;296:953-963.

Cohen EJ, Fulton JC, Hoffman CJ, et al. Trends in contact lens-associated corneal ulcers. *Cornea* 1996;15:566-570.

Cohen EJ, Laibson PR, Arentsen JJ, Clemons CS. Corneal ulcers associated with cosmetic extended wear soft contact lenses. *Ophthalmology* 1987;94:109-114.

Donshik PC. Giant papillary conjunctivitis. *Trans Am Ophthalmol Soc* 1994;92:687-744.

El-Maghraby A, Salah T, Waring GO 3rd, et al. Randomized bilateral comparison of excimer laser in situ keratomileusis and photorefractive keratectomy for 2.50 to 8.00 diopters of myopia. *Ophthalmology* 1999;106:447-457.

Erturk H, Ozcetin H. Phakic posterior chamber intraocular lenses for the correction of high myopia. *J Refract Surg* 1995;11:388-391.

Excimer laser photorefractive keratectomy (PRK) for myopia and astigmatism. American Academy of Ophthalmology. *Ophthalmology* 1999;106:422-437.

Farooqui MA, Al-Muammar AR. Topography-guided CATz versus conventional LASIK for myopia with the NIDEK EC-5000: A bilateral eye study. *J Refract Surg* 2006;22:741-745.

Fechner PU, Singh D, Wulff K. Iris-claw lens in phakic eyes to correct hyperopia: preliminary study. *J Cataract Refract Surg* 1998;24:48-56. 66.

Fechner PU, van der Heijde GL, Worst JG. The correction of myopia by lens implantation into phakic eyes. *Am J Ophthalmol* 1989;107:659-663.

Fink AM, Gore C, Rosen E. Cataract development after implantation of the Staar Collamer posterior chamber phakic lens. *J Cataract Refract Surg* 1999,25.278-282.

Goss DA: Variables related to the rate of childhood myopia progression. *Optom Vis Sci* 1990;67(8):631–636.

Imayasu M, Petroll WM, Jester JV, et al. The relation between contact lens oxygen transmissibility and binding of Pseudomonas aeruginosa to the cornea after overnight wear. *Ophthalmology* 1994;101:371-388.

Iribarren R, Iribarren G, Castagnola MM, et al. Family history and reading habits in adult-onset myopia. *Curr Eye Res* 2002;25(5):309–315.

Joslin CE, Tu EY, McMahon TT, et al. Epidemiological characteristics of a Chicago-area Acanthamoeba keratitis outbreak. Am J Ophthalmol 2006;142:212-217.

Joslin CE, Tu EY, Shoff ME, et al. The association of contact lens solution use and acanthamoeba keratitis. *Am J Ophthalmol* 2007;144:169-180. 56

Khor WB, Aung T, Saw SM, et al. An outbreak of Fusarium keratitis associated with contact lens wear in Singapore. *JAMA* 2006;295:2867-2873.

Koidou-Tsiligianni A, Alfonso E, Forster RK. Ulcerative keratitis associated with contact lens wear. *Am J Ophthalmol* 1989;108:64-67.

Ladage PM, Yamamoto K, Ren DH, et al. Effects of rigid and soft contact lens daily wear on corneal epithelium, tear lactate dehydrogenase, and bacterial binding to exfoliated epithelial cells. *Ophthalmology* 2001;108:1279-1288.

Laibson PR, Cohen EJ, Rajpal RK. Conrad Berens Lecture. Corneal ulcers related to contact lenses. *CLAO J* 1993;19:73-78.

Landesz M, Worst JG, Siertsema JV, van Rij G. Correction of high myopia with the Worst myopia claw intraocular lens. *J Refract Surg* 1995;11:16-25.

Lee HK, Choe CM, Ma KT, Kim EK. Measurement of contrast sensitivity and glare under mesopic and photopic conditions following wavefront-guided and conventional LASIK surgery. *J Refract Surg* 2006;22:647-655.

Liu Z, Pflugfelder SC. The effects of long-term contact lens wear on corneal thickness, curvature, and surface regularity. *Ophthalmology* 2000;107:105-111.

MacRae SM, Matsuda M, Phillips DS. The long-term effects of polymethylmethacrylate contact lens wear on the corneal endothelium. *Ophthalmology* 1994;101:365-370.

MacRae SM, Matsuda M, Shellans S, Rich LF. The effects of hard and soft contact lenses on the corneal endothelium. *Am J Ophthalmol* 1986;102:50-57.

MacRae SM, Matsuda M, Shellans S. Corneal endothelial changes associated with contact lens wear. *CLAO J* 1989;15:82-87.

Macsai MS, Varley GA, Krachmer JH. Development of keratoconus after contact lens wear. Patient characteristics. *Arch Ophthalmol* 1990;108:534-538.

Maguen E, Tsai JC, Martinez M, et al. A retrospective study of disposable extended-wear lenses in 100 patients. *Ophthalmology* 1991;98:1685-1689.

Marcus SB, Rubin ML. Correction of ametropia with spectale lenses. Chapter 36. Duane's Ophthalmology on CD-Rom. Tasman W and Jaeger EA, editors. Philadelphia: *Lippincott Williams & Wilkins,* 2006 edition.

Margolis TP, Whitcher JP. Fusarium-A new culprit in the contact lens case. *JAMA* 2006;296:985-987.

Milder B, Rubin ML. Anisometropia. In The fine art of prescribing glasses. 3rd ed. Gainesville: *Triad Publishing Company,* 2004:225–226.

Mimouni F, Colin J, Koffi V, Bonnet P. Damage to the corneal endothelium from anterior chamber intraocular lenses in phakic myopic eyes. *Refract Corneal Surg* 1991;7:277-281.

Mondino BJ, Weissman BA, Farb MD, Pettit TH. Corneal ulcers associated with daily-wear and extended-wear contact lenses. *Am J Ophthalmol* 1986;102:58-65.

Moore MB, McCulley JP, Luckenbach M, et al. Acanthamoeba keratitis associated with soft contact lenses. *Am J Ophthalmol* 1985;100:396-403.

Mutti DO, Mitchell GL, Moeschberger ML, et al. Parental myopia, near work, school achievement, and children's refractive error. *Invest Ophthalmol Vis Sci* 2002;43(12):3633–3640.

Nilsson SE, Montan PG. The annualized incidence of contact lens induced keratitis in Sweden and its relation to lens type and wear schedule: results of a 3-month prospective study. *CLAO* J 1994;20:225-230.

Nilsson SE, Montan PG. The hospitalized cases of contact lens induced keratitis in Sweden and their relation to lens type and wear schedule: results of a three-year retrospective study. *CLAO J* 1994;20:97-101.

Nourouzi H, Rajavi J, Okhovatpour MA. Time to resolution of corneal edema after long-term contact lens wear. *Am J Ophthalmol* 2006;142:671-673.

Pallikaris IG, Kymionis GD, Astyrakakis NI. Corneal ectasia induced by laser in situ keratomileusis. *J Cataract Refract Surg* 2001;27:1796-1802.

Parssinen O, Hemminki E, Klemetti A: Effect of spectacle use and accommodation on myopic progression: final results of a three-year randomized clinical trial among schoolchildren. *Br J Ophthalmol* 1989; 73(7):547–551.

Poggio EC, Abelson M. Complications and symptoms in disposable extended wear lenses compared with conventional soft daily wear and soft extended wear lenses. *CLAO J* 1993;19:31-39.

Poggio EC, Abelson MB. Complications and symptoms with disposable daily wear contact lenses and conventional soft daily wear contact lenses. *CLAO J* 1993;19:95-102.

Poggio EC, Glynn RJ, Schein OD, et al. The incidence of ulcerative keratitis among users of daily-wear and extended-wear soft contact lenses. *N Engl J Med* 1989;321:779-783.

Pop M, Payette Y. Risk factors for night vision complaints after LASIK for myopia. *Ophthalmology* 2004;111:3-10.

Rapuano CJ, Sugar A, Koch DD, et al. Intrastromal corneal ring segments for low myopia: a report by the American Academy of Ophthalmology. *Ophthalmology* 2001;108:1922-1928.

Ren DH, Petroll WM, Jester JV, et al. The relationship between contact lens oxygen permeability and binding of Pseudomonas aeruginosa to human corneal epithelial cells after overnight and extended wear. *CLAO J* 1999;25:80-100.

Ren DH, Yamamoto K, Ladage PM, et al. Adaptive effects of 30-night wear of hyper-O(2) transmissible contact lenses on bacterial binding and corneal epithelium: a 1-year clinical trial. *Ophthalmology* 2002;109:27-39; discussion 39-40. 57

Sanders DR, Brown DC, Martin RG, et al. Implantable contact lens for moderate to high myopia: phase 1 FDA clinical study with 6 month follow-up. *J Cataract Refract Surg* 1998;24:607-611.

Saragoussi JJ, Othenin-Girard P, Pouliquen YJ. Ocular damage after implantation of oversized minus power anterior chamber intraocular lenses in myopic phakic eyes: case reports. *Refract Corneal Surg* 1993;9:105-109.

Saw SM, Ooi PL, Tan DT, et al. Risk factors for contact lens-related fusarium keratitis: a case-control study in Singapore. *Arch Ophthalmol* 2007;125:611-617.

Schallhorn SC, Farjo AA, Huang D, Boxer Wachler BS, Trattier WB, Tanzer DJ, Majmudar PA, Sugar A; American Academy of Ophthalmology. Wavefront-guided LASIK for the correction of primary myopia and astigmatism, a report by the American Academy of Ophthalmology. *Ophthalmology* 2008;115(7):1249-1261.

Schallhorn SC, Kaupp SE, Tanzer DJ, et al. Pupil size and quality of vision after LASIK. *Ophthalmology* 2003;110:1606-1614.

Schein OD, Buehler PO, Stamler JF, et al. The impact of overnight wear on the risk of contact lens-associated ulcerative keratitis. *Arch Ophthalmol* 1994;112:186-190.

Schein OD, Glynn RJ, Poggio EC, et al. The relative risk of ulcerative keratitis among users of daily-wear and extended-wear soft contact lenses. A case-control study. Microbial Keratitis Study Group. *N Engl J Med* 1989;321:773-778.

Schein OD, McNally JJ, Katz J, et al. The incidence of microbial keratitis among wearers of a 30-day silicone hydrogel extended-wear contact lens. *Ophthalmology* 2005;112:2172-2179.

Seiler T, Koufala K, Richter G. Iatrogenic keratectasia after laser in situ keratomileusis. *J Refract Surg* 1998;14:312-317.

Stehr-Green JK, Bailey TM, Brandt FH, et al. Acanthamoeba keratitis in soft contact lens wearers. A case-control study. *JAMA* 1987;258:57-60.

Stehr-Green JK, Bailey TM, Visvesvara GS. The epidemiology of Acanthamoeba keratitis in the United States. *Am J Ophthalmol* 1989;107:331-336.

Stern G, Zam S. The pathogenesis of contact lens-associated pseudomonas aeruginosa corneal ulceration. 1. The effect of contact lens coatings on adherence of pseudomonas aeruginosa to soft contact lenses. *Cornea* 1986;5:41-45.

Suchecki JK, Ehlers WH, Donshik PC. A comparison of contact lens-related complications in various daily wear modalities. *CLAO J* 2000;26:204-213.

Thebpatiphat N, Hammersmith KM, Rocha FN, et al. Acanthamoeba keratitis: a parasite on the rise. *Cornea* 2007;26:701-706.

Tuan KM, Liang J. Improved contrast sensitivity and visual acuity after wavefront-guided laser in situ keratomileusis: in-depth statistical analysis. *J Cataract Refract Surg* 2006;32:215-220.

U.S. Food and Drug Administration. Advice for patients with soft contact lenses: new information on risk of serious fungal infection. Available at: http://www.fda.gov/cdrh /medicaldevicesafety/atp/041006-keratitis.html. Accessed November 21, 2006.

Update: Fusarium keratitis--United States, 2005-2006. *MMWR Morb Mortal Wkly Rep* 2006;55:563-564.

Wilhelmus KR, Robinson NM, Font RA, et al. Fungal keratitis in contact lens wearers. *Am J Ophthalmol* 1988;106:708-714.

Wilson LA, Ahearn DG. Association of fungi with extended-wear soft contact lenses. *Am J Ophthalmol* 1986;101:434-436.

Wilson LA, Sawant AD, Ahearn DG. Comparative efficacies of soft contact lens disinfectant solutions against microbial films in lens cases. *Arch Ophthalmol* 1991;109:1155-1157.

Chapter XII

Myopia and Progression

Abstract

Various types of modalities to attempt to slow myopia progression and axial elongation are presented in this chapter. The high prevalence of myopia and its prominence as a public health problem emphasize the importance of finding effective treatments that slow myopia progression and axial elongation. High myopia is associated with sight threatening retinal complications and interventions to slow myopia progression in children would seem to be beneficial. Treatments that have been investigated include various types of spectacle lenses and contact lenses, as well as pharmaceutical agents such as atropine and pirenzepine.

A number of previous studies have evaluated the efficacy of several interventions to reduce the progression of myopia (Gwiazda, 2009; Saw et al., 2002; Syniuta and Isenberg, 2001). It is also well recognized in prescribing practices that uncorrected refractive error during childhood can result in the development of amblyopia and strabismus (Adler and Millodot, 2006).

Prevention of Myopia Progression

Most myopic refractive errors develop and progress during childhood and adolescence. Treatments proposed to prevent or reduce the progression of myopia include optical correction, use of cycloplegic eyedrops, pressure-lowering eyedrops, contact lenses, and visual training. Information about the effects of nutritional changes on the progression of myopia is largely anecdotal and no scientifically valid studies are available.

1. Optical Correction

Optical correction in the form of bifocal eyeglasses, multifocal eyeglasses, or removal of distance eyeglasses when performing close work, has been recommended in an attempt to reduce accommodation, since accommodation has been implicated in the progression of myopia. Studies examining distance eyeglasses alone have failed to demonstrate any overall effects on the progression of human myopia (Ong et al.,1999).

Single Vision Lenses

An active emmetropization mechanism regulated by optical defocus is supported by results of numerous studies (reviewed in Wallman and Winawer, 2004). Strong evidence is provided by compensatory ocular growth seen in response to lens-induced defocus in animal models (Hung et al., 1995). Based on these results, it has been suggested that spectacle intervention in myopic children with the commonly prescribed single vision lenses (SVLs) might lead to increased progression and axial elongation. Patterns of lens wear in myopic patients can vary from full-time wear, to the use of lenses for distance viewing only, to non-wear of prescribed lenses. Limited data are available on myopia progression by pattern of lens wear, though pilot data suggest that progression is similar for the different patterns (Ong et al., 1999).

Under-correction of myopia with SVLs is a treatment option advocated by some clinicians.

Only one masked, randomized clinical trial has been conducted to evaluate this treatment (Chung et al., 2002). Ninety-four of 106 (89%) myopic children aged 9-14 years completed two years of spectacle wear in SVLs, half randomized to full correction and half to under-correction by approximately 0.75 D. Two-year progression in the fully corrected group was 0.77 D, significantly less than the 1.0 D in the under-corrected group ($p < 0.01$).

Bifocals and Progressive Addition Lenses

The use of bifocals or progressive addition lenses (PALs), sometimes called no-line bifocals, for slowing the progression of myopia has produced relatively small treatment effects overall, on the order of 0.15 to 0.50 D over 1.5 to 3 years (Leung and Brown, 1999; Edwards et al., 2002; Fulk et al., 2000; Gwiazda et al., 2003; Gwiazda et al., 2004;Hasebe et al., 2008), although treatment effects are reported to be larger in certain subgroups of myopic children.

The largest of the treatment trials with this type of lens was the Correction of Myopia Evaluation Trial (COMET), a multi-center, randomized, double-masked clinical trial to evaluate whether PALs slow the rate of progression of myopia compared to conventional SVLs (Gwiazda et al., 2003). COMET enrolled 469 children aged 6 -11 years who were ethnically diverse (46% white, 26% African-American, 14% Hispanic, and 8% Asian) and had baseline myopia between −1.25 D and −4.50 D. The primary outcome measure was progression of myopia by cycloplegic autorefraction with tropicamide. Retention was excellent, with 462/469 (98.5%) of the children completing the three-year visit. Adjusted mean myopia increased from baseline to 3 years by 1.28 ± 0.06 D in the PAL group and 1.48 ± 0.06 D in the SVL group. The overall adjusted 3-year treatment effect of 0.20 ± 0.08D was statistically significant ($p = 0.004$) but not clinically meaningful. All of the treatment effect occurred in the first year. Additional analyses showed that there were significant 3-year treatment effects in children with larger lags of accommodation in combination with near esophoria (0.64D ± 0.21), shorter reading distances (0.44D ± 0.20), or lower baseline myopia (0.48D ± 0.15) that became larger from 1 to 3 years of follow-up (Gwiazda et al., 2004). These results support a role for retinal defocus in myopia progression and suggest that myopic children with large accommodative lags and near esophoria may benefit from wearing PALs.

A study similar to COMET was conducted in Japan (Hasebe et al., 2008). A unique feature of this investigation of PALs vs. SVLs for slowing myopia progression in 6-12 year old children was the use of a crossover design. Children with myopia from −1.25 to −6.0 D were randomly chosen to wear one type of spectacle lens for the first half of the study, and then midway through the 3-year period of follow-up they were switched to the other eyeglass type. Results showed a statistically significant treatment benefit of PALs vs SVLs of 0.17 D at 18 months. At the end of the second 18-month period, after children wore the other lens type, progression in the group wearing PALs first was 0.29 D less than in the group with SVLs first, leading to the suggestion that early intervention with PALs may work better than SVLs in this age and refractive error range. As in COMET, children with larger accommodative lags had a larger treatment effect than those with smaller lags (0.61 D vs. 0.15 D), and children who were esophoric or orthophoric at near had a larger treatment effect than those who were more exophoric (0.55 D vs. 0.18 D).

SVLs vs MLs

Findings of a systematic review and meta-analysis based on high quality randomized controlled trials (RCTs) to assess the effect of multifocal lenses (MLs) versus the effect of single vision Lenses (SVLs) on myopic progression in children indicated that MLs slowed myopia progression by a mean of 0.25D in school-aged children compared with the use of SVLs. This effect appeared to be greater in children with greater levels of myopia at baseline and in Asians. Remaining questions to be clarified by future RCTs include determining an optimal treatment period, how long the effect can last after intervention stops, and whether customized near addition lenses are more effective (Li et al., 2011).

2. Topical Cycloplegic Agents

Administration of atropine eyedrops has long been proposed as a treatment to prevent progression of myopia. Atropine inhibits accommodation, which may exert forces on the eye that result in axial elongation. In animal studies, atropine also appears to inhibit growth factors acting to elongate the eye independent of accommodation (Oishi and Lauber, 1988; Tigges et al., 1999; Lind et al., 1998).

The results of randomized, controlled clinical trials conducted in Taiwan and Singapore (three of which were masked) provide reasonable evidence that administration of atropine eyedrops retards the progression of myopia in school children (Shih et al., 1999; Shih et al.,2001; Yen et al., 1989; Chua et al., 2006). In one study, a range of atropine concentrations was utilized; 0.1%, 0.25%, and 0.5%. All reduced progression of myopia compared with the control group. The 0.5% concentration was the most effective (Shih et al., 1999).

Atropine eyedrops were first proposed as a treatment of myopia in the 1920s (Gimbel, 1973). Since then, there have been numerous studies on this subject (Kelly et al., 1975; Bedrossian et al., 1979; Brodstein et al., 1984; Brenner, 1985; Chou et al., 1997; Romano and Donovan, 2000; Kennedy et al., 2000; Chiang et al., 2001; Syniuta and Isenberg, 2001; Lee et al., 2006; Fan et al., 2007). However, evidence from randomized control trials has become available only over the last 2 decades (Yen et al., 1989; Shih et al., 1999; Shih et al., 2001; Chua et al., 2006; Liang et al., 2008; Tong et al., 2009). These trials confirm that atropine eyedrops are effective in the control of myopia in a dose-related manner (Yen et al., 1989; Shih et al., 1999; Shih et al., 2001; Chua et al., 2006; Liang et al., 2008; Tong et al., 2009). Atropine for the Treatment of Myopia 1 (ATOM1), a randomized trial, involving 400 children aged 6 to 12 years found that, over 2 years, atropine 1% showed myopia progression (mean±standard deviation) to -0.28±0.92 diopters (D) in children, compared with -1.20±0.69 D in the placebo group ($P < 0.001$) (Chua et al., 2006). Shih et al. (Shih et al., 1999) showed that the myopic progression in Taiwanese children was -0.004±0.63, -0.47±0.91, and -0.47±0.91 D/year in the 0.5%, 0.25%, and 0.1% atropine groups, respectively, compared with -1.06±0.61 D/year in their tropicamide (control) group. Liang et al. (Liang et al., 2008), in a smaller study of 65 children, demonstrated myopic progression of -0.15±0.15, -0.38±0.32, and -0.21±0.23 D/year in the 0.5%, 0.25%, and 0.25% atropine plus auricular pressure groups, respectively.

More recently, it has also been shown that atropine eyedrops are effective in populations in the West where children generally have less rapid rates of progression of myopia than in Taiwan (Chiang et al., 2001; Syniuta and Isenberg, 2001; Kennedy et al., 2000). It is now also known that the beneficial effects remain once the use of atropine is discontinued. Potential risks of long-term atropine use are uncertain and include the risk of light toxicity to ocular structures, the potential for local allergic and systemic reactions, and the effect on accommodative amplitudes following discontinuation of atropine. However, it has recently been reported that daily atropine usage over 2 years for the treatment of myopia has no significant effect on retinal function as demonstrated by recordings of multifocal electroretinograms in children (Luu et al., 2005). Other potential disadvantages include the possible need for bifocal or multifocal eyeglasses (depending on the concentration of atropine administered), photosensitivity and glare, and the inconvenience of using daily eyedrops. Although atropine is used in many countries in Asia for slowing the progression of myopia, it is rarely used in the United States for this purpose. The side effects associated with atropine (e.g., photophobia, cycloplegia) are considered by many clinicians to be unacceptable for long-term therapy.

Muscarinic transmission in retinal cells is believed to be involved in the visual control of refractive development. Experimental studies have revealed that the non-selective muscarinic antagonist, atropine, reduces the progression of axial myopia in humans via a nonaccommodative mechanism (Stone et al., 1991; McBrien et al., 1993). Kennedy et al. showed that topically applied atropine solution (1%) on a daily basis reduced the mean annual rate of myopia progression from approximately 0.77D per year to 0.05D per year during the treatment period (Kennedy et al., 2000). However, the actual mechanisms involved in the process are still unclear. Although the beneficial effect of atropine in reducing progression of myopia in humans has been reported in a number of studies (Kennedy et al., 2000; Shih et al., 1999; Yen et al., 1989), the effects of atropine treatment on retinal function have been studied previously (Luu et al., 2005). The multifocal electroretinogram (mfERG), first described by Sutter and Tran (Sutter and Tran, 1992), has proved to be a sensitive technique in the detection of retinal dysfunction and has shown that atropine usage over 2 years for the treatment of myopia causes no significant retinal dysfunction. There are, however, at least two potential chronic side effects associated with the long term use of atropine. Firstly, accumulation of atropine over a period of time might be toxic to the neural retina. Secondly, constant pupillary dilatation will increase the amount of light entering the eye and could theoretically cause photic damage to the retina. Photic retinopathy has been reported from a variety of light sources and intensities including solar exposure, welding arc, laser light, operating microscope, ophthalmoscope and fundus camera exposure (Lessel et al., 1991; Lawwill et al., 1977). Infants and adolescents are at a greater risk of photic retinopathy because of their clear ocular media (Lawwill et al., 1977).

Cyclopentolate 1% administered nightly was evaluated in one study in school children in Taiwan. It was found to slow the rate of progression of myopia compared with controls (mean myopic progression of -0.6 D/year compared with -0.9 D/year, which is statistically significant), but not as much as atropine did (mean myopic progression of -0.2 D/year) (Yen et al., 1989). Tropicamide 1% was evaluated in a study of monozygotic twins, and no significant difference in progression of myopia was noted compared with controls (Schwartz, 1981).

Recently, pirenzepine hydrochloride has been evaluated in two multicenter, double-masked, placebo-controlled parallel studies to slow the progression of myopia in school-aged children. Unlike atropine, which affects both accommodation and mydriasis, pirenzepine has a relatively selective effect on accommodation. The United States study examined 174 children age 8 to 12 years (Siatkowski et al., 2004), and the Asian study examined 353 children age 6 to 13 years (Tan et al., 2005). Both studies found 2% pirenzepine ophthalmic gel effective and relatively safe in slowing myopia progression over a one-year treatment period.

Because of uncertainty about long-term safety and optimal dosage, administration of atropine eyedrops or pirenzepine hydrochloride to reduce myopic progression in children is recommended only in research trials (Chua et al., 2006; Siatkowski et al., 2004; Tan et al., 2005).

3. Pressure-Lowering Eyedrops

Lowering IOP has been suggested as a pharmacologic intervention that might reduce progression of myopia, presumably by reducing internal pressure on the ocular wall. One prospective clinical trial comparing administration of 0.25% timolol maleate with the use of single-vision eyeglasses failed to show any retardation of progression of myopia (Jensen, 1991; Jensen, 1988).

4. Contact Lenses

Soft contact lens use was evaluated in a randomized clinical trial in the United States (Horner et al., 1999). No statistically significant difference in the rate of myopia progression could be demonstrated between the contact lens group and the group using single-vision eyeglasses.

It has long been postulated that rigid contact lens use could slow the progression of myopia in children (Jensen, 1964; Morrison, 1960). Previous studies published were limited by methodological difficulties (Stone, 1973; Stone, 1976; Grosvenor and Goss, 1988;

Grosvenor et al., 1989; Perrigin et al., 1990; Andreo, 1990). A two-year randomized clinical trial evaluating the effect of rigid contact lenses on myopia progression in school children was conducted in Singapore (Katz et al., 2003), and another study concurrently in the United States (Walline et al., 2001). The study of 428 Singaporean children ages 6 to 12 years found that rigid gas permeable contact lenses did not slow the rate of myopia progression over 2 years, even among children who used them regularly and consistently (Katz et al., 2003). The United States study compared the effects of rigid gas permeable contact lenses and soft contact lenses on myopia progression in 116 children age 8 to 11 years. They found that rigid contact lens wearers progressed less than soft contact lens wearers, and that the corneal curvature of the soft lens group steepened more than the rigid lens group, but the axial growth was not statistically significantly different between the groups. Because some of the effect was likely influenced by transient corneal curvature changes, the authors concluded that the results indicate that rigid gas permeable contact lenses should not be prescribed primarily for myopia control (Walline et al., 2004).

Although it has been suggested that orthokeratology can slow the progression of myopia in children, there is no randomized controlled trial evidence to support this (Katz et al., 2003; Cho et al., 2005). A two-year pilot study was conducted to determine whether orthokeratology can effectively reduce and control myopia in children. Thirty-five Hong Kong children age 7 to 12 years undergoing orthokeratology treatment were compared with 35 children wearing single-vision eyeglasses from an earlier study (control). The study found a statistically significant change in axial length for the orthokeratology group and the control group (0.29 ± 0.27 mm and 0.54 ± 0.27 mm respectively). However, there are substantial variations in changes in eye length among children and there is no way to predict the effect for individual subjects (Cho et al., 2005). Because of lack of efficacy and associated risks, orthokeratology is not recommended for prevention of myopia progression in children (Katz et al., 2003; Cho et al., 2005).

Many early investigations of rigid gas permeable contact lenses (RGP) for myopia control suffered from lack of randomization and a high drop out rate from the contact lens group (Perrigin et al.,1990; Khoo et al., 1999). In an attempt to eliminate the high loss to follow-up found in previous studies, a recent randomized clinical trial, the Contact Lens and Myopia Progression (CLAMP) study, implemented a run-in period to ensure good compliance with rigid contact lens wear (Walline et al.,2004). One hundred and sixteen children who successfully completed the run-in period were randomized to wear either RGP or soft contact lenses for three years. Results showed a statistically significant difference in 3-year myopia progression in the RGP vs. soft lens group (-1.56 ± 0.95 D for RGP wearers vs. -2.19 ± 0.89 D for the soft lens group, $p<0.001$). Most of the slowed progression with RGP lenses was found in the first year. Corneal curvature steepened significantly less over three years in the RGP group (0.62 ± 0.60 D compared to the soft lens group (0.88 ± 0.57 D, $p=0.01$), again with most of the difference found in the first year. Three year axial elongation was not significantly different between treatment groups. These results, taken together, suggest that the slowed myopia progression was mainly due to corneal flattening, which may be reversible with discontinuation of RGP lens wear. In the absence of differences in axial elongation and with most of the treatment effect occurring in the first year, the authors of the CLAMP study concluded that RGP lenses should not be prescribed mainly for myopia control.

The Longitudinal Orthokeratology Research in Children (LORIC) was a pilot study conducted in Hong Kong to determine if overnight wear of specially designed RGP contact lenses slowed axial elongation and the progression of myopia (Cho et al., 2005). Thirty-five children wore these lenses for two years, and their results were compared to those from an historical control group of children wearing SVLs. Change in axial length rather than refractive error is typically used as the outcome measure because of corneal flattening produced by the lenses. Results of the study showed that over the 2-year period axial length in the orthokeratology group increased by 0.29 mm vs. 0.54 mm for the control group, a significant difference. A well-designed study on what is now called corneal refractive therapy with sufficient subject numbers and random assignment still needs to be conducted to more fully evaluate this type of treatment for slowing myopia progression.

Anecdotal reports and evidence from pilot studies have suggested that the use of soft contact lenses speeds up myopia progression (Fulk et al., 2003). However, a recent randomized trial investigating the effect of soft contact lenses on myopia progression in children reported no significant difference in progression between soft contact lens and spectacle wearers (Walline et al., 2008).

5. Other Treatments

Methylxanthine

Trier et al. (Trier et al., 2008), in a 36-month pilot study, tested whether 7-methylxanthine (7-mx), a metabolite of caffeine and theobromine and adenosine antagonist, was useful against elongation progression in childhood myopia. There is today no treatment that efficiently and without side effects controls the progression of myopia (Saw et al., 2002). Topically applied muscarine antagonists, like the nonselective antagonist atropine, and the M1 selective antagonist pirenzepine have been shown to reduce myopia progression and axial eye growth (Fan et al., 2007; Siatkowski et al., 2008; Tan et al., 2005). The mechanism of action of atropine and pirenzepine has not been established, but it is assumed that it is independent of their action on accommodation, and that it may depend on receptors in the retina or the sclera (Yin et al., 2004). Reduced accommodation and dilation of the pupil, however, remain a problem both with atropine and to a lesser degree with pirenzepine. Treatment of young rabbits with a metabolite of caffeine and theobromine, 7-methylxanthine (7-mx), increases the thickness of the posterior sclera, increases the content of collagen-related amino acids in posterior sclera, and at the same time increases the diameter of the collagen fibrils in the posterior sclera (Trier et al., 1999). Recently, 7-mx has been shown to reduce the amount of myopia and eye elongation induced by form deprivation in guinea pigs and to counteract the thinning of posterior sclera and of collagen fibrils induced by form deprivation (Cui et al., 2008).

Theobromine and its metabolite, 7-mx, both have very low toxicity (Tarka, 1982; Tarka et al., 1991) and no carcinogenic effects (IARC, 1991).

Methylxanthines in non-toxic doses block adenosine receptors (ADOR) competitively. Adenosine in the concentrations found under physiological conditions activates primarily A1 and A2A adenosine receptors (ADORA1 and ADORA2A) on the cell surface. ADORA1s are widely distributed in the CNS, whereas ADORA2As are found mainly in the dopamine-rich regions of the brain (Fredholm et al., 1999). Adenosine has a general homeostatic role in the regulation of cell metabolism, but also a specific neuromodulatory role with ADORA1s having an inhibitory role and ADORA2As having a facilitatory role in the release of neurotransmitters such as dopamine, noradrenalin, acetylcholine, glutamate, and serotonin (Cunha, 2001). ADORA1s and ADORA2As have been localized in the ciliary body and the retina and ADORA2As in the retinal pigment epithelium of adult rats (Kyanta et al., 1997) and humans (unpublished results, Zhongshan Ophthalmic Center). Both ADORA1s and ADORA2As are expressed in human scleral fibroblasts (Cui et al., 2008).

Experimental myopia in animals has been linked to changes in retinal dopamine and acetylcholine neurotransmission (Liu et al.,2007; Iuvone, 1991; McBrien et al., 2001; Gao et al., 2006; Ouyang et al., 2003; Cottriall et al., 1996). Both of these neurotransmitters are modulated by ADORs (Cunha, 2001; Salmi et al., 2005; Oliveira and Correia-de-Sa, 2005; Marks et al., 2003; Ei Yacoubi et al., 2001; Moo-Puc et al., 2001). The mechanism by which 7-mx affects eye elongation and myopia progression could therefore theoretically involve modulation of muscarinic acetycholine or dopamine receptors. On the other hand, it is also possible that ADORs are directly involved in the control of eye growth. Because of receptor adaptation, the effects related to blocking of ADOR1s are attenuated during chronic treatment with non-selective ADOR antagonists like 7-mx, whereas effects related to blocking of ADORA2As are unchanged (Shi and Daly, 1999; White and Nguyen, 2002; Quarta et al., 2004).

Adenosine liberated from the retina is believed to activate ADORA2s on the retinal pigment epithelium and augment the standing potential (SP) (Gallemore et al., 1998). The effect on the SP might therefore give us a measure of the potency of a specific methylxanthine as a blocker of adenosine receptors. The receptor affinity of 7-mx is three to five times higher than theobromine (Müller et al., 1993). Correspondingly, the lightrise of SP in humans is more reduced by 7-mx than by theobromine (unpublished results, K Trier, 2004). Interestingly, high ametropia in children is associated with retinal electrophysiological abnormalities, a finding consistent with the hypothesis that the retina is involved in the process of emmetropization (Flitcroft et al., 2005).

Orthokeratology

Orthokeratology has been practiced for decades, yet since its use of a temporary alteration of the corneal shape does not correct the intrinsic cause of myopia and since it is associated with potential complications such as infective keratitis, its use in children is still controversial (Van Meter et al., 2008; McLeod, 2007). Although few studies have investigated the effect of undercorrection to slow down the progression of early-onset myopia, it had recently reported that undercorrection exhibited no beneficial effect on its reduction, and the response for prescribing undercorrected glasses was in broad agreement of such report (Adler and Millodot, 2006; Chung et al., 2002).

Traditional Chinese Interventional Treatments

Traditional Chinese medicine practioners frequently use various forms of acupuncture (i.e; fine needle insertion, acupressure, surface electricity, and laser stimulation) for preventing progression of myopia in children. Facial "Qi Qong" eye exercises were created in the 1950s in China. It was postulated that massaging the various acupuncture pressure points around the eye improves venous blood circulation, relaxes the muscles, and reduces eye strain. These eye exercises are part of the school routine in many parts of China, and teachers guide the children in the performance of these eye exercises as often as twice a day for 10 minutes. The evidence from two non randomised studies conducted in Singapore and Taiwan were inconclusive (Rajan et al., 1998; Shih et al.,1995). In another nonrandomized clinical trial of 242 adolescent eyes in 295 people in Beijing, small pieces of adhesive pressure plaster grains of *Semen impatiens* were evaluated. Significant treatment effects were claimed (Liu et al., 1994). The data from two RCTs do not support a clear conclusion for either benefit or harm of the treatments (Wei et al., 2011; AAO, 2013).

Other Considerartion

Previous studies have shown that the mean rate of myopia progression in Asian children is greater than in age-matched European children (Gwiazda et al., 2003; Saw et al., 2005; Lam et al., 1999; Grosvenor et al., 1987) This is in agreement with findings of a meta-analysis which determined the mean rate of myopia progression in Asian children to be approximately 0.20 D per year faster than their age-matched European counterparts (Donovan et al., 2012).

In contrast to the 0.87 dioptres per year annualized progression rate for Asians found in a meta-analysis (Donovan et al., 2012), a large, longitudinal survey (Zhao et al., 2002) estimated the mean annual progression rate of myopic Chinese school children aged 5 to 13 years old at baseline to be 0.35 dioptres per year. However this study differed from those used in a meta-analysis (Donovan et al., 2012) as the sample was population-based rather than recruited from schools or brought into a study by parents, and the participants were from a semi-rural rather than an urban area of China. Meta-analysis (Donovan et al., 2014) revealed higher myopia progression rates in urban Asians compared with urban Europeans. Younger children demonstrated greater annual rates of progression of myopia and females had slightly greater mean progression rates than males.

Undercorrection

Although few studies have investigated the effect of undercorrection to slow down the progression of early-onset myopia, it had recently reported that undercorrection exhibited no beneficial effect on its reduction, and the response for prescribing undercorrected glasses was in broad agreement of such report (Adler and Millodot, 2006; Chung et al., 2002).

Prevention

Treatments have been reported that purport to prevent progression of refractive errors, particularly myopia. Evidence reported in the peer-reviewed literature, including from randomized clinical trials, is currently insufficient to support a recommendation for intervention.

References

Adler D, Millodot M. The possible effect of undercorrection on myopic progression in children. *Clin Exp Optom* 2006;89:315-321.

American Academy of Ophthalmology Preferred Practice Pattern Clinical Questions. Acupuncture to slow myopia in children. American Academy of Ophthalmology. San Francisco, CA 2013.

American Academy of Ophthalmology. Radial keratotomy for myopia. American Academy Ophthalmology. *Ophthalmology* 1993;100(7):1103-1115.

Andreo LK. Long-term effects of hydrophilic contact lenses on myopia. *Ann Ophthalmol* 1990;22:224-227, 229.

Bedrossian RH. The effect of atropine on myopia. *Ophthalmology* 1979;86(5):713-719.

Chiang MF, Kouzis A, Pointer RW, Repka MX. Treatment of childhood myopia with atropine eyedrops and bifocal spectacles. *Binocul Vis Strabismus Q* 2001;16:209-215.

Cho P, Cheung SW, Edwards M. The longitudinal orthokeratology research in children (LORIC) in Hong Kong: a pilot study on refractive changes and myopic control. Curr Eye Res 2005;30:71-80.

Chua WH, Balakrishnan V, Chan YH, et al. Atropine for the treatment of childhood myopia. *Ophthalmology* 2006;113:2285-2291.

Chua WH, Balakrishnan V, Chan YH, Tong L, Ling Y, Quah BL, Tan D. Atropine for the treatment of childhood myopia. *Ophthalmology* 2006;113:2285–2291. [PubMed: 16996612]

Chung K, Mohidin N, O'Leary DJ. Undercorrection of myopia enhances rather than inhibits myopia progression. *Vis Res* 2002;42:2555–2559.

Cottriall CL, McBrien NA. The M1 muscarinic antagonist pirenzepine reduces myopia and eye enlargement in the tree shrew. *Invest Ophthalmol Vis Sci* 1996;37:1368–1379.

Cui D, Trier K, Chen X et al. Effects of 7-methylxanthine on form deprived myopia in guinea pig. In ARVO annual meeting, Ft. Lauderdale, FL; 2008.

Cui D, Trier K, Chen X, et al. Distribution of adenosine receptors in human sclera fibroblasts. *Mol Vis* 2008;14:523–529.

Cunha RA. Adenosine as a neuromodulator and as a homeostatic regulator in the nervous system: different roles, different sources and different receptors. *Neurochem Int.* 2001;38:107–125.

Donovan L, Sankaridurg P, Ho A, Naduvilath T, Smith III EL, Holden BA. Myopia Progression Rates in Urban Children Wearing Single-Vision Spectacles. *Optom Vis Sci* 2012 January ; 89(1): 27–32. doi:10.1097/OPX.0b013e3182357f79.

Edwards MH, Li RW, Lam CS, Lew JK, Yu BS. The Hong Kong progressive lens myopia control study: study design and main findings. *Invest Ophthalmol Vis Sci* 2002; 43:2852-2858. [PubMed: 12202502]

Fan DSP, Lam DSC, Chan CKM, et al. Topical atropine in retarding myopia progression and axial length growth in children with moderate to severe myopia: A pilot study. *Jpn J Ophthalmol* 2007;51:27–33.

Flitcroft DI, Adams GG, Robson AG, et al. Retinal dysfunction and refractive errors: an electrophysiological study of children. *Br J Ophthalmol* 2005;89:484–488.

Fredholm BB, Bättig K, Holmen J, et al. Actions of caffeine in the brain with special reference to factors that contribute to its widespread use. *Pharmacol Rev* 1999;51:83–133.

Fulk GW, Cyert LA, Parker DE, West RW. The effect of changing from glasses to soft contact lenses on myopia progression in adolescents. *Ophthalmic Physiol Opt* 2003;23:71–77. [PubMed: 12535059]

Fulk GW, Cyert LA, Parker DE. A randomized trial of the effect of single-vision vs. bifocal lenses on myopia progression in children with esophoria. *Optom Vis Sci* 2000;77:395-401.

Gallemore RP, Hughes BA, Miller SS. Light-induced responses of the retinal pigment epithelium. In: Marmor MF, Wolfensberger TJ, editors. The retinal pigment epithelium. New York: *Oxford University Press;* 1998. p. 175–198.

Gao Q, Liu Q, Ma P, et al. Effects of direct intravitreal dopamine injections on the development of lid-suture induced myopia in rabbits. *Graefes Arch Clin Exp Ophthalmol.* 2006;244:1329-1335.

Grosvenor T, Goss DA. The role of bifocal and contact lenses in myopia control. *Acta Ophthalmol Suppl* 1988;185:162-166.

Grosvenor T, Perrigin DM, Perrigin J, Maslovitz B. Houston Myopia Control Study: a randomized clinical trial. Part II. Final report by the patient care team. *Am J Optom Physiol Opt* 1987; 64:482–498. [PubMed: 3307440]

Grosvenor T, Perrigin J, Perrigin D, Quintero S. Use of silicone-acrylate contact lenses for the control of myopia: results after two years of lens wear. *Optom Vis Sci* 1989;66:41-47.

Gwiazda J, Hyman L, Hussein M, Everett D, Norton TT, Kurtz D, Leske MC, Manny R, Marsh-Tootle W, Scheiman M. A randomized clinical trial of progressive addition lenses versus single vision lenses on the progression of myopia in children. *Invest Ophthalmol Vis Sci* 2003; 44:1492–1500. [PubMed: 12657584]

Gwiazda J. Treatment options for myopia. *Optom Vis Sci* 2009,86.624-628.

Gwiazda JE, Hyman L, Norton TT, Hussein ME, Marsh-Tootle W, Manny R, Wang Y, Hasebe S, Ohtsuki H, Nonaka T, Nakatsuka C, Miyata M, Hamasaki I, Kimura S. Effect of progressive addition lenses on myopia progression in Japanese children: a prospective, randomized, doublemasked, crossover trial. *Invest Ophthalmol Vis Sci* 2008;49:2781-2789. [PubMed: 18579755]

Horner DG, Soni PS, Salmon TO, Swartz TS. Myopia progression in adolescent wearers of soft contact lenses and spectacles. *Optom Vis Sci* 1999;76:474-479.

Hung LF, Crawford ML, Smith EL 3rd. Spectacle lenses alter eye growth and the refractive status of young monkeys. *Nat Med* 1995;1:761–765. [PubMed: 7585177]

IARC. Monographs on the evaluation of the carcinogenic risk of chemicals to man. Geneva: WHO, International Agency for Research on Cancer, 1972-present; 1991. p. 51–357.

Iuvone PM, Tigges M, Stone RA, et al. Effects of apomorphine, a dopamine receptor agonist, on ocular refraction and axial elongation in a primate model of myopia. *Invest Ophthalmol Vis Sci* 1991;32:1674–1677.

Jensen H. Myopia progression in young school children. A prospective study of myopia progression and the effect of a trial with bifocal lenses and beta blocker eye drops. *Acta Ophthalmol Suppl* 1991;(2000):1-79.

Jensen H. Myopia progression in young school children. *Acta Ophthalmologica Suppl* 1991;69:1–79.

Jensen H. Timolol maleate in the control of myopia. A preliminary report. *Acta Ophthalmol Suppl* 1988;185:128-129.

Jessen GN. Contact lenses as a therapeutic device. *Am J Optom Arch Am Acad Optom* 1964;41:429-435.

Katz J, Schein OD, Levy B, et al. A randomized trial of rigid gas permeable contact lenses to reduce progression of children's myopia. *Am J Ophthalmol* 2003;136:82-90.

Kennedy RH, Dyer JA, Kennedy MA, et al. Reducing the progression of myopia with atropine: a long term cohort study of Olmsted County students. *Binocul Vis Strabismus Q* 2000;15:281-304.

Khoo CY, Chong J, Rajan U. A 3-year study on the effect of RGP contact lenses on myopic children. *Singapore Med J* 1999; 40:230–237. [PubMed: 10487074]

Lam CS, Edwards M, Millodot M, Goh WS. A 2-year longitudinal study of myopia progression and optical component changes among Hong Kong schoolchildren. *Optom Vis Sci* 1999; 76:370–380. [PubMed: 10416931]

Lessel M, Thaler A, Heilig P, et al. Intraoperative retinal light damage reflected in electrophysiologic data. *Doc Ophthalmol* 1991;76:323–333.

Leung JT, Brown B. Progression of myopia in Hong Kong Chinese schoolchildren is slowed by wearing progressive lenses. *Optom Vis Sci* 1999;76:346-354. [PubMed: 10416928]

Li et al. Multifocal versus single vision lenses intervention to slow progression of myopia in school-age children: A meta-analysis. *Surv Ophthalmol* 2011; 56:451-460.

Lind GJ, Chew SJ, Marzani D, Wallman J. Muscarinic acetylcholine receptor antagonists inhibit chick scleral chondrocytes. *Invest Ophthalmol Vis Sci* 1998;39:2217-2231.

Liu H, Lu Y, Dong Q, et al. Treatment of adolescent myopia by pressure plaster of semen impatientis on otoacupoints. *J Trad Chin Med* 1994;14:283-286.

Liu Q, Wu J, Wang X, et al. Changes in muscarinic acetylcholine receptor expression in form deprivation myopia in guinea pigs. *Mol Vis* 2007;13:1234-1244.

Luu CD, Lau AM, Koh AH, Tan D. Multifocal electroretinogram in children on atropine treatment for myopia. *Br J Ophthalmol* 2005;89:151-153.

Marks GA, Shaffery JP, Speciale SG, et al. Enhancement of rapid eye movement sleep in the rat by actions at A1 and A2a adenosine receptor subtypes with a differential sensitivity to atropine. *Neuroscience* 2003;116:913–920.

McBrien NA, Cottriall CL, Annies R. Retinal acetylcholine content in normal and myopic eyes: a role in ocular growth control? *Vis Neurosci* 2001;18:571-580.

McBrien NA, Moghaddam HO, Reeder AP. Atropine reduces experimental myopia and eye enlargement via a nonaccommodative mechanism. *Invest Ophthalmol Vis Sci* 1993;34:205–215.

McLeod SD. Overnight orthokeratology and corneal infection risk in children. *Arch Ophthalmol* 2007;125:688-689.

Moeschberger ML. Ocular predictors of the onset of juvenile myopia. *Invest Ophthalmol Vis Sci* 1999;40:1936-1943. [PubMed: 10440246]

Moo-Puc RE, Góngora-Alfaro JL, Alvarez-Cervera FJ, et al. Caffeine and muscarinic antagonists act in synergy to inhibit haloperidolinduced catalepsy. *Neuropharmacology* 2003;45:493–503.

Morrison RJ. The use of contact lenses in adolescent myopic patients. *Am J Optom Arch Am Acad Optom* 1960;37:165-168.

Müller CE, Shi D, Manning M, et al. Synthesis of paraxanthine analogs (1,7-disubstituted xanthines) and other xanthines unsubstituted at the 3-position: structure-activity relationship at adenosine receptors. *J Med Chem* 1993;36:3341–3349.

Oishi T, Lauber JK. Chicks blinded with formoguanamine do not develop lid suture myopia. *Curr Eye Res* 1988;7:69-73.

Oliveira L, Correia-de-Sa P. Protein kinase A and Ca(v)1 (L-Type) channels are common targets to facilitatory adenosine A2A and muscarinic M1 receptors on rat motoneurons. *Neurosignals* 2005; 14:262–272.

Ong E, Grice K, Held R, et al. Effects of spectacle intervention on the progression of myopia in children. *Optom Vis Sci* 1999;76:363-369.

Ouyang CH, Chu RY, Hu WZ. Effects of pirenzepine on lensinduced myopia in the guinea-pig. *Zhonghua Yan Ke Za Zhi* 2003;39:348–351.

Perrigin J, Perrigin D, Quintero S, Grosvenor T. Silicone-acrylate contact lenses for myopia control: 3-year results. *Optom Vis Sci* 1990;67:764-769.

Quarta D, Ferré S, Solinas M, You ZB, Hockemeyer J, Popoli P, Goldberg SR. Opposite modulatory roles for adenosine A1 and A2A receptors on glutamate and dopamine release in the shell of the nucleus accumbens. Effect of chronic caffeine exposure. *J Neurochem* 2004;88:1151–1158.

Rajan U, Tan FT, Chee D, et al. Accupressure point massage for myopia. VII International Conference on Myopia Program and Abstracts. Taipei, Taiwan. *Myopia International Research Foundation,* 57, 1998.

Saw SM, Gazzard G, Au Eong KG, Tan DT. Myopia: attempts to arrest progression. *Br J Ophthalmol* 2002;86:1306-1311.

Saw SM, Tong L, Chua WH, Chia KS, Koh D, Tan DT, Katz J. Incidence and progression of myopia in Singaporean school children. *Invest Ophthalmol Vis Sci* 2005; 46:51–57. [PubMed: 15623754]

Schallhorn SC, Farjo AA, Huang D, Boxer Wachler BS, Trattier WB, Tanzer DJ, Majmudar PA, Sugar A; American Academy of Ophthalmology. Wavefront-guided LASIK for the correction of primary myopia and astigmatism: a report by the American Academy of Ophthalmology. *Ophthalmology 2008*;115(7):1249-1261.

Schwartz JT. Results of a monozygotic cotwin control study on a treatment for myopia. *Prog Clin Biol Res* 1981;69 Pt C:249-58.

Shi D, Daly JW. Chronic effects of xanthines on levels of central receptors in mice. *Cell Mol Neurobiol* 1999;19:719–32.

Shih YF, Chen CH, Chou AC, et al. Effects of different concentrations of atropine on controlling myopia in myopic children. *J Ocul Pharmacol Ther* 1999;15:85-90.

Shih YF, Hsiao CK, Chen CJ, Chang CW, Hung PT, Lin LL. An intervention trial on efficacy of atropine and multi-focal glasses in controlling myopic progression. *Acta Ophthalmol Scand* 2001; 79:233–236. [PubMed: 11401629]

Shih YF, Lin LL, Hwang CY, et al. The effects of Qi-Qong ocular exercise on accommodation. *Chin J Physiol* 1995;38:35–42.

Siatkowski RM, Cotter S, Miller JM, Scher CA, Crockett RS, Novack GD. Safety and efficacy of 2% pirenzepine ophthalmic gel in children with myopia: a 1-year, multicenter, double-masked, placebo-controlled parallel study. *Arch Ophthalmol* 2004; 122:1667–1674. [PubMed: 15534128]

Siatkowski RM, Cotter SA, Crockett RS, Miller JM, Novack GD, Zadnik K. Two-year multicenter, randomized, double-masked, placebo-controlled, parallel safety and efficacy study of 2% pirenzepine ophthalmic gel in children with myopia. *J J AAPOS* 2008; 12:332–339.

Stone J. Contact lens wear in the young myope. *Br J Physiol Opt* 1973;28:90-134.

Stone J. The possible influence of contact lenses on myopia. *Br J Physiol Opt* 1976;31:89-114.

Stone RA, Lin T, Laties AM. Muscarinic antagonist effects on experimental chick myopia. *Exp Eye Res* 1991;52:755–758.

Sutter EE, Tran D. The field topography of ERG components in man—I. The photopic luminance response. *Vis Res* 1992;32:433–446.

Syniuta LA, Isenberg SJ. Atropine and bifocals can slow the progression of myopia in children. *Binocul Vis Strabismus Q* 2001;16:203-208.

Tan DT, Lam DS, Chua WH, Shu-Ping DF, Crockett RS. One-year multicenter, double-masked, placebo-controlled, parallel safety and efficacy study of 2% pirenzepine ophthalmic gel in children with myopia. *Ophthalmology* 2005;112:84–91. [PubMed: 15629825]

Tarka SM Jr, Morrissey RP, Apgar JL. Chronic toxicity/carcinogenicity studies of the cocoa powder in rats. *Food Chem Toxicol* 1991;29:7–19.

Tarka SM Jr. The toxicology of cocoa and methylxanthines: a review of the literature. *Crit Rev Toxicol* 1982;9:275–312.

Tigges M, Iuvone PM, Fernandes A, et al. Effects of muscarinic cholinergic receptor antagonists on postnatal eye growth of rhesus monkeys. *Optom Vis Sci* 1999;76:397-407.

Tong L, Huang XL, Koh AL, Zhang X, Tan DT, Chua WH. Atropine for the treatment of treatment of childhood myopia. *Ophthalmology* 2006; 113:2285-2291. [PubMed: 16996612]

Tong L, Huang XL, Koh AL, Zhang X, Tan DT, Chua WH. Atropine for the treatment of treatment of childhood myopia: effect on myopia progression after cessation of atropine. *Ophthalmology* 2009; 116:572-579.

Trier K, Munk Ribel-Madsen S, Cui D, Brøgger Christensen S. Systemic 7-methylxanthine in retarding axial eye growth and myopia progression: a 36-month pilot study. *J Ocul Biol Dis Infor* 2008;1(2-4):85-93.

Van Meter WS, Musch DC, Jacobs DS, et al. Safety of overnight orthokeratology for myopia: a report by the American Academy of Ophthalmology. *Ophthalmology* 2008;115:2301-2313.e1.

Walline JJ, Jones LA, Mutti DO, Zadnik K. A randomized trial of the effects of rigid contact lenses on myopia progression. *Arch Ophthalmol* 2004;122:1760-1766.

Walline JJ, Jones LA, Sinnott L, Manny RE, Gaume A, Rah MJ, Chitkara M, Lyons S. A randomized trial of the effect of soft contact lenses on myopia progression in children. *Invest Ophthalmol Vis Sci* 2008;49:4702–4706. [PubMed: 18566461]

Walline JJ, Mutti DO, Jones LA, et al. The contact lens and myopia progression (CLAMP) study: design and baseline data. *Optom Vis Sci* 2001;78:223-233.

Wallman J, Winawer J. Homeostasis of eye growth and the question of myopia. *Neuron* 2004;43:447-468. [PubMed: 15312645]

Wei ML, Liu JP, Liu M. Acupuncture for slowing the progression of myopia in children and adolescents (Review). Cochrane Database of Systematic Reviews 2011, Issue 9. Art. No: CD007842.DOI:10.1002/14651858.CD007842.pub2.

White PJ, Nguyen TT. Chronic caffeine treatment causes changes in cardiac Adenosine receptor function in rats. *Pharmacology* 2002;65:129–135.

Yen MY, Liu JH, Kao SC, et al. Comparison of the effect of atropine and cyclopentolate on myopia. *Ann Ophthalmol* 1989;21:180–182, 187.

Yin GC, Gentle A, McBrien NA. Muscarine antagonist control of myopia: A molecular search for the M1 receptor in chicks. *Mol Vis.* 2004;10:787–793.

Zadnik K. Myopia development in childhood. *Optom Vis Sci* 1997;74:603-608.

Zhao J, Mao J, Luo R, Li F, Munoz SR, Ellwein LB. The progression of refractive error in schoolage children: Shunyi district, China. *Am J Ophthalmol* 2002; 134:735-743. [PubMed: 12429251]

Glossary

Aberration - Difference in focus or magnification as a result of difference in refraction of different wavelengths composing white light.

Aberrations - Chromatic (color) Aberrations: is the change in light direction in materials with different refractive index due to the different wavelengths of light. A simple plus lens will bend blue light rays more than red rays, leading to the optical aberration known as chromatic aberration. The blue rays come to focus closer to the lens than the red rays. Chromatic aberration occurs strongly in the human eye; with almost 3.00D difference in the focus of the far ends the visible spectrum. This is the basis of the red-green test used for refinement of the sphere power in clinical refraction. Chromatic dispersion is caused because each wavelength of light has its own index of refraction. Shorter wavelengths (blue) deviate the most in materials with higher index of refraction. Aberration can be modified by changing the shape of the lens or changing the refractive index of the lens or changing the aperture size (results in fewer marginal rays) or changing the position of the aperture. In general, it is not possible to eliminate all aberration at once. Minimize one may worsen the other; therefore we need to prioritize and minimize the most irritating aberrations. Aberrations are all object/image distance dependent.

Accommodation - The change in the curvature of the lens that helps to focus images of objects close the eye. It is the mechanism by which the eye changes refractive power by altering the shape of its crystalline lens. During accommodation, the ciliary muscle contracts allowing the zonular fibers to relax. This relaxation causes the equatorial edge of the lens to move away from the sclera during accommodation resulting in increased lens convexity (roundness). This increase in roundness primarily occurs on the front surface of the lens.

Add - The portion of the multifocal lens (usually the lower part) that provides near vision.

Ametropia - The refractive state of an eye that is unable to focus correctly due to refractive error. Ametropia refers to the absence of emmetropia. In axial ametropia, the eyeball is either unusually long (myopia) or short (hyperopia). In refractive ametropia, the length of the eye is statistically normal, but the total power of the eye is abnormal.

Amplitude of Accommodation - also known as the accommodative response, is the maximum increase in diopter power obtainable by an eye. The amplitude of accommodation is measured monocularly.

Angiography, fluorescein, ocular - Photographic visualization of the passage of fluorescein through the intraocular vessels after intravenous injection.

Anisocoria - A condition in which the pupils are of unequal size.

Anterior chamber angle - The junction of the cornea and the iris, from which aqueous humor leaves the eye.

Anterior chamber - The small compartment between the cornea and the iris that is filled with a clear, transparent fluid called aqueous humor. The anterior chamber (frontispiece) is bounded anteriorly by the cornea, posteriorly by the front surface of the iris and lens, and peripherally by the anterior chamber angle. The anterior chamber is deepest in its central portion (3 mm) and shallowest at the peripheral insertion of the iris. In humans, its volume is approximately 0.20 ml.

Anterior segment - The front of the eye; includes the structures between the front surface of the cornea and the vitreous.

Aphakia - Absence of the lens, usually because of cataract extraction.

Aqueous humor - Is secreted by the nonpigmented epithelium of the ciliary processes into the posterior chamber and flows through the pupil into the anterior chamber.

A-scan ultrasonography - A diagnostic procedure in which sound waves travelling in a straight line are used to reveal the position of, and distances between, structures within the eye and orbit. Also called A-mode ultrasonography.

Aspheric lens - radius changes from the center to the outside (becomes less curved usually)

Astigmatism - The refractive error of an eye whose corneal surface curvature is greater in one meridian than another; both distant and near objects appear blurred and distorted. Astigmatism occurs when incident light rays do not converge at a single focal point.

Axial Myopia - Occurs when the power of the eye is 60D but the eye is longer than 22.6mm. Every millimeter of axial elongation causes approximately 3D of myopia.

Axial ray - A light ray that strikes the venter of a lens of any shape and passes undeviated through the lens material. Also called principal ray.

Axis - The meridian perpendicular to the meridian with curvature in a cylindrical lens.

Balancing - A procedure performed on both eyes at once to ensure that the optical correction determined by refractometry for distance vision does not include an uneven overcorrection or undercorrection. Also called binocular balancing.

Base curve - The curve of the lens surface, usually the outer or front side of the lens, from which the other curves necessary for sight correction are calculated.

Base - The bottom.

Bifocal lenses - One that has two powers: usually one for correcting distance vision and one for correcting near vision.

Binocular balancing - See Balancing.

Binocular vision - The blending of the separate images seen by each eye into one image; occurs when both eyes are directed toward a single target and perfectly aligned.

Biomicroscope - Microscope for examining the eye; consists essentially of a dissecting microscope combined with a light source that projects a rectangular light beam that can be changed in size and focus. Also called Slit lamp.

B-mode ultrasonography - See B-scan ultrasonography

Bruch membrane - Tissue between the choriocapillaris and the retinal pigment epithelium.

B-scan ultrasonography - A diagnostic procedure that provides two-dimensional reconstruction of ocular and orbital tissues, using radiating sound waves. Also called B-mode ultrasonography.

Cataract - Opacity of the crystalline lens

Concave lens - A piece of glass or plastic in which one or both surfaces are curved inward. Also called negative lens or minus lens.

Concave mirror effect - The lighting effect of a retinoscope that produces convergent rays.

Contrast Sensitivity - Contrast indicates the variation in brightness of an object. When an eye chart uses perfectly black ink on perfectly white paper, 100% contrast is achieved. Acuity charts approximate 100% contrast. Acuity charts are helpful for characterizing central visual acuity. However, they are less helpful for examining visual function away from fixation. Contrast sensitivity is tested using alternating light and dark bars at varying intensity. The number of light bands per-unit length or per-unit angle is called the spatial frequency.

Conus of optic disk - Condition in which the choroid and retinal pigment epithelium do not extend to the optic disk, allowing the sclera to be observed ophthalmoscopically at its margin.

Converge - To come together.

Convergence (in prism diopters) - required for an ametrope to bi-fixate a near object is equal to the dioptric distance from the object to the center of rotation of the eyes, multiplied by the subject's intra-pupillary distance in centimeters. Convergence (Δ) = 100/working distance (cm) x Pupillary Distance (cm).

Convex lens - A piece of glass or plastic in which one or both surfaces are curved outward. Also called positive lens or plus lens.

Critical Angle - occurs when going from a denser to a rarer medium. There is a point where a' = 90° and all light is therefore internally reflected. The angle of incidence (a) that produces this condition is termed the Critical Angle (CA). Total internal reflection occurs when the angle exceeds CA. As n increases, CA decreases. The angle can be determined using Snell's law as follows: $n \sin i_c = n' \sin 90°$ where: i_c = the critical angle and the refracted angle is 90°, $\sin i_c = n'/n \times 1$

Cross cylinder - A special lens consisting of two cylinders of equal power, one minus and one plus, with their axes set at right angles to each other; used for determining the axis and power of an astigmatic correction. See Jackson Cross Cylinder

Cycloplegia - Paralysis of accommodation. Temporary paralysis of the ciliary muscle (preventing accommodation) and of the iris sphincter muscle (preventing dilation of the pupil).

Cycloplegic refraction - Refractometry performed with the use of a drug that temporary paralyzes the ciliary muscle, thus blocking accommodation.

Cylindrical lens - A lens that has curvature in only one meridian.

Cylindrical lens - Different powers in different meridians

Depth of field - is the same principle for objects as the depth of focus is for images. When an optical system such as the camera is focused on an object, nearby objects are also in focus, inside the camera's depth of field. Objects outside of the depth of field will be out of focus.

Depth of focus - describes the image location range where the image is clear when focused by an optical system. Outside this range, the image will be significantly blurry. However, within this few millimeter range, the image appears quite sharp.

Diopter - A diopter is a unit of accommodative amplitude; it describes the vergence of a waveform and describes the vergence at a specific distance from the source; and it is also defined as the power of the lens. A diopter is the reciprocal of the distance in meters.

Duochrome Test - Chromatic aberration of the eye results in green light being focused in front of the retina, yellow light at the retinal plane, and red light behind the retina. Therefore, when red is brighter, it indicates that more minus is needed to move the focus of red light further behind the retina? When green is brighter, more plus is needed to move the green light to focus further into the posterior chamber.

Emmetropia - The refractive state of an eye that is able to focus correctly. Refractive condition in which no refractive error is present with accommodation at rest.

Far point of the eye - Is the object point imaged by the eye onto the retina in an unaccommodated eye. If a corrective lens is used to correct for myopia, the lens has its secondary focal point coincident with the far point of the eye. The far point of the emmetropic eye is at infinity. Myopia exists if, without accommodation, a point at infinity is imaged in front of the retina (in the vitreous). The stimulus on the retina is therefore not a point, but a blur circle. Moving the object closer to the myopic eye, until the image is a point focus on the retina, establishes the far point of the eye. Hyperopia exists, if without accommodation, an object point at infinity is imaged neither in the vitreous nor on the retina, but theoretically, behind it.

Fogging - Method to determine refractive error in which accommodation is relaxed by means of convex spheres that make the patient artificially myopic.

Fusion - The blending by the brain of the separate images received by the two eyes so that a single view is perceived even when the eyes move.

Geometric optics - The area of optics that deals with the transmission of light as rays and is concerned with the effect of lenses on light and the production of images.

Horizontal and vertical meridians - The radial meridians that divide the circular visual field mapping device into quarters.

Hyperopia - Farsightedness; the eye is too short for its optical system. Hyperopia refers to light striking the retina before converging at its focal point.

Image - Visual impression of an object formed by a lens or mirror.

Informed consent - The process by which, after discussion with the physician about the risks and benefits of a proposed procedure, the patient agrees to undergo a treatment.

Interpupillary distance (IPD or PD) - The distance from the center of the pupil of one eye to the center of the pupil of the other eye.

Interval or Conoid of Sturm - The interval is a conical image space bound by the two focal lines of a spherocylinder lens. At the center of the Conoid of Sturm is the Circle of Least Confusion. The Circle of Least Confusion is the dioptric midpoint of a cylindrical lens and is defined as the spherical equivalent of the cylindrical lens. This is where the horizontal and vertical dimensions of the blurred image are approximately equal. The goal of a spherical refractive correction is to choose a lens that places the Circle of Least Confusion on the retina. The smaller the Interval of Sturm, the smaller is the blur circle (Circle of Least Confusion).

Jackson Cross Cylinder (JCC) - Cross cylinders are combinations of two cylinders whose powers are numerically equal and of opposite sign and whose axes are perpendicular to each other. The Jackson Cross Cylinder is usually mounted in a ring with a handle at 45 degrees from the axis so that a twirl of the handle changes the cross cylinder to a second position. Example: +0.25x90/–0.25x180 to –0.25x90/+0.25x180 When the JCC is placed in contact with a spherocylinder, it displaces both focal lines simultaneously in opposite directions, expanding the initial Interval of Sturm in the first position and contracting it in the second. However, there will be no displacement of the Circle of Least Confusion, only the diameter of the circle will increase in the first and decrease in the second position of the JCC. When a +/-0.50 JCC is placed on a lensometer, with the red axis at 0 and 180 degrees, the lensometer will read the power as -0.50 +1.00 x 090. But, remembering that the JCC has no spherical power, only cylindrical power. For this reason, we can more accurately write the power of the JCC as –0.50 x 180 combined with +0.50 x 90

Keratometer - An instrument used to measure the curvature/refractive power of the cornea. It accomplishes this by measuring the radius of curvature of the central cornea. The central cornea can be thought of as a high powered convex spherical mirror. Also called ophthalmometer.

Keratometry - The measurement of corneal curvature.

Laser - The word Laser is an acronym for light amplification by stimulated emission of radiation. Stimulated emission of a photon of electromagnetic radiation is the basic physical principle that makes lasers possible.

Law of Reflection. - A = a' where A = angle of incidence and a' equals the angle of reflection. The angle of incidence and the angle of reflection are both measured from a normal to the surface. The normal is at 90° to the surface the light is hitting.

Legal blindness - A best corrected visual acuity of 20/200 or less or a visual field reduced to 20° or less in the better-seeing eye.

Lens - Part of the optical focusing system of the eye, immediately behind the iris. Also called crystalline lens.

Lensometer - The lensometer measures the vertex power of the lens. The vertex power is the reciprocal of the distance between the back surface of the lens and its secondary focal point. This is also known as the back focal length. For this reason, a lensometer does not really measure the focal length of a lens. The true focal lengths are measured from the principal planes, not from the lens surface. The lensometer works on the Badel principle with the addition of an astronomical telescope for precise detection of parallel rays at neutralization. The Badel principal is Knapp's law applied to lensometers. A lensometer is really an optical bench consisting of an illuminated moveable target, a powerful fixed lens, and a telescopic eyepiece focused at infinity. The key element is the field lens that is fixed in place so that its focal point is on the back surface of the lens being analyzed. A lensometer measures the back vertex power of the spectacle lens. However, when measuring a bifocal addition, the spectacles must be turned around in the lensometer so that the front vertex power is measured. This is because the distance portion of the spectacle lenses is designed to deal with essentially parallel light. However, the bifocal addition is designed to work on diverging light, originating from a standard working distance of 40 centimeters. This diverging light from the near object is made parallel by the bifocal lens. The parallel light then enters the distance lens where it is refracted with the expected optical affect to give the patient clear vision. In this way, the bifocal exerts its effect on the light from the object before it passes through the rest of the lens. For strong bifocal corrections, there would be a significant difference in the bifocal strength measurement when using the front versus back vertex measurement.

Macula - Macula or macula lutea (from Latin macula, "spot" + lutea, "yellow") is the specialized area of the retina close to the center of the back of the eye that provides detailed central vision. It is an oval-shaped highly pigmented yellow spot near the center of the retina of the human eye. It has a diameter of around 6 mm and is often histologically defined as having two or more layers of ganglion cells. Near its center is the fovea, a small pit that contains the largest concentration of cone cells in the eye and is responsible for central, high resolution vision.

Manifest refraction - Refractometry performed without the use of cycloplegic drugs.

Measuring Accommodation*:* Tests of accommodation are performed monocularly. When measuring the accommodative amplitude, it is assumed that you are testing an emmetropia, or someone who is corrected with spectacles, so that their far point is at infinity. Target size, target illumination, and speed of target approach will affect the measurement of the amplitude of accommodation. The push up method works well for emmetropes, or fully corrected ametropes.

Media opacities - The general term used to describe a variety of conditions that cloud, obscure, or otherwise affect the ocular media and, ultimately, may disrupt vision.

Medium - is any material that transmits light. Light travels at different speeds in different media. Light travels faster in a vacuum and slower through any material. A medium's refractive index (n) = speed of light in a vacuum (c)/speed of light in a particular medium (v). Refractive indices are always equal to or greater than 1.0. The index tells us how much light has slowed down when entering a refractive media. Denser media have higher n values; rarer media have smaller n values.

Meridian - Plane.

Minus lens - A minus lens always reduces vergence; defines a focal point; and diverges image rays to produce a virtual image of an object at infinity to the left of the minus lens

Minus lens - See concave lens.

Miotic - A drug that causes the iris sphincter muscle to contract, producing miosis (pupillary constriction), which reduces the amount of light entering the eye.

Mires - The perpendicular crossed lines in a lensmeter.

Multifocal - See bifocal lens, trifocal lens.

Mydriasis - Dilation of the pupil

Mydriatic - A drug that dilates the pupil.

Myopia - Optical condition in which parallel rays of light come to focus in front of the retina. Nearsightedness; the eye is too long for its optical system. Myopia refers to defocus due to light coming to focus anterior to the retinal plane.

Myopic crescent - Term applied to a conus of the optic disk in myopia.

Near add - See add

Near point of the eye - Is found when the uncorrected refractive error of the eye is added to the accommodative ability of the eye. If the amplitude of accommodation is 10D, the near point is 10cm in front of the eye (specifically, 10cm in front of the vertex of the cornea which is used as a convenient reference point)

Near visual acuity - The ability to see clearly at a normal reading distance.

Negative lens - See concave lens.

Neovascularization - The abnormal growth of new blood vessels.

Neutralization point - The lens power that is the approximate correction for a refractive error.

Neutralization - See lensometry

Nodal point - The point in the eye where light entering or leaving the eye and passing through the nodal point, is undeviated. This allows similar triangles to be used to determine the retinal image size of an object in space. For example, to determine the retinal image size of a Snellen letter (viewed at 6 meters), the following formula would be used: Retinal image height/Snellen letter height = 17mm/6000mm

Nodal points - Locations in an optical system toward and from which are directed corresponding incident and transmitted rays that make equal angles with the optic axis.

Objective refractometry - See retinoscopy

Ocular media - The three transparent optical structures that transmit light: cornea, lens, and vitreous.

OD (oculus dexter) - Latin for right eye.

Opacification - Clouding of the lens, occurs in many people over age 65.

Opaque - Refers to a substance that completely blocks light.

Ophthalmic registered nurse - A registered nurse with special training in problems related to the eye; frequently functions as a surgical assistant to an ophthalmologist, a director of an ophthalmic surgery service, or a director of clinical services.

Ophthalmologist - A medical doctor (physician) who specializes in the prevention, diagnosis, and medical as well as surgical treatment of vision problems and diseases of the eye.

Ophthalmology - The medical and surgical speciality concerned with the eye and its surrounding structures, their proper function, eye disorders, and all aspects of vision.

Ophthalmometer - See keratometer.

Ophthalmoscope - An instrument for examining directely or indirectely the vitreous and fundus.

Ophthalmoscope, Direct – image is upright. Magnification is based on the total refractive power of the eye. Using the basic magnification formula of M = F/4, an emmetropic eye of +60.00D would provide +60/4 = +15X. An aphakic eye of +40.00D would provide +40/4 = +10X.

Ophthalmoscope, Indirect – the image of the fundus becomes the object of the condensing lens, which then forms an aerial image that is larger and inverted. The two plus lenses (the eye and the condensing lens) determine the magnification of the aerial image. For the emmetropic eye, using the formula $M_A = (-)D_{Eye}/C_{ondensing\ lens} = (-)60/D_{(condensing\ lens)}$, we find that a 20D condensing lens results in (-)60/20 = -3X. As the power of the condensing lens decreases, the magnification increases. Axial magnification increases exponentially, based on the formula *Axial magnification:* $M_A = (M)^2$.

Optic chiasm - The point behind the eyes in the brain where the two optic nerves merge and the axon fibers from the nasal retina of each eye cross to the opposite side.

Optic disc - The location where the central retinal artery enters and the central retinal vein, as well as the nerve fibers, exits. Also called optic nerve head.

Optic nerve head - See optic disc

Optic nerve - The nerve that carries electric impulses to the brain's visual cortex, where they are integrated to produce the sensation of sight.

Optic radiation - The nerve cell that transmits visual information from the lateral geniculate body to the visual cortex.

Optic tract - The part of the brain between the optic chiasm and the lateral geniculate body.

Optical center - The point of optimal vision; the single point of a lens through which light may pass without being bent or changed.

Optical centers, distance between - See distance between optical centers.

Optical coherence Tomography (OCT) - uses diode laser light in the near-infrared spectrum (810 nm) to produce high-resolution cross-sectional images of the retina using coherence interferometry. It allows cross-sectional imaging of the retina and optic disc based on the interference patterns produced by low coherence light reflected from retinal tissues. It is a noninvasive, rapid, objective, and reproducible method for evaluating the retinal nerve fiber layer (RNFL).

Optician - An independent professional licensed to dispense eyeglasses and contact lenses from the prescription of an ophthalmologist or optometrist.

Optics - The branch of physical science that deals with the properties of light and vision. Optics is the study of light or, more broadly, the study of the electromagnetic spectrum.

Optometrist - An independent practitioner trained in the prescription of eyeglasses and contact lenses as well as in the detection of eye disease.

Optotypes - Test symbols of graduated size for measuring visual acuity.

Optotypes, Snellen - See Snellen chart.

Orthokeratology - A method of molding the cornea with contact lenses to improve unaided vision.

OS (oculus sinister) - Latin for left eye.

Pachymeter - An instrument, attached to a slit lamp, that measures the distance between the corneal endothelium. Sometimes spelled pachometer.

Pachymetry - The measurement of corneal thickness by the use of a pachymeter. Sometimes spelled pachometry.

Parallax - An optical distorsion that occurs when the measure's line of sight is not parallel to that of the patient.

Parallel - Refers to rays that travel side by side in the same direction, neither diverging nor converging.

Paraxial - Refers to parallel light rays from a distant source that enter the lens at any point other than the center.

PD - See interpupillary distance.

Perimetry - The measurement of the expanse and sensitivity of peripheral vision and the visual field to pinpoint possible defects.

Peripheral vision - The visual perception of objects and space that surround the direct line of sight.

Photoreceptor - A light-sensitive cell.

Physical optics - The area of optics that describes the nature of light in tems of its wave properties.

Physiologic blind spot - The sightless "hole" in the normal visual field corresponding to the optic disc.

Physiology - The function and operation of an organism.

Pinhole occlude - The hand-held device that completely covers one eye and allows the other to view a chart through a tiny central opening, often used to confirm a diagnosis of refractive error.

Plus lens - See convex lens.

Plus lenses - always add vergence; define a focal point; and converge image rays to produce a real image of an object at infinity to the right of a plus lens.

PMMA - See polymethylmethacrylate lenses.

Polymethylmethacrylate (PMMA) lenses - Contact lenses that provide oxygen by means of a tear pump only; no oxygen or carbon dioxide diffuses through the lens.

Positive lens - See convex lens.

Posterior segment examination - See funduscopic examination.

Posterior segment - The rear portion of the eye; includes the vitreous and the retina. The posterior chamber (frontispiece) is bounded anteriorly by the iris, peripherally by the ciliary processes, and posteriorly by the anterior lens capsule and its zonule. Its volume in adults is about 0.06 ml.

Power Transposition - *Converting plus to minus cylinder and vice versa.* To convert plus to minus cylinder and vice versa, add sphere power to cylinder power = new sphere power, change sign of cylinder power, change axis by 90 degrees. **Examples:** +2.50 +3.50 x 95 = +6.00 – 3.50 x 005 ; –2.75 – 2.00 x 010 = -4.75 + 2.00 x 100

Power - See vergence power.

Prentice's Rule - determines how much deviation you get by looking off center of a lens. There is no prismatic power at the optical center of the lens. Deviation in prism diopters (PD) = h (cm) x F where F = power of the lens and h = distance from the optical center of the lens.

Presbyopia - The progressive loss of the accommodative ability of the lens, due to natural processes of aging. Presbyopia is a condition that develops with aging and results in insufficient accommodation for near work in a patient whose distance refractive error is fully corrected.

Principal axis - The pathway of a light ray that strikes the center of a lens of any shape and passes undeviated through the lens material.

Principal meridians - The meridians of maximum and minimum corneal curvature.

Principal ray - See axial ray.

Prism Diopter (Δ) - is defined as a deviation of 1 cm at 1 meter. For angles under 45° (or 100 Δ), each degree (°) of angular deviation equals approximately 2 Δ.*(Approximation Formula).*

Prism diopter - The unit of measure of the refraction power of a prism.

Prism - A triangular piece of glass or plastic with flat sides, an apex, and a base.

Prismatic effect - An optical distortion in which images are displaced from their normal position; can occur if the distance between optical centers (DBC) does not correspond to the interpupillary distance (IPD).

Prisms - are defined as a transparent medium that is bound by two plane sides that are inclined at an angle to each other. Prisms are used to deviate light, but do not change the vergence and for this reason, they do not focus light. With prisms, light is bent towards the base. The image of an object formed by a prism is a virtual image. The image will appear displaced towards the apex of the prism.

Progressive-addition multifocals - Multifocals in which no discrete, visible line divides the distance and near segments; rather, the optical power is added progressively in a transitional zone. Also called progressive^-add multifocals.

Pseudophakia - The use of an intraocular lens to correct the vision of an aphakic patient.

Pupil - The opening in the center of the iris that enlarges (admitting more light) and reduces (admitting less light).

Range of Accommodation denotes the linear distance (expressed in centimeters or meters) over which the accommodative power allows an individual to maintain clear vision. The range lies between the near point of accommodation and the far point of accommodation. This is considered the most useful clinical measurement of accommodation. It helps answer the question as to whether an individual's accommodative range comfortably encompasses his visual needs. Clinically, accommodative ranges are measured from the anterior corneal surface (reference position). Optically, for the purist, that reference should be the primary principle plane of the eye, 1.4 mm behind the anterior corneal surface.

Refinement - The second step in refractometry, requiring patient participation and responses, which confirms the information produced by retinoscopy. Also called subjective recfractometry.

Refracted - Refers to a light ray that bends when it passes at an angle from one transparent medium to another.

Refraction - (1) In physics, the bending of light ray as it passes through substances of different densities. Refraction is the bending of light between media and is a function of the incident angle. This is based on Snell's Law and is not dependent on the speed of light. Snell's Law is the relationship between the incident and refracted angles of the light ray. (2) In eye care, the process of measuring a patient's refractive error and the clinical judgment to determine the optical correction needed. Refraction is the bending of light between media and is a function of the incident angle.

Refractive error - Refractive error (ametropia) is a disorder that occurs when parallel rays of light entering the non-accommodating eye are not focused on the retina. A nonpathologic deficiency in the eye's optical system.

Refractive index - The ratio of the speed of light in a vacuum to its speed through a specific substance.

Refractive Myopia - Occurs when the power of the eye exceeds 60D and the length of the eye is 22.6mm. This is due to steeper corneal curvatures or higher lenticular powers.

Refractive state - The relative ability of the refractive components of the eye to bring objects into focus on the retina.

Refractometry - The measurement of refractive error with a variety of instruments and tehniques.

Refractor - An instrument for determining a corrective lens prescription; stores a range of trial lenses than can be dialed into position. Also called phoropter.

Regular astigmatism - The most common form of astigmatism, in which the cornea resembles a football standing on one end or on its side.

Resting Level of Accommodation: In the absence of visual stimuli, the eye assumes an accommodative posture approximately 1D inside the far point, at the so-called "dark focus". This phenomenon helps explain "night" myopia and "empty field" myopia. Activation of the sympathetic nervous system is apparently involved in driving the accommodative state from the resting level to the far point in ordinary seeing.

Retinoscope - A retinoscope allows the clinician to objectively determine the spherocylindrical refractive error; irregular astigmatism, and also evaluate opacities and irregularities of the cornea and lens. Most retinoscope today use a streak projection system. This streak of light is reflected from a mirror. Additionally, the streak can be moved in relation to a convex lens in the device by way of the sleeve. This allows the light to leave the device as if it were coming from a point behind the retinoscope (plano mirror setting) or as if it were coming from a point between the examiner and the patient (concave mirror setting). For Copeland retinoscopes, the plano position is with the sleeve up, while the Welch Allyn retinoscope is in the plano position with the sleeve down. Normally, the examiner will use their right eye to perform retinoscopy on the patient's right eye and their left eye for the patient's left eye. The examiner should align themselves just off-center to minimize lens reflections and to allow the patient to visualize the distance target to relax their accommodation. The patient should be instructed to look at a distance target such as a large Snellen letter (20/200-20/400).

Retinoscopy - Objective method of determining the refraction of the eye by observing the movements of the reflection of light from the eye (skiascopy).

Spherical Equivalent - Dioptric midpoint of a sphero-cylindrical lens. ½ cylinder power + sphere power. This is also known as the Circle of Least Confusion. When one wishes to utilize only partial correction of the astigmatism, it is still desirable to keep the circle of least confusion on the retina. This is why we use the spherical equivalent formula to maintain the circle of least confusion on the retina.

Spherical lens - Power and radius is the same in all meridians

Telescopes - Are afocal optical systems consisting of two lenses, separated in space, in air. There are two types of telescopic systems, Keplerian and Galilean.

Visual axis - Straight line connecting an object seen with the fovea.

Vitreous cavity - The vitreous cavity is the largest cavity of the eye. It is bounded anteriorly by the lens, zonule, and ciliary body and posteriorly by the retina and optic nerve. It has a volume of 4.5 ml.

Author's Contact Information

Dr. Dieudonne Kaimbo Wa Kaimbo,
Professor
Ophthalmology and Biophysics
University of Kinshasa
226b, Colonel Mondjiba, Gombe,
BP 16540 Kinshasa 1
Tel: +243 9 98238928
Email: dieudonne_kaimbo@yahoo.com

Index

#

20th century, 128
21st century, 181
7-mx, 285, 286

A

Aberration, 121, 295
abuse, 4, 25
Acanthamoeba, 267, 270, 273, 274, 275, 276, 277
access, 141
accommodation, 1, 5, 6, 13, 31, 103, 123, 164, 165, 168, 173, 176, 177, 178, 179, 181, 183, 184, 185, 186, 187, 188, 189, 190, 191, 192, 193, 196, 197, 198, 199, 200, 262, 263, 264, 265, 276, 279, 280, 281, 283, 285, 292, 295, 297, 298, 300, 303, 304, 305
acetylcholine, 191, 286, 290
acid, 4, 15, 133
acne, 267
acrylate, 168, 289, 291
activity level, 22
actuality, 167
acupuncture, 287
acute angle closure glaucoma, 13, 193
acute glaucoma, 132, 138
adaptation, 123, 264, 286
adenoma, 204, 219
adenosine, 115, 285, 286, 288, 290, 291
adhesion, 228, 234, 236, 238, 247
adjustment, 21, 23, 162, 165, 167, 180, 191, 207, 229
adolescents, 283, 289, 293
adults, 3, 24, 28, 29, 30, 34, 178, 191, 192, 194, 204, 206, 209, 211, 217, 218, 220, 222, 226, 231, 243, 247, 248, 250, 254, 255, 258, 303
advancement, 235
adverse effects, 14, 193
aesthetic, 101
aetiology, 6, 246
African-American, 280
age, vii, 3, 5, 6, 11, 16, 18, 20, 21, 22, 23, 24, 25, 26, 27, 28, 29, 31, 34, 35, 133, 134, 137, 145, 149, 152, 153, 154, 155, 156, 160, 161, 166, 183, 191, 192, 193, 194, 196, 197, 205, 206, 208, 209, 210, 217, 220, 222, 225, 228, 230, 231, 232, 234, 242, 243, 244, 245, 246, 248, 250, 260, 265, 281, 283, 284, 287, 290, 301
age-related macular degeneration, 205
aggregation, 28, 34, 201
aging population, 208
agonist, 11, 290
AIDS, 11
Air Force, 116
Airy disk, 115, 116
alcohol abuse, 4
alcohol use, 172
allergic reaction, 200
allergy, 196
alters, 190
amblyopia, 5, 142, 186, 192, 201, 202, 203, 218, 220, 224, 279
ametropia, xi, 1, 18, 30, 151, 276, 286, 295, 304
amino, 285
amino acid, 285
amplitude, 130, 131, 164, 176, 177, 189, 191, 192, 197, 200, 265, 295, 298, 300
anatomy, v, vii, 2, 37, 140, 142, 163, 168, 251, 257
angiogenesis, 14, 159
angiography, 230, 242, 249, 250
angle closure glaucoma, 4, 193, 194, 218
Anisocoria, 296
Anisometropia, 33, 219, 262, 276
annual rate, 282, 287
Anterior chamber, 216, 296

Anterior segment, 296
anticholinergic, 191, 193, 194
anticholinergic effect, 194
apex, 120, 303
Aphakia, 296
aqueous humor, 296
argon, 226
aripiprazole, 4
Aristotle, 127
arrest, 291
arteries, 149
arterioles, 147, 207, 234
artery, 202, 203, 224, 301
Asia, 17, 18, 19, 21, 25, 156, 157, 213, 282
Asian countries, 17, 18, 19, 214
assessment, 28, 116, 172, 216, 225, 258
assessment tools, 216
astigmatism, 3, 10, 23, 118, 121, 133, 168, 179, 180, 185, 188, 189, 190, 197, 200, 205, 216, 248, 272, 275, 277, 291, 296, 304, 305
astrocytes, 201
asymmetry, 212
asymptomatic, 166, 201, 202, 261, 262
ataxia, 197
atmosphere, 131, 138
atmospheric pressure, 109
atoms, 130
atrophy, 3, 131, 144, 227, 228, 230, 231, 232, 233, 236, 239, 240, 241, 242, 243, 246, 247, 248, 251, 253, 254, 255, 256, 257, 258
Atropine, 194, 281, 288, 290, 292
automation, 181
autopsy, 201
autosomal dominant, 8, 13, 16, 201, 245
autosomal recessive, 8, 245
avoidance, 265
axons, 134, 201, 211

B

bacteria, 267
Bangladesh, 17, 28
Barbados, 18, 34, 208, 213, 214, 215, 219, 221, 225
barium, 108
basal cell nevus syndrome, 203
base, 17, 18, 19, 21, 26, 112, 120, 139, 162, 164, 165, 166, 167, 177, 206, 207, 208, 209, 211, 212, 213, 228, 247, 266, 287, 303
basic research, xi
beams, 141, 181
Beijing, 16, 18, 19, 21, 22, 23, 24, 34, 213, 214, 215, 226, 228, 229, 245, 248, 255, 260, 287
Belgium, ix
bending, 177, 304
beneficial effect, 282, 286, 287
benefits, 162, 168, 171, 261, 298
benign, 241, 268
beta blocker, 290
bias, 152
bilateral, 9, 12
Binocular balancing, 178, 296
biomechanics, 221
biomolecules, 145
birefringence, 143
birth weight, 32
blame, 264
blind spot, 167, 215, 302
blindness, xi, 8, 9, 11, 12, 13, 16, 19, 21, 27, 28, 30, 34, 205, 211, 212, 218, 221, 222, 224, 225, 226, 228, 243, 244, 249, 250, 251, 252, 253, 254, 255, 257, 259, 260, 299
blood, 7, 134, 144, 147, 149, 208, 215, 220, 229, 236, 242, 243, 249, 287, 301
blood circulation, 287
blood flow, 7, 147, 149, 208, 215, 220, 242, 249
blood pressure, 229
blood supply, 7, 134, 236, 242
blood vessels, 144, 243, 301
body mass index (BMI), 25, 26, 229
brain, 116, 134, 141, 194, 196, 286, 289, 298, 301, 302
brain damage, 196
Britain, 28, 251

C

caffeine, 285, 289, 291, 293
calcium, 140
calcium carbonate, 140
caliber, 207, 220
calibration, 160
candidates, 190
capillary, 149, 208
capsule, 131, 135, 136, 303
carbon, 303
carbon dioxide, 303
carcinogenicity, 292
cataract, vii, 3, 4, 6, 12, 25, 30, 121, 125, 130, 133, 134, 135, 136, 137, 140, 145, 146, 148, 149, 155, 205, 206, 208, 209, 212, 218, 220, 221, 222, 223, 226, 257, 272, 273, 296
cataract extraction, 135, 296
caucasian population, 7, 215
caucasians, 19
CDC, 217
cell death, 8

cell metabolism, 286
cell surface, 285
central nervous system (CNS), 14, 196, 197, 201, 217, 219, 286
cerebrospinal fluid, 219, 222, 240, 253
changing environment, 25
chemicals, 6, 108, 267, 289
Chicago, 149, 199, 275
childhood, 3, 20, 191, 193, 200, 205, 216, 254, 255, 262, 275, 279, 285, 288, 292, 293
children, ix, 3, 5, 6, 10, 11, 13, 14, 16, 18, 19, 20, 21, 22, 23, 24, 26, 28, 29, 30, 31, 32, 33, 35, 141, 152, 153, 154, 155, 156, 158, 160, 166, 178, 179, 191, 192, 193, 194, 195, 196, 197, 199, 200, 204, 205, 221, 227, 231, 244, 250, 254, 255, 256, 258, 266, 276, 279, 280, 281, 282, 283, 284, 285, 286, 287, 288, 289, 290, 291, 292, 293
Chile, 31
China, 16, 17, 18, 19, 21, 23, 29, 33, 35, 159, 211, 212, 215, 226, 228, 243, 244, 252, 256, 259, 287, 293
chinese medicine, 287
cholinesterase, 4
choroid, vii, 7, 143, 144, 229, 230, 231, 236, 239, 240, 241, 242, 247, 251, 255, 297
choroiditis, 259
chromosome, 8, 9, 10, 13, 15, 16, 20, 29, 30, 33, 158, 159, 160, 237, 245
chronic glaucoma, 204, 221
ciliary muscle, 3
circulation, 7, 147, 223, 231, 242, 287
cty, 9, 250
clarity, 5, 101, 183, 185
classes, 121
classification, 200, 216, 228, 233, 235, 246
cleaning, 269, 270
clinical application, 120
clinical judgment, 177, 264, 304
clinical presentation, xi, 200
clinical trials, 3, 213, 230, 245, 273, 281, 288
closure, 4, 9, 10, 13, 14, 15, 137, 159, 193, 194, 216, 219, 239, 253
clustering, 32
coatings, 139, 277
cocoa, 292
coding, 12
coherence, 11, 139, 148, 228, 235, 238, 242, 247, 249, 250, 251, 252, 253, 255, 256, 257, 258, 259, 260, 302
collaboration, ix
collagen, 6, 7, 9, 11, 14, 132, 133, 142, 143, 158, 232, 255, 285
color, 8, 125, 131, 137, 143, 144, 166, 231, 240, 295
color blindness, 8
coma, 163, 168
commercial, 141
common findings, 231
communication, 149
community, 6, 254, 264
compensation, 144
competition, 266
complement, 230
compliance, 284
complications, vii, xi, 3, 6, 12, 32, 171, 224, 227, 231, 239, 245, 248, 257, 258, 261, 267, 269, 273, 277, 279, 286
components of, 152
composition, 8, 108, 144, 171
computer, 157
conception, 235
concordance, 20
conduction, 201
configuration, 201, 219
confrontation, 172
congenital cataract, 121
conjugate, 102
conjunctiva, 172
conjunctivitis, 267, 270, 273, 275
connective tissue, 8, 211
conoid, 298
consensus, 1, 208
consent, 298
conservation, 139
construction, 101
contact lenses, 28, 166, 267, 274, 290, 303
contamination, 270, 274
contour, 139, 158, 233
contrast sensitivity, 134, 135, 136, 275, 278
control group, 281, 284, 285
controlled trials, 281
controversial, 25, 272, 286
convention, 106, 107
convergence, 20, 106, 164, 165, 168, 177, 191, 266, 297
cooperation, 191
cornea, vii, 1, 2, 3, 26, 118, 121, 122, 123, 130, 132, 133, 134, 137, 139, 142, 148, 154, 161, 162, 172, 179, 180, 190, 266, 267, 270, 271, 274, 275, 277, 296, 299, 300, 301, 302, 304, 305
corneal transplant, 136
corneal ulcer, 270, 274, 277
correlation, 2, 23, 26, 27, 145, 156, 159, 169, 206, 209, 210, 219, 233, 247, 248, 251, 253, 254
cortex, 145, 302
corticosteroids, 267
cosmetic, 162, 262, 266, 271, 275

cost, 243
covering, 142
cracks, 3, 227, 228, 229, 230, 233, 242, 246, 247, 248, 256, 259
cross cylinder, 197, 297, 299
crossed polaroids, 142, 148
cross-sectional study, 22, 248
crown, 108
crystalline, 2, 5, 131, 134, 140, 142, 145, 146, 149, 152, 153, 154, 155, 160, 161, 271, 273, 295, 297, 299
crystals, 138, 140, 141, 142
cycles, 127, 146
cycloplegia, 4, 175, 178, 184, 191, 192, 193, 194, 195, 196, 197, 199, 263, 282
cycloplegic refraction, 178, 190, 193, 197, 199, 200, 297
cylinder, 112, 185, 197, 297, 299
cyst, 238
cystoid macular edema, 4

D

daily living, 245
database, 157
defects, 3, 9, 148, 158, 167, 201, 204, 211, 212, 213, 215, 227, 228, 254, 257, 270, 302
deficiency, 304
deformability, 212
degradation, 6, 168
delirium, 194
demyelination, 203, 217
Department of Health and Human Services, 217
deposits, 268, 270, 271
depression, 167
deprivation, 6, 10, 15, 31, 155, 160, 202, 255, 285, 290
depth, 2, 11, 103, 122, 123, 127, 138, 146, 147, 152, 153, 154, 158, 161, 167, 172, 183, 216, 231, 232, 242, 251, 252, 255, 258, 278, 297
detachment, 3, 6, 10, 166, 169, 214, 228, 231, 232, 234, 235, 236, 237, 238, 239, 242, 247, 249, 251, 252, 254, 255, 257, 258, 259
detection, 149, 171, 173, 230, 282, 299, 302
developing countries, 17
developmental process, 237
deviation, 115, 120, 182, 191, 242, 282, 303
diabetes, 4, 145, 149, 207, 216, 217, 220, 221, 229
diabetic retinopathy, 145, 203, 205, 218, 220, 221, 222, 223, 226, 252
diagnosis, 216
Diamox, 4
diastole, 147
differential equations, 127
diffraction, 115, 116, 117, 126, 136, 137, 138
diffuse reflection, 100
diffusion, 210
dilation, 172, 197, 285, 297, 300
diode laser, 302
diopter, 298, 303
disability, 1, 29, 136, 147, 149
discomfort, 175, 193, 268
discrimination, 173, 186, 190
discs, 204, 213, 215, 219, 226, 239
diseases, vii, 172, 205, 206, 218, 235, 252, 256, 301
disequilibrium, 9
disinfection, 269
dislocation, 273
disorder, 1, 203, 234, 304
dispersion, 108, 116, 273, 295
displacement, 4, 162, 164, 165, 168, 299
distilled water, 108
distortions, 262
distribution, 2, 4, 121, 128, 151, 152, 154, 155, 161, 201
divergence, 103, 106, 162, 164, 263
diversity, 259
dizygotic, 10, 20, 29, 156
dizygotic twins, 10, 20, 29, 156
DNA, 14, 159
doctors, 125
DOI, 30, 217, 223, 293
dopamine, 6, 11, 15, 23, 26, 286, 289, 290, 291
dosage, 194, 195, 196, 283
dose-response relationship, 212
down syndrome, 194, 196
drawing, 105
drugs, 4, 14, 178, 190, 191, 193, 194, 300
DSC, 11, 252, 289
dysphoria, 266

E

East Asia, 17, 18, 19, 21, 22, 24, 25, 216, 244, 259
edema, 4, 121, 133, 134, 136, 137, 138, 252, 267, 270, 271, 276
editors, 16, 276, 289
education, 20, 21, 24, 25, 27, 32, 33, 34, 159, 205, 214, 259
educational attainment, 25
effusion, 4, 13
egg, 6
Ehlers-Danlos syndrome, 14
electric current, 127
electric field, 127, 130
electricity, 127, 287

electromagnetic, 99, 127, 128, 129, 299, 302
electromagnetic waves, 99
electrons, 128, 129, 130, 145, 251
electroretinography, 243
element, 99
elementary school, 156
elongation, 1, 2, 3, 6, 11, 21, 23, 29, 155, 229, 231, 235, 239, 240, 242, 243, 245, 247, 248, 279, 280, 281, 284, 285, 286, 290, 296
emission, 145, 299
Emmetropia, 159, 298
Emmetropization, 10, 14, 32, 158, 159
endothelium, 132, 276, 302
energy, 127, 128, 129, 139, 145
energy conservation, 139
engineering, 30, 148
enlargement, 102, 202, 213, 239, 240, 247, 288, 290
environment, 12, 20, 25, 134, 155, 156, 157, 161, 187, 234, 238
environmental change, 25
environmental effects, 5
environmental factors, 7, 9, 20, 25, 31, 156, 211, 245
environments, 156
epidemic, 13, 25, 31
epidemiologic, 211, 214
epidemiologic studies, 211, 214
epidemiology, vii, ix, 13, 26, 28, 158, 205, 222, 243, 251, 255, 277
epiretinal membrane, 228, 236, 237, 238, 247, 253, 256
epithelia, 271
epithelial cells, 7, 132, 138, 242, 275, 277
epithelium, 21, 137, 138, 143, 144, 228, 236, 239, 240, 241, 242, 243, 247, 267, 275, 277, 286, 289, 296, 297
equality, 186, 187
equipment, 178
esotropia, 161, 184, 191, 192, 194, 265
ethnic groups, 23, 152
ethnic Indians, 206
ethnicity, 5, 11, 19, 23, 24, 29, 30, 161, 171
etiology, xi, 8, 25, 155, 157, 169, 175, 200, 267
Europe, 17
evidence, 7, 8, 15, 16, 20, 24, 32, 33, 127, 149, 151, 155, 157, 160, 167, 206, 208, 212, 245, 246, 259, 272, 280, 281, 284, 285, 287
evolution, 234, 258
examinations, 25, 184, 191, 201, 236, 262, 270, 271
excitation, 148
exclusion, 27
exercise, 292
exons, 14
exotropia, 265
exposure, 23, 145, 155, 207, 267, 283, 291
extracellular matrix, 6, 8
extraction, 135, 168, 169
eye, v, 6, 9, 10, 12, 14, 16, 19, 21, 25, 27, 28, 29, 30, 31, 32, 33, 34, 37, 143, 147, 148, 151, 154, 156, 159, 172, 175, 178, 199, 204, 205, 206, 207, 208, 209, 210, 211, 212, 213, 214, 215, 216, 217, 218, 219, 220, 221, 222, 223, 224, 225, 226,228, 229, 232, 233, 243, 244, 246, 248, 250, 251, 252, 254, 255, 256, 258, 259, 260, 269, 274, 275, 288, 291, 292
eyedrops, 283

F

fabrication, 111, 266
FAD, 145
families, 8, 15, 28, 33, 157, 158, 245
family history, 12, 245
family studies, 155, 156
Far point, 176, 298
fever, 4, 194, 195
fiber, vii, 4, 21, 132, 133, 134, 137, 142, 143, 144, 148, 201, 202, 203, 215, 216, 219, 232, 239, 240, 241, 295, 301, 302
fiber bundles, 144
fibroblasts, 286, 288
fibrosis, 246
field curvature, 101, 115
field defect, 3, 167, 204, 211, 212, 213, 215
filament, 181
films, 278
filters, 135, 144, 185
fixation, 142, 164, 167, 191, 192, 297
flame, 100
flexibility, 234
fluctuations, 123, 131
fluid, 131, 132, 133, 134, 137, 138, 147, 230, 235, 240, 257, 296
fluorescence, 145, 149
Fogging, 187, 198, 298
Food and Drug Administration (FDA), 269, 272, 273, 277, 278
force, 4, 130, 190, 192, 235
formal education, 20
formation, 99, 121, 133, 137, 209, 231, 234, 237, 238, 239, 241, 247, 255, 256, 272, 273
formula, 104, 109, 111, 116, 180, 301, 305
fovea, 167, 231, 237, 242, 300, 305
fragments, 138
frames, 266
France, 148
friction, 126

Fundus, 144, 227, 247, 254
funduscopic examination, 303
fungal infection, 278
fungi, 267, 278
fusion, 166

G

galaxies, 147
Galilean telescope, 114, 123
ganglion, 21, 203, 211, 300
gel, 283, 292
gene expression, 7
genes, 7, 8, 11, 12, 25, 156, 157, 237, 253
genetic disease, 237
genetic disorders, 7
genetic factors, vii, 7, 8, 20, 21, 24, 155, 156, 214
genetic linkage, 8
genetic predisposition, 25
genetics, 15, 16, 34, 218, 260
genome, 8, 10, 13, 159
genomic regions, 8
geometric optics, 125, 298
geometrical optics, vii, 99, 100, 101, 115
geometry, 125, 127
Germany, 11, 12, 30, 245, 254
gifted, 157
glasses, vii, 14, 15, 33, 141, 163, 164, 166, 182, 184, 186, 187, 188, 207, 264, 266, 276, 286, 287, 289, 291
glaucoma, vii, 3, 4, 6, 10, 13, 15, 29, 34, 121, 132, 137, 138, 147, 148, 149, 167, 193, 194, 204, 205, 210, 211, 212, 213, 214, 215, 216, 217, 218, 219, 220, 221, 222, 223, 224, 225, 229, 239, 240, 241, 242, 249, 251, 253, 256, 257, 258, 273
glaucoma, 210, 211, 213, 214, 215, 216, 217, 218, 220, 221, 222, 223
glial cells, 201
glucose, 145
glue, 141
glutamate, 286, 291
glycine, 14
grades, 161, 163, 167, 232, 233
grading, 208, 233, 246
granules, 144
graph, 116, 117, 119
gratings, 117, 135
Greeks, 1, 262
growth, 2, 6, 8, 11, 14, 15, 16, 25, 26, 153, 154, 155, 158, 159, 161, 207, 229, 280, 281, 284, 285, 286, 289, 290, 292, 293, 301
growth factor, 6, 207, 281
Guangzhou, 24, 35, 219
guidelines, 216, 262, 269, 271

H

hallucinations, 196
halos, 121, 264
hardness, 245
hazards, 193
haze, 132
health, 171, 206, 222, 225, 243, 270, 279
health care, 171
height, 6, 25, 26, 27, 33, 35, 102, 104, 105, 229, 231, 262, 301
hemianopsia, 167
hemoglobin, 144
hemorrhage, 121, 155, 202, 203, 230
heredity, 16, 155, 157, 264
heritability, 32, 156, 157
heterogeneity, 158, 213
high school, 3, 31, 126
higher education, 25, 214
Hispanic population, 17
Hispanics, 228
history, vii, 10, 11, 35, 136, 155, 156, 157, 160, 171, 172, 176, 183, 196, 198, 208, 209, 210, 233, 238, 245, 246, 249, 252, 267, 269, 275
Hong Kong, 10, 18, 24, 28, 244, 248, 254, 258, 284, 285, 288, 289, 290
human, 5, 6, 8, 12, 16, 29, 145, 147, 148, 149, 155, 158, 159, 163, 219, 224, 240, 250, 251, 277, 279, 286, 288, 295, 300
Hunter, 201, 219
hygiene, 267, 269
hyperopia, 4, 5, 18, 23, 24, 28, 151, 152, 155, 175, 179, 180, 191, 192, 206, 210, 214, 216, 265, 275, 295, 298
hypertension, 207, 218, 223, 225
hypoplasia, 157
hypothesis, 23, 25, 158, 210, 211, 237, 286
hypoxia, 207, 231, 269, 271
hypoxia-inducible factor, 231
hysteria, 192

I

iatrogenic, 265
Iceland, 140
ideal, 99, 101, 102, 104, 106, 110, 115, 117, 165, 181
idealization, 114
identification, 148, 173, 211
identity, 171

idiopathic, 14, 32, 238, 249, 258
idiosyncratic, 4, 194
illumination, 122, 123, 135, 145, 149, 173, 176, 262, 264, 300
image, 1, 2, 6, 99, 100, 101, 102, 103, 104, 105, 106, 107, 108, 109, 110, 112, 113, 114, 115, 116, 117, 118, 119, 121, 122, 123, 124, 135, 136, 139, 140, 146, 148, 149, 162, 163, 164, 165, 166, 167, 168, 183, 185, 186, 233, 236, 242, 263, 295, 296, 297, 298, 300, 301, 302, 303
image analysis, 149
imagery, 263
imagination, 103
imaging systems, 102, 104
implants, 168, 273
improvements, 168
impulses, 302
in vivo, 219, 231
incidence, 6, 10, 12, 21, 27, 28, 30, 34, 109, 110, 120, 139, 140, 171, 210, 220, 222, 225, 231, 232, 237, 244, 248, 249, 254, 259, 260, 261, 267, 268, 276, 277, 297, 299
income, 21
independent variable, 205
India, 9, 17, 18, 19, 28, 211, 212, 215, 217, 223, 244
Indians, 206, 256
indirect measure, 204
individuals, 1, 2, 5, 6, 17, 158, 177, 179, 184, 192, 202, 211, 212, 214, 215, 228, 243, 244, 245, 246, 248, 262, 267, 268, 271
Indonesia, 17, 18, 32
induction, 14, 155, 272
infancy, 10, 14, 32, 154, 158
infants, 5, 158, 182, 193, 194, 196, 197, 199, 219, 283
infarction, 134
infection, 290
inflammation, 132, 267
informed consent, 298
inheritance, 12, 157, 252, 264
inhibitor, 14, 23, 159
initiation, 171
injections, 252, 289
injuries, 172
insertion, 240, 269, 272, 287, 296
insulin, 4, 13, 145
integrity, 147, 202
intelligence, 33
interface, 139, 141, 228, 248, 255, 257
interference, 126, 128, 130, 137, 138, 139, 142, 143, 147, 148, 250, 302
intervention, 14, 33, 280, 281, 283, 288, 290, 291
intraocular, 6, 10, 11, 15, 30, 34, 109, 121, 122, 135, 139, 140, 143, 149, 167, 168, 193, 194, 214, 218, 219, 225, 229, 241, 253, 271, 273, 274, 275, 276, 277, 295, 304
intraocular pressure, 11, 15, 30, 34, 121, 143, 167, 193, 194, 214, 218, 225, 229, 241
investment, 186
iodine, 141
ipsilateral, 224
IQ scores, 26
Iran, 32
Ireland, 13, 23
iridocyclitis, 273
iris, 4, 118, 121, 125, 126, 143, 144, 172, 191, 194, 273, 296, 297, 299, 300, 303, 304
iritis, 132
ischemia, 203, 207
Islam, 10
Israel, 27, 244, 249
issues, 7, 263
Italy, 250, 262

J

Japan, 17, 18, 19, 25, 34, 211, 212, 215, 228, 243, 281
Jordan, 23

K

Keplerian telescope, 114, 123
keratoconjunctivitis, 267
Keratoconus, 122, 203, 274
Keratometry, 180, 271, 299
keratoplasty, 168, 271
kindergarten, 33
kindergarten children, 33
Korea, 17, 18, 24, 215

L

laboratory studies, 5
lactate dehydrogenase, 275
lakes, 132, 136
laminar, 215
laser ablation, 272
lasers, 249, 255, 257, 258, 299
Latin America, 243
Latinos, 9, 33, 215, 225, 251
laws, 110, 125
leakage, 230
legs, 173

Lensometry, 178, 182, 198
lesions, 121, 122, 135, 144, 201, 202, 203, 228, 231, 232, 234, 236, 254, 256
leucine, 12
level of education, 26, 205
light, vii, xi, 1, 5, 23, 26, 99, 100, 101, 102, 103, 104, 106, 107, 108, 109, 110, 111, 113, 114, 115, 116, 117, 118, 119, 120, 121, 122, 123, 125, 126, 127, 128, 129, 130, 131, 132, 133, 134, 135, 136, 137, 138, 139, 140, 141, 142, 143, 144, 145, 146, 147, 148, 149, 151, 162, 163, 164, 173, 175, 177, 179, 181, 185, 190, 196, 211, 263, 269, 272, 282, 283, 290, 295, 296, 297, 298, 299, 300, 301, 302, 303, 304, 305
light beam, 126, 127, 130, 139, 179, 296
light conditions, 5, 272
light scattering, 129, 131, 132, 133, 134, 143, 146, 148
light units, 135, 136
liquids, 108
localization, 230
loci, 8, 9, 11, 13, 15, 28, 29, 33, 158, 159, 245
locus, 8, 9, 10, 13, 16, 29, 35, 159, 160, 245, 256
LogMAR, 174
longitudinal study, 23, 30, 207, 290
Luo, 16, 207, 221, 293
lying, 240

M

Macula, 300
macular degeneration, 6, 19, 34, 205, 217, 220, 222, 230
magnetic field, 127
magnetism, 127
magnification, 102, 103, 113, 301
magnitude, 18, 123, 126, 129
majority, 7, 155, 204, 213
Malaysia, 19, 29, 32
malingering, 192
mammals, 6
man, 289, 292
management, vii, xi, 120, 171, 200, 253, 255, 261, 266
mapping, 9, 298
Marfan syndrome, 4, 7, 9, 13
mass, 229
materials, 167, 178, 266, 295
matrix, 6, 8, 10
matrix metalloproteinase, 10
matter, 107, 120, 129, 136, 181, 264
measurements, 9, 11, 26, 128, 137, 139, 147, 149, 151, 152, 158, 160, 162, 172, 175, 176, 177, 180, 182, 190, 198, 217, 242, 251, 252, 254, 272, 299, 300, 302, 304
media, 108, 110, 111, 121, 131, 137, 139, 140, 148, 149, 181, 191, 192, 283, 300, 301, 304
media opacities, 300
median, 149
medical, vii, xi, 18, 34, 131, 137, 168, 171, 172, 175, 177, 178, 235, 237, 261, 269, 301
medication, 12, 175, 199
medicine, 287
medium, 164, 300
melanin, 143, 144, 229
melanoma, 203, 222
mellitus, 145
membranes, 202, 203, 229, 230, 238, 258
meridian, 8, 119, 153, 155, 180, 188, 197, 204, 296, 297
meta-analysis, 18, 211, 212, 281, 287, 290
metabolism, 145, 286
metals, 108
meter, 107, 126, 137, 181, 188, 263, 303
methodology, 19, 20
mice, 291
microscope, 118, 141, 146, 283, 296
microstructure, 236
migraine headache, 4
migration, 201
military, 26, 159
miosis, 123, 190, 193, 300
miscommunication, 186
mixing, 100, 148
models, 23, 25, 102, 181, 231, 280
modifications, 233, 246
molecular weight, 133
molecules, 129, 130
momentum, 125
Mongolia, 17, 18
monozygotic twins, 156, 283
morphology, 147, 202, 205, 219, 221, 253, 254
morphometric, 253
motivation, 168
muscles, 6, 287
mutation, 9, 12, 13, 14
Mydriasis, 300
myelin, 201
myopathy, 228

N

NAD, 145
naming, 173
National Health and Nutrition Examination Survey (NHANES), 25, 211, 217

nausea, 167
Near add, 300
nearsightedness, xi, 1, 300
negative relation, 21
neonates, 155
neovascularization, 3, 14, 15, 16, 203, 217, 228, 229, 232, 234, 242, 243, 248, 249, 250, 252, 253, 254, 255, 256, 258, 259, 260, 267
Neovascularization, 202, 222, 229, 243, 301
Nepal, 31
nerve, vii, 7, 21, 131, 134, 142, 144, 148, 157, 167, 172, 201, 202, 203, 204, 211, 212, 213, 214, 215, 216, 217, 218, 219, 220, 221, 222, 224, 229, 233, 236, 239, 240, 241, 242, 301, 302
nerve fibers, vii, 21, 142, 144, 201, 202, 203, 216, 217, 218, 219, 220, 221, 222, 224, 240, 301
nervous system, 196, 201, 288
Netherlands, 211, 212, 215, 218
neuritis, 203
neurons, 201
neuropathy, 203, 210, 213, 218, 224, 229, 241, 254
neurotransmission, 286
neurotransmitters, 286
neutral, 5
nevus, 203
New Zealand, 13
nicotinamide, 145
Niels Bohr, 129
normal aging, 241
normal curve, 2
normal development, 161
normal distribution, 152
Northern Ireland, 23, 28, 31
Norway, 30
nuclei, 130
nucleus, 129, 137, 140, 145, 291
nutrients, 7, 207, 210, 242
nutrition, 223

O

object, 101, 103
object ray, 101, 103
occlusion, 192, 201, 202, 203, 224, 229, 252
ocular diseases, 206, 224
oedema, 12
oil, 194
oligodendrocytes, 201
opacification, 135, 148
opacity, 136, 209, 217, 220
open angle glaucoma, 210, 212, 218, 221, 222, 224
ophthalmic medical assistants, 177
ophthalmologist, ix, 136, 166, 177, 178, 190, 200, 301, 302
ophthalmoscopy, 118, 123, 124, 149, 183, 194, 197, 232, 242
optic chiasm, 302
optic nerve, 7, 21, 131, 144, 149, 157, 167, 172, 201, 204, 211, 212, 213, 214, 215, 217, 219, 229, 233, 239, 240, 242, 253, 256, 301, 302, 305
optic nerve head, 301
optic neuritis, 203, 224
optical properties, 102, 108, 125
optical systems, 99, 100, 101, 114, 116, 305
opticians, 10, 16
optics, v, 10, 16, 27, 99, 124, 125, 159, 161, 169, 176, 199, 200, 263, 302
orbit, 14, 32, 129, 172, 296
organic disease, 218
organism, 303
ornithine, 15
oscillation, 130
overlap, 111, 112, 185, 205
oxidation, 145
oxygen, 203, 207, 231, 266, 267, 269, 275, 277, 303
oxyhemoglobin, 144

P

Pacific, 7
pain, 269
Pakistan, 244
pallor, 233, 246
Paraguay, 218
parallax, 302
parallel, xi, 1, 103, 104, 105, 106, 107, 113, 119, 120, 126, 140, 151, 162, 189, 241, 263, 283, 292, 299, 300, 302, 304
paralysis, 191, 297
parasite, 277
paraxial, 110, 111, 302
parents, 11, 20, 23, 26, 34, 155, 156, 157, 194, 287
participants, 20, 207, 213, 214, 244, 287
pathogenesis, vii, 6, 8, 21, 201, 211, 220, 234, 236, 237, 243, 246, 268, 277
pathology, 121, 155, 171, 202, 243, 248
pathophysiology, 211, 218
pathways, 7, 8, 99
patient care, 10, 29, 289
perfusion, 217
peripheral vision, 302
permeability, 277
permit, 162, 195, 264
pharmaceutical, 264, 279
phenotype, 8, 25, 31

phenylephrine, 194
Philadelphia, 14, 16, 169, 199, 200, 257, 274, 276
photodetector, 139
photographs, 118, 146
photons, 99, 128, 130, 145
photophobia, 202, 220, 282
photorefractive keratectomy, 271, 272, 275
photosensitivity, 282
physical activity, 11, 22
physical characteristics, 27, 101
physical optics, 99, 148, 302
physics, 126, 127, 128, 148, 304
physiological, 2
physiology, 2, 200
pigmentation, 144, 196, 214, 241
pigs, 285, 290
pilot study, 15, 244, 255, 284, 285, 288, 289, 292
pitch, 125, 147
placebo, 282, 283, 292
plaque, 202, 203, 222, 241
plastics, 142, 266
plausibility, 207
playing, 23, 157
pleasure, 157
PMMA, 266, 303
point of origin, 162
Poland, 28
polarization, 140, 141, 148
polymers, 266
polymethylmethacrylate, 168, 276, 303
polymorphism, 8, 12, 15
polystyrene, 147
pools, 133, 138
population, 4, 8, 9, 10, 11, 12, 13, 15, 17, 18, 19, 20, 21, 23, 24, 25, 26, 27, 28, 29, 30, 31, 32, 33, 34, 134, 152, 159, 161, 204, 206, 207, 208, 209, 211, 212, 213, 215, 217, 218, 219, 220, 221, 222, 223, 224, 225, 226, 227, 228, 231, 232, 239, 244, 245, 247, 249, 250, 251, 252, 253, 254, 255, 259, 265, 287
population density, 20
population group, 23
positive correlation, 27, 145
posterior cortex, 145
posterior segment, 303
preparation, 214
presbyopia, 165, 175, 225, 262, 265, 273, 274, 303
preschool, 3, 10
preschool children, 3, 10
preservation, 122
pressure gradient, 215, 222
pressure groups, 282
preterm infants, 196
prevalence rate, 5
prevention, 7, 23, 208, 284, 301
primary school, 22
primate, 11, 290
principal meridians, 303
principles, 99, 128, 130, 141, 177, 178, 183, 262
prism, 303
private schools, 21
PRK, 272, 275
probability, 23, 128, 232
prognosis, 16, 220, 223, 229, 230, 246, 248, 252, 260
progression, v, 216, 224, 238, 246, 248, 264, 279, 284, 288, 290
progression of myopia, 290
project, 33, 136, 217
propagation, 101
protection, 266
protective factors, 223
proteins, 9, 131, 133, 145
Pseudomonas aeruginosa, 268, 269, 275, 277
ptosis, 155
puberty, 10, 158
public health, 206, 243, 279
public schools, 21
pupil, 115, 277, 304

Q

quality of life, 211, 216, 222, 245
quanta, 128, 129
quantum theory, 128, 129

R

race, 161, 171, 221
racial differences, 20
radial keratotomy, 122
radial scattering, 137
radiation, 127, 128, 148, 203, 299, 302
radiotherapy, 203, 222
radius, 4, 111, 154, 180, 296, 299, 305
random assignment, 285
rapid eye movement sleep, 290
rare earth elements, 108
rash, 194, 195
rate of change, 183
ray sketching, 106
ray tracing, 106
rays, 101, 103, 104, 106, 108, 118, 148
reactions, 172, 193, 195, 196, 200, 282
reading, 134, 140, 147, 157, 158, 165, 166, 173, 175, 176, 177, 192, 263, 265, 275, 280, 300

reasoning, 102, 110
receptors, 21, 131, 285, 286, 288, 291
recession, 147
recognition, 173
recombination, 14
recommendations, 269, 274
reconstruction, 297
recovery, 160, 183, 273
recreational, 261
reflectivity, 230
reflexes, 179
refraction, 10, 27, 109, 151, 152, 154, 159, 169, 172, 176, 177, 183, 184, 187, 190, 192, 195, 197, 198, 199, 200, 304
refractive errors, 14, 15, 27, 28, 30, 32, 33, 34, 35, 217, 225
refractive index, 25, 29, 108, 109, 110, 111, 113, 116, 132, 134, 137, 138, 139, 140, 142, 143, 163, 167, 208, 295, 300, 304
refractive surgery, 271
refractometry, 178, 182, 297, 300, 304
refractors, 181
regression, 23, 25, 229
regression analysis, 229
regression model, 25
relaxation, 4, 177, 187, 188, 295
relevance, 155
relief, 183
remyelination, 217
repair, 238, 258
replication, 9
requirements, 183, 184, 261, 264
researchers, 227, 237
resection, 204
residues, 145
resistance, 196, 266
resolution, 5, 116, 136, 137, 139, 144, 173, 175, 234, 239, 247, 257, 258, 276, 300, 302
respiration, 145
response, 6, 116, 117, 155, 179, 181, 183, 194, 213, 280, 286, 287, 292, 295
responsiveness, 155
retardation, 283
retina, xi, 1, 2, 6, 7, 10, 23, 101, 102, 116, 121, 122, 123, 134, 137, 139, 140, 144, 145, 148, 149, 151, 161, 163, 164, 172, 173, 177, 179, 181, 183, 185, 189, 190, 201, 207, 220, 221, 222, 224, 227, 229, 231, 234, 235, 236, 238, 239, 242, 243, 247, 250, 251, 253, 255, 257, 258, 259, 260, 263, 282, 285, 286, 298, 300,301, 302, 303, 304, 305
retinal detachment, 3, 6, 13, 14, 32, 166, 214, 232, 234, 235, 236, 237, 238, 239, 242, 247, 249, 250, 251, 253, 255, 256, 257, 258, 259
retinal disease, 136
retinal image, 104, 301
retinoblastoma, 202
retinopathy, 19, 21, 27, 145, 203, 205, 220, 222, 227, 228, 229, 233, 246, 249, 251, 255, 259, 283
retinoscopy, 178, 179, 188, 192, 198, 200, 305
rings, 138, 142
risk, vii, 6, 8, 13, 20, 21, 22, 25, 26, 27, 30, 31, 34, 155, 157, 206, 207, 208, 209, 210, 211, 212, 213, 214, 216, 217, 218, 219, 220, 222, 223, 224, 225, 231, 232, 245, 249, 250, 253, 256, 259, 267, 268, 270, 272, 277, 278, 282, 283, 289, 290
risk factors, vii, 13, 21, 22, 25, 27, 30, 31, 34, 207, 208, 211, 216, 217, 218, 219, 220, 222, 223, 224, 225, 245, 249, 250, 253, 256, 259, 272
room temperature, 109
root, 1, 117
rosacea, 267
routes, 99
rules, 115
rural areas, 16, 34
rural population, 25, 28, 218, 223

S

safety, 142, 266, 268, 283, 292
scatter, 100, 122, 130, 131, 133, 135, 143, 149
scattering, 100, 121, 130, 131, 132, 133, 134, 135, 136, 137, 143, 146, 147
school, 3, 10, 11, 13, 14, 16, 20, 21, 22, 24, 25, 28, 29, 30, 31, 32, 33, 35, 126, 152, 155, 156, 157, 158, 182, 205, 222, 244, 256, 262, 276, 281, 283, 284, 287, 290, 291
school achievement, 13, 22, 31, 158, 276
school work, 262
schooling, 27
science, 142, 263, 266, 302
sclera, 7, 12, 15, 125, 132, 143, 144, 148, 172, 204, 207, 211, 215, 229, 233, 239, 240, 241, 251, 256, 285, 288, 295, 297
sclerosis, 1, 21, 131, 208, 209
scope, 118, 180
scotoma, 121, 235, 243
secretion, 231
selenium, 245
self-assessment, 172
semen, 290
sensation, 193, 196, 302
sensitivity, 134, 135, 136, 148, 149, 167, 194, 243, 262, 269, 290, 297, 302
serotonin, 286
services, 301
sex, 11, 21, 26, 29, 161, 205, 221, 229, 237, 245

shape, 6, 9, 109, 111, 112, 121, 122, 156, 181, 236, 240, 241, 256, 260, 267, 286, 295, 296, 303
shortage, 236
showing, 26, 152, 211, 230
siblings, 156
side effects, 171, 193, 261, 282, 285
signaling pathway, 7
signals, 201, 217
signs, 107, 194, 196, 228, 271
sine wave, 117
Singapore, 17, 18, 19, 22, 24, 28, 30, 31, 32, 33, 34, 35, 157, 159, 205, 206, 207, 208, 209, 211, 215, 219, 220, 221, 223, 224, 225, 226, 247, 248, 250, 256, 259, 275, 277, 281, 284, 287, 290
single-nucleotide polymorphism, 8
skin, 193, 194, 195
slit lamp, 121, 131, 132, 146, 148, 296, 302
smoking, 172
Snellen chart, 135, 136, 137, 302
society, 243
solution, 131, 132, 133, 148, 165, 166, 194, 195, 196, 268, 269, 270, 274, 275, 282
South Africa, 31
South Asia, 18
South Korea, 30, 217
Southeast Asia, 22, 24
Spain, 244, 257
spatial frequency, 297
species, 129, 155
spectroscopy, 148
speculation, 240
speech, 197
speed of light, 108, 127, 300, 304
sphincter, 191, 297, 300
stability, 271, 273
stabilization, 6
standard deviation, 157, 242, 282
state, 2, 5, 15, 109, 127, 129, 132, 136, 145, 146, 161, 176, 179, 181, 184, 187, 189, 191, 193, 198, 241, 245, 265, 268, 273, 295, 298, 304
sterile, 269, 270
stigma, 100
stigmatic image, 114
stimulation, 5, 177, 191, 287
stimulus, ix, 298
storage, 269
strabismus, 141, 192, 224, 266, 279
stress, 264, 265
stretching, 2, 227, 229, 232, 239, 240, 242, 247, 250
striae, 10
stroma, 132, 143, 267
structural protein, 9
structure, 7, 14, 27, 129, 139, 141, 142, 159, 217, 230, 241, 242, 256, 291
subgroups, 280
subjectivity, 175
subluxation, 4
substitution, 13, 14
sulfa drugs, 4
sulfate, 8, 141, 196
sulfonamide, 4, 13
Sun, 238, 258, 259
surgical removal, 136
surrogates, 22
susceptibility, 9, 10, 11, 15, 29, 33, 157, 160, 211, 212, 213, 215, 217, 229, 245, 246
suture, 273, 289, 291
Sweden, 33, 142, 215, 276
swelling, 235, 269
symmetry, 99, 165
sympathetic nervous system, 304
symptoms, 121, 136, 164, 172, 175, 178, 183, 192, 196, 236, 261, 262, 269, 271, 272, 276
syndrome, vii, 4, 7, 8, 11, 14, 157, 159, 194, 196, 201, 203, 204, 205, 217, 218, 219, 220, 222, 224, 225
synthesis, 6, 11
syphilis, 4

T

Taiwan, 15, 18, 19, 20, 24, 28, 30, 228, 248, 250, 252, 281, 282, 283, 287, 291
target, 116, 134, 135, 136, 176, 179, 181, 186, 296, 299, 300, 305
Task Force, 274
teachers, 287
techniques, vii, 177, 178, 183, 185, 190, 193, 200, 271
technology, 168
telangiectasia, 202
temperature, 109, 128, 195
tension, 147, 218, 221, 223, 249, 256
terminals, 20
testing, 135, 137, 148, 149, 161, 173, 176, 188, 189, 190, 193, 265, 300
TGF, 11, 12
therapy, 13, 15, 171, 192, 201, 202, 230, 259, 264, 282, 285
thinning, 5, 6, 21, 143, 153, 155, 160, 212, 229, 231, 233, 239, 241, 246, 247, 267, 285
Tibet, 218
time frame, 197
TIR, 110

tissue, 8, 132, 134, 139, 147, 207, 211, 215, 222, 234, 235, 242
titanium, 266
toddlers, 182
tonometry, 183
topical anesthetic, 193, 200
torsion, 204
total internal reflection, 110
toxicity, 12, 194, 195, 196, 282, 285, 292
toxicology, 292
training, 264, 279, 301
transmission, 9, 139, 140, 149, 185, 269, 282, 298
transparency, 134, 139, 149
transparent medium, 130, 303, 304
transplant, 136
Transverse magnification, 102, 107
trauma, 4, 132, 133
treatment, vii, xi, 4, 6, 14, 15, 16, 192, 194, 197, 200, 201, 211, 218, 221, 230, 243, 250, 253, 258, 259, 265, 273, 280, 281, 282, 283, 284, 285, 286, 287, 288, 290, 291, 292, 293, 298, 301
trial, 10, 11, 13, 14, 15, 29, 31, 33, 107, 121, 178, 180, 183, 184, 186, 187, 197, 198, 200, 259, 276, 277, 280, 282, 283, 284, 285, 287, 289, 290, 291, 292, 304
Trial frame, 184, 186
Tropicamide (Mydriacyl), 197
truck drivers, 5
tumor, 14, 159
tumor growth, 14, 159
Turkey, 23
twins, 12, 20, 156, 245, 283
two-dimensional space, 204
type 1 diabetes, 220
typhoid, 4
typhoid fever, 4
tyrosine, 145

U

ultrasonography, 154, 231, 296, 297
ultrasound, 139
ultrastructure, 253
uniform, 133, 137, 181
united, 9, 17, 18, 21, 24, 28, 30, 33, 34, 116, 156, 161, 211, 215, 217, 218, 220, 223, 224, 225, 227, 254, 258, 267, 269, 273, 277, 278, 282, 283, 284
United Kingdom (UK), 148, 159, 227
United States (USA), 9, 17, 18, 21, 24, 28, 30, 33, 34, 116, 149, 156, 161, 211, 215, 217, 218, 220, 223, 224, 225, 254, 258, 267, 269, 273, 277, 278, 282, 283, 284
universe, 125, 127, 147
urban, 9, 16, 20, 21, 22, 24, 25, 28, 29, 31, 34, 213, 217, 218, 226, 259, 287
urban areas, 22
urban population, 25, 31, 217
urine, 108

V

vacuum, 108, 127, 300, 304
valine, 14
valuation, 117, 172
variable factor, 143
variables, 153, 205
variations, 17, 33, 224, 250, 272, 284
vascularization, 271
vasculature, 147, 149, 172
vein, 202, 203, 229, 252, 301
velocity, 127, 147, 258
vergence, 106, 107, 112
vertebrates, 161
vertex, 262
vertex distance, 262
vertical dimensions, 298
vessels, 3, 144, 147, 204, 229, 231, 237, 239, 240, 241, 243, 247, 295
vibration, 140, 141, 142
video games, 157
vision, vii, 5, 7, 9, 11, 14, 17, 18, 19, 24, 31, 32, 33, 114, 121, 122, 133, 136, 138, 141, 144, 148, 149, 155, 159, 161, 162, 163, 164, 165, 166, 175, 176, 177, 183, 184, 186, 187, 188, 190, 192, 195, 197, 198, 202, 204, 205, 206, 210, 216, 221, 222, 224, 226,228, 234, 237, 242, 243, 244, 246, 250, 251, 253, 254, 255, 258, 261, 262, 263, 264, 266, 267, 269, 270, 272, 277, 280, 281, 283, 284, 289, 290, 295, 296, 299, 300, 301, 302, 304
visual acuity, 1, 2, 121, 127, 133, 134, 135, 137, 138, 149, 159, 163, 171, 172, 173, 175, 182, 183, 187, 188, 189, 192, 193, 197, 198, 199, 216, 229, 232, 242, 243, 246, 250, 252, 254, 261, 262, 270, 272, 278, 297, 299, 300, 302
visual environment, 155
visual field, 3, 121, 123, 163, 167, 172, 211, 212, 213, 215, 216, 217, 218, 221, 222, 225, 243, 244, 249, 259, 298, 299, 302
visual stimuli, 5, 304
visual system, 5, 172
visualization, 144, 230, 242, 251, 295
vitreous hemorrhage, 121, 155, 203

W

watches, 179
water, 108, 109, 112, 113, 127, 130, 131, 132, 141, 245, 269, 270
wavelengths, 108, 125, 126, 128, 129, 131, 137, 143, 144, 145, 148, 185, 295
weakness, 247
wear, 168, 207, 267, 268, 269, 270, 271, 273, 274, 275, 276, 277, 278, 280, 281, 284, 285, 289, 292
welding, 283
Western countries, 19, 228
Western Europe, 28, 30, 218, 220, 254
wires, 127
Wisconsin, 220
work activity, 33, 159
work environment, 157
workers, 144, 196
World Health Organization (WHO), 9, 289
worldwide, vii, xi, 5, 17, 18, 19, 20, 21, 24, 25, 205, 211, 214, 223, 228, 243
worry, 101

X

X chromosome, 157, 237, 245

Y

yield, 103, 122, 127, 144, 163
young adults, 3, 28, 191
young people, 10